Criminal on the Road

A STUDY OF SERIOUS MOTORING OFFENCES AND THOSE WHO COMMIT THEM

T. C. WILLETT
B.Sc.(Soc.), Ph.D.

With a Foreword by

HERMANN MANNHEIM

TAVISTOCK PUBLICATIONS

PUBLISHED UNDER THE AUSPICES OF THE INSTITUTE FOR THE STUDY AND TREATMENT OF DELINQUENCY

First published in 1964
by Tavistock Publications (1959) Limited
of 11 New Fetter Lane, London, E.C.4
and printed in Great Britain
by Cox & Wyman Limited
Fakenham

OC01621650

TO MY WIFE

Contents

Contents

Contents

Foreword

by

HERMANN MANNHEIM

The avalanche of modern motor traffic has changed the surface of the earth and produced a host of entirely new problems for scores of professions. Technicians, engineers, industrialists, town planners, economists, sociologists, psychologists, psychiatrists, lawyers, doctors, artists, writers, and last but not least criminals have been forced to forget much of what they had learnt and to go to school again. Criminologists cannot expect to be left untouched by this process. They have often been charged with turning a blind eye on the revolution brought about by the motor car, and they have in any case not been quicker than others to adapt themselves to an unprecedented situation. Nevertheless, it would be unfair to say that they have been entirely asleep. In several countries, notably the United States, West Germany, and Scandinavia, much important research on various aspects of the subject has been published in the years since the second world war, and as far as possible it has been summarized in the present volume. As the list of references shows, this country has so far lagged behind, but much of the leeway has been made up by Dr Willett. Here, as so often, the main difficulty lies in the multitude and vast dimensions of the new problems and the scarcity of funds and of workers competent to tackle them as members of a research team.

Moreover, criminology is, and is likely to remain, an unpopular subject. Public opinion as a rule accuses it of trying to whitewash and to pamper the criminal. In two cases, however, the charge is different: whenever criminologists turn their attention to the white-collar criminal or the traffic offender, public opinion makes a *volte-face* and accuses them of being unduly harsh and punishment-minded. It is in fact the prevailing popular theory that these unfortunate victims of the motor age have been brought into the sphere of the criminal law and the criminal courts only by a deplorable combination of legal tricks and social and moral misjudgements which should be put right without delay.

The author of the present volume has courageously tackled a large number of the problems involved, and some of the facts brought to light in his research are entirely out of harmony with the picture of the motoring offender as it exists in the mind of the man in the street. To make his investigation realistic he limits it to serious offences showing at least two of the following features: deliberate intent, harm to persons or property, and dishonesty. He then presents a number of hypotheses to be tested by empirical research, all of which have some bearing on the popular image of this category of offenders: e.g. that the 'serious motoring offender' is a respectable and otherwise entirely law-abiding citizen, whose personality and background in no way predispose him to lawbreaking in general; who neither regards himself as a criminal nor is so regarded by the community; who usually has a non-manual occupation and is the driver of a private car; his punishment is much more lenient than that of other categories of offender, but once found guilty and punished he is not likely to repeat his offence.

The empirical research is preceded by a careful analysis of the law, of the role played by the police, and of the statistical tables presented in the book. In Parts II and III, which form the real backbone of the work, first a sample of 653 serious motoring offenders and their offences, committed in one of the English Home Counties, is examined in great detail, using the police files as the main source of information. This documentary part is supplemented by personal interviews with forty-three offenders. The author frankly admits that the resulting material is 'a mixture of fact and impression', but even so it is of profound interest, especially in the light of the concluding chapter. Some of the hypotheses which the author set out to test have been confirmed by the evidence, e.g. as was to be expected, in most cases neither the offender nor the police nor the public applied any social stigma to these offences. On the other hand, it was found that about 23 per cent of the offenders had previous convictions for non-motoring offences; therefore, the author concludes, his hypothesis that the serious motoring offender is otherwise a respectable, law-abiding citizen becomes somewhat doubtful, and the same applies to the other hypotheses that there is nothing in the offender's personality and background that predisposes him to break the law and that most of these offenders come from non-manual occupations.

There are many other important issues arising from Dr Willett's pioneer research which are likely to become the subject of prolonged controversies on the part of interested parties and among other research workers. This Foreword is not the place to enter into such disputes, but only to draw attention to the importance of the present study.

Preface

Since becoming interested in criminology some ten years ago I have been intrigued by the difficulty in defining it and in delineating its frontiers, as exemplified by the controversies surrounding the questions 'what is crime?' or 'what is delinquency?'

In discussions of these basic questions it is noticeable how often motoring offences are cited as prime examples of the problem of classifying deviant or antisocial behaviour. Here, it seems, is a borderland along the frontiers of criminology; a kind of 'no-man's-land' of behaviour, in which deliberately antisocial actions and actions which are inadvertently careless merge almost imperceptibly into an amorphous range of transgressions that we try to rationalize by calling them 'technical offences'. Moreover, it is a borderland which few, if any, criminologists have been moved to explore, perhaps because they have been unable to conceive of the motoring offence *per se* as 'crime'. This is the impression one gets from the relative lack of interest in motoring offences as criminological phenomena.

Yet it is possible that the study of motoring offences might illuminate some important sectors of criminology which have hitherto resisted examination. For we do not yet know much about the so-called 'normal persons' who people the social environment and supply the pressures to which criminal behaviour is a response. Hence the controversies about whether 'criminals' are abnormal persons in a normal environment, or normal persons reared in an abnormal environment, and about the standards of behaviour to be expected of the 'reasonable man'. Such questions will be unanswerable until it is known what distinctions there are, if any, between criminals and others who are not criminals, besides the mere fact that the former are caught and the others are not. Some insight has already been offered by Miller (1960) in his stimulating discussion of delinquent traits in normal persons, complementing the pioneer work done by Sutherland and Cressey (1955) in their study of white-collar crime, but there is still much to be done in this field. And if motoring offences do in fact bridge the gap between the criminal and the 'quasi-criminal', or even form one of its conceptual piers, then a study of the offences and the characteristics of those who commit them might be a useful contribution to knowledge.

There is another reason for choosing this subject. Safety and discipline

xiii

Preface

on the roads are unlikely to come about by reliance on the law and its enforcement; some change in the public attitude is required, and indeed is essential. It may be that the prevalence of motoring offences is, as Sutherland and Cressey (1955, p. 89) have suggested of crime in general, due to the fact 'that the law has been extended much more rapidly than the general mores, and when the law is not supported by the general mores it is relatively impotent and is violated frequently'. If this is so, the public would understandably find neither difficulty nor shame in identifying with even serious motoring offenders, and 'there but for the grace of God go I' is an expression that is common enough to suggest that this is what they do.

Given such an identification, it would not be surprising if serious motoring offences – and all other motoring offences also – were to continue to increase *ad infinitum*, thereby weakening respect for the law, claiming a disproportionate amount of police effort, and killing or injuring many more victims than any other kind of illegal activity. But if it can be shown that the identification – especially with the offender – could also be an identification with criminality, then it might help to bring about the change in attitude that is essential if driving, or any other use of the roads, is to become reasonably safe and pleasant. There is thus a hope that this study may be something more than an addition to academic knowledge.

In acknowledging the help I have received in the carrying out of this study, which was submitted as a doctoral thesis, I would mention a special indebtedness to my teacher, Dr Terence Morris, for his inspiration and guidance, without which the work could not have been accomplished. I am indebted also to Mr J. E. Hall Williams for assistance with legal aspects of the study; and to the Staff of the London School of Economics and of the University of London, particularly for the grant from the University Central Research Fund.

For making possible the operational part of the research I thank the Chairman of Quarter Sessions and the chief constable and police officers of the county in which the study was undertaken. I am grateful also to Mr Lodge and Mr Klein of the Home Office Research Unit, to Mr Willcock of the Social Survey, and to Dr Smeed and Dr Garwood of the Road Research Laboratory, all of whom provided me with valuable information. And for their help with the legal sections of the work and with the translation of certain material I thank Mr Ronald Bernstein, Mr T. G. Field-Fisher, Mr A. Kynric Lewis, Mr W. Lough, and Mr H. R. Spencer. I am indebted to Mr Bastick for preparing the graphs.

I would also like to acknowledge the kindness of Dr Ross McFarland, Dr Alan Canty, Dr Edward J. Kelleher, and the Rev. J. H. L. Waterson for

Preface

sending me literature and for allowing me to quote at length from their work. And I thank the Editor of *The Autocar* for permission to quote from leading articles in his journal.

But acknowledgements would be incomplete without mentioning the 'serious motoring offenders' who so kindly gave me their confidence and their time, and so often their hospitality also. I sincerely hope that I have not abused these privileges in my attempt to remain objective. Finally, I would express gratitude to my wife for her forbearance during four difficult years, for checking all the data, and for making the research possible at all.

University of Reading   T. C. WILLETT

PART ONE

Legal and Social Background

I

Orientation

This book deals primarily with two basic questions. First, is there any justification for regarding motoring offences as 'crimes' on a par with other criminal offences such as, for example, larceny? Second, and in consequence, are motoring offenders and their offences valid subjects for criminological study?

A sound answer to these questions must depend on careful definition of the terms involved: of 'crime', 'the criminal', 'criminology', and 'the motoring offence'. Yet it is unusual to take much trouble over definitions when dealing with questions like this; indeed, the majority of laymen and some criminologists do not hesitate to give an emphatic 'no' to both questions without much thought. The unwisdom of so impetuous an answer will be evident when the problems surrounding these definitions are looked at more closely.

Let us first consider the perennial question 'what is crime', so beloved of those who conduct criminological and legal discussions. It is perennial because it is fundamentally important to criminology as the term that delineates the body of knowledge in which that discipline claims to specialize. It is attractive also, because it can be relied upon to provoke acute controversy.

Most discussions about the definition of crime turn upon two conceptions: the 'legal' and the 'sociological'. The legal definition, which Sutherland and Cressey (1955, p. 4) called the 'conventional view', is that 'criminal behaviour is behaviour in violation of the criminal law. No matter what the degree of immorality, reprehensibility or indecency of an act it is not a crime unless it is prohibited by the criminal law.' Another view is that of Goodhart (1953, p. 84) who quotes Kenny's dictum that a crime 'can only be defined as an act which is punished by the State', hence 'attempts to define criminal law in terms of morality are bound to fail'. This is a very broad definition, including as it does such extremes of unlawful behaviour as capital murder on the one hand, and keeping a dog without a licence on the other. Lawyers would not quarrel with this kind of definition if it were used in an academic sense, but it is unusual to find criminologists

3

subscribing to it. Among those who do are Sutherland and Cressey (op. cit. p. 220), who cast beyond the traditional area of criminal activity, with its focus on crimes of violence against persons and property, towards areas of behaviour which had hitherto escaped the stigma of 'criminal' despite the social damage they did, e.g. the 'white-collar' crimes of illegal price fixing, and violations of the United States anti-trust laws by businessmen. Another representative is Hartung (1950), who studied the white-collar criminal activities of dealers in the wholesale meat industry in Detroit, which were accepted practices in a respectable trade. In criticizing Hartung's work, Burgess (1950) wrote that it was as unrealistic to classify these people as criminals and their acts as crimes as it would be if the stigma had been applied to 'traffic violators'; if, Burgess says, we are to take such a comprehensive view of crime, then all persons violating traffic regulations and health ordinances, etc., would be criminals and so, therefore, would the majority of citizens. He points out the importance of distinguishing between acts that are *universally* damned as criminal, and those to which the public are willing accomplices (in so far as they turn a blind eye to the offences), and he denies the usefulness of the latter as evidence of crime 'except in a technical legal sense'. But, as Hartung replied, on what other but a technical legal basis could an offender be adjudged criminal? In the courts of the United Kingdom and the United States, apparently none. And Hartung goes on to ask if there is any reason why traffic violators should not be regarded as criminals. There are few authorities, however, who would go so far as this, though Wootton (1959, p. 25) has done so in calling the motorist 'the typical criminal of today'.

On the contrary, we find many distinguished criminologists and lawyers taking an opposite line: the sociological or pragmatic view.

In discussing Hartung's work, Burgess (1950, pp. 33–4) recalled Ross's distinction between 'criminal' and 'criminaloid' offences, the latter being 'new offences resulting from recent legislation and regulation'; and he implies that to confuse the two is to bring the law into contempt. The same point was made by Lord Devlin in a speech to the Magistrates' Association (October 1960), when he spoke of 'grappling with the social and legal problems inseparable from the ownership of motor cars by the millions'. He claimed that 'the criminal law has lost much of the respect which it ought to have because we have failed to distinguish when we could have done so between what is sinful and disgraceful, and what is failure to measure up to a required standard of discipline'. Lord Devlin also made a distinction between 'real crimes' committed by the 'wicked', and 'quasi-criminal' offences committed by the 'errant', and he deplored the stigmatizing of the

4

Orientation

motorist who is 'merely errant' as a criminal: a term that should be applied only to the wicked if it were to have any social meaning. Mannheim (1946, p. 5) takes a similar position when he defines crime as essentially behaviour that is antisocial, and excludes that which is not manifestly antisocial from the criminal category. He makes the difficulty of defining crime in such terms abundantly clear when he points out that there is much antisocial behaviour that is not legally an offence, just as there are many offences that are not antisocial. Indeed, as Hartung (1950) says, where are we to stop in defining behaviour as criminal if we go beyond the limits of the law? Presumably at the limits of that range of attitudes which Sumner (1906) called 'the mores': the attitudes that refer to moral behaviour. And the position seems to be that Mannheim, Burgess, and others who take the sociological view regard 'crime' and 'criminal' as terms appropriate to behaviour that may or may not be illegal but is, by consensus, immoral and antisocial.

There would be no difficulty at all about this if there *were* consensus about what is and what is not antisocial and immoral behaviour, and similarly as to what is and what is not crime and criminal. But, unfortunately, no such consensus seems to exist, as Silvey (1961) demonstrates in a discussion of the relationship between public opinion and criminal law. He quotes a BBC audience research survey in which informants were given a list of offences and were asked which they considered 'the *worst* crime, the most serious crime'; the results were as follows:

Offence	Percentage of respondents
Indecent assault on women or children	25
Cruelty to children	21
Planned murder for money	20
Killing a policeman to escape arrest	9
Being drunk in charge of a car	6
Robbery with violence	6
Rape	6
Causing death by dangerous driving	6

As Silvey remarks, the lack of agreement is the most surprising feature of the results: for example, not more than a quarter of the respondents agree over any one offence, and the distribution of opinion is very wide. It is also interesting, and perhaps significant, that indecent assault (which can include quite trivial offences) is considered to be more serious than capital murder or causing death by dangerous driving.

To make matters even more confusing, the term criminal is not always

5

used when a crime has been committed, even if the act is one that would unhesitatingly be called a crime by most people, e.g. larceny or infanticide. It is improbable that a person who commits such an offence *only once* would be called a criminal, for it would appear that the term criminal is much more emotionally loaded than the term crime; hence the too ready application of the label criminal to the motoring offender seems to be extreme. Indeed it may be that Lord Somers spoke for Everyman when he said in the Lords that 'there is too much of the view that the motorist is a criminally minded man out for himself and without any thought for anyone else. Most people are motorists now, and the British race is not criminally minded' (*The Times*, 11 June 1959).

However, it is hard for an objective observer to find much justification for Lord Somers's complaint, since it is unusual to hear anyone expressing himself so violently about motoring offenders. One exception is Cardinal Cushing, Archbishop of Boston, who was quoted in *The Pedestrian* (Spring 1961) as being 'forced to the conclusion that the seriously enacted provisions of the law for the safety of the highways are binding under pain of sin. Reckless speeding, drunken driving, weaving in and out of line without regard for road markings and contemptuous violation of traffic signals . . . these are sins before God no less than other offences punished by State law.' Another exception is Waterson (1961), Vicar of Stoke D'Abernon, who writes about religion and road safety in similar terms to those of Archbishop Cushing. Waterson refers to Lord Devlin's distinction between errant and wicked driving, and he draws attention to the moral problem implicit in the latter, and to the illogical refusal of the public to conceive of such conduct as sinful. He infers that men and women dislike facing the facts about these offences because their own consciences are so tender about 'the strong inclination in driving a motor car to revert to a more primitive level of personality', as in the case of 'a lorry driver who was tried for manslaughter after he had deliberately rammed a private car and killed its occupants because he was sick of being dazzled by other people's headlights, and swore to eliminate the next that bothered him'. Waterson has much to say that is of relevance and interest, and his work will be referred to later; but, for the moment, let us keep his views to the context of this section and quote especially his comment that the sin of Lord Devlin's wicked driver is 'considerably Original'!

Much more typical of the general attitude to motoring offences is the view of the Standing Joint Committee of the Automobile Association and the Royal Automobile Club, as expressed in their *Memorandum to the Royal Commission on the Police* (1960): 'It is desirable that the manner in which the police deal with *motorists* who commit minor offences should be very different from the attitude towards *persons* who commit serious *criminal* offences' (author's italics). The use of the term 'persons' may be accidental, yet it seems to be deliberate; perhaps it means 'persons, including motorists', and if so one's suspicions are unfounded. Be that as it may, *The Times* (4 January 1961) commented in a leading article dealing with this particular part of the *Memorandum* that 'many drivers unfortunately create the impression that they do not regard anything they do on the highway as in the accepted sense criminal – and that they are prepared to do anything they have a sporting chance of getting away with'. Indeed it is true to say that the *Memorandum* avoids *any* reference to criminality, saying later in its recommendations that 'it is desirable for the police to concentrate on enforcement action against motorists who commit serious offences' – not, it may be noted, serious *criminal* offences – 'rather than on prosecutions for minor offences of a technical nature'.

So it seems that there is an understandable tendency to tread warily when applying the terms crime and criminal to motoring offences and to those who commit them. This is so even among the police, where one would expect to find a precise usage of both terms. Most of the officers with whom the writer talked defined crime as the group of indictable offences that threaten the security and the safety of the person or property or both; but most of them excluded motoring offences from the criminal category.

To the police the criminal seems to be an individual whom they can identify with what they call 'the criminal class', i.e. someone whose main job is unlawful activity. They found no difficulty in so categorizing most offenders against the person with violence, or against property, but there was much confusion about others, especially sex offenders and those who take vehicles without the owner's consent. About motoring offenders there was no doubt shown whatsoever in most cases: nearly all officers took the sociological line and put them in a different class from the criminal. As a chief constable put it: 'Of course you will find that all motoring offenders but a handful are normal respectable citizens who are no more criminal than you or me.' On the whole their offences were not stigmatized as crimes, though they were condemned sometimes as gross misbehaviour. However, some detailed questioning and discussion about certain motoring offences raised doubts among police officers as to whether they should be called criminal: for example, driving while disqualified, and failing to stop after an accident in which the damage had been other than trivial. There was some hesitation also in regard to questions about the criminality of dangerous driving when there was evidence of aggression and selfishness. But

7

Legal and Social Background

perhaps the most significant indication of the attitude to the motoring offender of those who administer the law is the frequency with which the practice of putting 'arrested' offenders, and those charged with indictable offences, in the dock is dispensed with; in many cases of drunken driving heard in court by the writer, the accused sat in a chair in front of the dock. A still more marked indication is the convention in motoring cases of withholding evidence of previous convictions for non-motoring offences; they are said to be irrelevant. The motoring offender is thus accorded a tolerance that is not given to many minor offenders; those charged with indecent exposure, petty larceny, and so on are put in the dock and treated with the full force of the criminal court procedure.

In this tolerance – and it is a surprising tolerance considering the nuisance that the motoring offender causes them – the police only reflect the public attitude. It will be shown later that motoring offenders suffer little or no disgrace for their transgressions when compared with minor sexual offenders and those convicted of trivial offences against property. Over 300 people were questioned during this research about the extent to which motoring offenders could be regarded as criminal, and none was prepared to apply this stigma unless leading questions were put to them. A most striking proof of this attitude is the custom among the police and the public of calling all incidents involving damage by or to vehicles 'accidents', thus implying that the event was not the consequence of any deliberate intention, but an unfortunate affair of pure chance. By contrast, we do not find the more impulsive offences of assault or shoplifting being called accidents; yet there is often more of an element of chance in them than there is in motoring cases such as the following, taken from *The Times* (1 February 1961):

DEATH OF BRIDE 'ON YOUTH'S SHOULDERS' · ACT OF GROSS FOLLY IN CAR

A learner driver, aged 17, who admitted causing the death of a young bride by dangerous driving, was fined £75 at Leicestershire Assizes yesterday and banned from driving for seven years. He was given a year to pay the fine.

Mr Justice Streatfeild told Alan Ross Kendall, a chemical process worker, of Chapman Street, Loughborough: 'You loaded your car with too many passengers, drove at excessive speed, deaf to appeals to slow down and almost contemptuous of a possible crash. As a result of what happened on your ghastly night out a man's 20-year-old bride of one week was snatched from him. Her death is on your shoulders and will be for the rest of your life.'

Mr Brian Bush, for the prosecution, said that on 5 November, Kendall took his father's car, without permission, to drive to a youth club dance. He arranged to give nine friends a lift home but a police officer intervened saying the car was not intended for so many.

There were four passengers in the car, which was driven at excessive speed on

8

Orientation

the main road towards Nottingham at Castle Donnington. One of the passengers, Miss Maureen Lowe, asked him to slow down but Kendall laughed and retorted: 'What's a crash?' Another girl passenger, Miss Violet Adcock, replied: 'When one car bangs into another.'

A few moments later the tragic crash occurred, Mr Bush said.

Mr John Ernest Merryman was driving in the opposite direction on the correct side of the road, his bride, Sonia, by his side. Kendall shot across a bend and hit the oncoming car head on.

The Judge said he was satisfied that this otherwise decent young lad had been showing off before his friends. It was an act of gross folly.

A letter printed in *The Autocar* (8 September 1961) is also of interest in this context:

CRIME ON THE ROAD?

Highway Menaces. Last night I witnessed something that many motorists must have noted, for it happens regularly. A car in front of me pulled out to overtake another car. He misjudged the distance and, in addition, the driver of the car being over-taken deliberately accelerated.

The point of no return was reached and the driver of the overtaking car by a hairsbreadth managed to cut in, just missing a collision with a car approaching him from the opposite direction. It was dusk and the driver of this car blazed his head-lamps straight into the eyes of the approaching driver as he drove at him on the wrong side of the road. I saw the car falter in its path and its driver must have been completely blinded as he aimed the car for the cut-in.

Now this, had it culminated in an accident, would have probably been fatal, due to the speeds involved. The overtaking driver was obviously in the wrong for not braking the moment he saw the car he was trying to pass was accelerating with him.

But this, in my opinion, is not the end of the story by any means. This business of glaring one's headlamps into the eyes of someone driving a car fast and straight at *you* is simply crazy. It just shows the length that some people will go 'to teach him a lesson'. Those drivers were almost the best educated corpses in the road at that instant.

The driver of the car being overtaken deserves special mention. This man I think is way ahead of the dangerous driving fraternity. What he did, from where I was sitting, was attempted murder. It was coolly and deliberately executed. Nothing slipshod. Only the poor power output of his engine failed him.

Sheffield.   BARRIE GREGORY.

Further evidence of the illogicality of calling all incidents 'accidents' is an analysis in *The Daily Telegraph* (15 January 1960) of the 'factors regarded by the police as contributing to accidents' in 1958. These include driving under the influence of drink, negligently turning round in the road, and overtaking improperly on the nearside. It is obvious that any one of these actions makes an incident not only possible, but probable; is it then sense to call the outcome an accident? The answer is as questionable as the practice of applying the term crime to particular offences without knowing by what standards the term is used. That is what most of the people questioned in this research did: they were ready to say whether or not they

9

thought an offence to be a crime; but they were nonplussed when asked by what standards they judged it to be one. The question 'what is crime' seemed never to have occurred to them. This may not be surprising, but it may be of some significance since it is very probable that the incidence of particular offences is related to the public's disapproval of them; hence they will tend to increase where there is little or no disapproval or where there is apathy. Perhaps one of the main reasons for the rise in motoring offences since 1945 is that the offender is not made by the community to feel that he has done anything seriously wrong.

To sum up this discussion on the definition of the terms crime and criminal – and it has been treated much too briefly to do it justice – one is faced by a choice between the legal standpoint, according to which even the smallest motoring offences are crimes and their perpetrators criminals, and the sociological standpoint, which adopts social rather than legal criteria.

Acceptance of the legal definition in a study of this kind would, I think, make it unacceptable as a serious piece of work in criminology. There would be a danger of it deteriorating into an academic 'stunt' or, at best, an exercise in self-evident fact-finding that would be of little or no interest to anyone. In any case, the range of offences that would have to be studied would make the scale of the research prohibitively large and expensive if the results were to mean anything.

Hence the sociological point of view will be taken in this work, in the sense that the terms crime and criminal are applicable realistically only to offences and to behaviour that the community would punish in some way – even if by no more than disapproval or condemnation – whatever were done by the official agencies of the law. To be more explicit, a crime is here defined as an offence that usually involves behaviour for which the perpe-trator would be castigated by the majority of people in a community, regardless of whether he had been caught by the police and dealt with in the courts. *And here it should be noted that the emphasis is laid on the behaviour that is involved in the commission of the offence rather than on the offence itself.* To risk academic disapproval in the interests of clarity, one might leave the last word with the writer of the popular song: 'It ain't what you do but the way that you do it.' However, the above definition does not mean much unless it is supplemented by an attempt to specify the kinds of behaviour that would be so castigated – and on this point the writer is laid open to every critic inside and outside the social sciences. In the absence of survey data an empirically derived hypothesis is put forward; it is suggested that it is behaviour that involves at least *two* of the following elements:

deliberate intent, harm to persons or property, and dishonesty; or, to put it more clearly, an intent to do wrong, an action that is very likely to hurt someone or someone's property, and a willingness to tell lies about the part played in the event, usually in order to escape conviction. Whether the individual behaving thus would be called a criminal or not depends on the subtle distinction between the use of that term as a noun and its use as an adjective. Perhaps all that can be said at this stage is that the use of the term by the layman as an adjective tends to lead to its use ultimately as a noun.

Needless to say, it is not easy to find motoring offences in which any two of the above elements could be present; if it were, the public attitude would be less apathetic than it is. Let us, however, consider the offences listed in the Home Office Returns of *Offences relating to Motor Vehicles* since these are the offences which might properly be called motoring offences; and here it should be noted that the so-called 'traffic offences' are a general group that includes all motoring offences and also offences in which horses, carts, barrows, steamrollers, and a variety of other road users are concerned.

Without stretching the imagination beyond the credible it would appear that no more than the following classes of offence could exhibit the criteria given above to a degree sufficient to earn the stigma of being serious, and hence potentially criminal; but this is, of course, a matter of opinion, and any choice must be controversial. However, for reasons to be given below, the following were chosen for study in this research:

Causing death by dangerous driving, and manslaughter
Driving recklessly or dangerously
Driving under the influence of drink or drugs
Driving while disqualified
Failing to insure against third-party risks
Failing to stop after, or to report, an accident.

The qualification 'to a degree sufficient to earn the stigma of being serious' is mentioned because, paradoxically, some quite trivial offences can and do show the criteria of deliberate intent, harmfulness, and dishonesty. For example, speeding is sometimes deliberate, and there is often a firm denial by the offender when he appears in court that he was exceeding the speed limit. Some idea of what might be happening daily during peak hours with regard to movement to and from London can be gained from a survey by members of a London firm, Univision Ltd, which was published by the *Observer* (31 July 1960). Four experienced observers noted certain kinds of motoring misbehaviour during the morning and evening rush hours on a five-mile stretch of the A4 trunk road on the outskirts of London for 158 consecutive weekdays during the period January to June, and they attributed the incidents proportionately to sixteen different classes of vehicle. For instance, they reported that of 293 chauffeur-driven Jaguar cars observed, 57 per cent were racing other vehicles, and the same was said of 20 per cent of 427 solo motor cycles; moreover 89 per cent of the Jaguars and 94 per cent of the solo motor cyclists were disregarding the speed limit of 40 miles per hour. Both Jaguars and motor cyclists also had a relatively poor record for disregarding red traffic lights and driving over 'zebra' pedestrian crossings when people were on them; and 90 per cent of the motor cyclists were observed to be 'weaving dangerously in and out of traffic'. Of the sixteen classes of vehicle, none came out unscathed but, on balance, it would seem that the drivers of buses and coaches were among the more law-abiding, next to the police patrols who, incidentally, showed poor 'lane discipline'. By far the 'worst' of the classes were the Jaguar drivers, whether chauffeurs or not, and the solo motor cyclists; private cars did not show up too badly except in failure to observe speed limits. An impressionistic survey, no doubt, but one that would probably meet with substantial agreement from motorists who know the road in question, as the present writer does.

It is not only the group of 'moving' offences that is difficult to categorize as serious or not; after some thought it will be evident that some parking offences can be extremely antisocial and deliberately so. It is not unknown to see drivers park their vehicles purposely to obstruct much-used exits, or to make it impossible for other vehicles parked before them to move. However, if such offences were included in what purports to be a criminological study, it is unlikely that it would be taken seriously.

Perhaps this is one of the reasons for the habitual omission of motoring crime from the majority of major criminological researches, to which Wootton (1959, p. 26) has called attention. Another reason was suggested by Mannheim (1960), when he wrote of the interest that could be stimulated among criminologists and sociologists in these offences; he stressed the great difficulty of research that would require a multi-disciplinary approach on a prohibitively large scale, and it might face 'many obstacles from powerful vested interests'.

SURVEY OF THE LITERATURE

Whatever the reason, a survey of the available literature suggests that there is yet much to be done if motoring offences and offenders are to be brought into proper criminological perspective. Such material as there is seems to fall into two main categories: first, the commentaries on the official statistics, in which individual offenders are not studied; and second, a number of monographs, mostly from other than criminological sources. The first group tell us quite a lot about the incidence of offences, but little or nothing about the offenders, for which it is necessary to rely on the small-scale studies in the second group.

In Britain very little has been produced in either category, and there is justification for the charge that our criminologists are not very interested; even the commentaries on statistics are scarce, and most of the other work that can be made relevant is from the study of accident prevention. This is not so in other countries such as Germany, Scandinavia, and especially the United States, where the motor vehicle seems to be as much a part of crime as it is of life itself – as indeed it may become here, if it has not done so already.

Of the British work, Wootton's (1959) has attracted the most attention in criminological and sociological circles. Although it falls in the category of a commentary on the official statistics, it goes rather further in that it takes a provocatively legal line of argument, accusing the motorist of being 'the typical criminal of today', whose entitlement to this doubtful distinction is obscured by his membership of the well-to-do classes in whose favour, according to Wootton, the law tends to operate.

Wootton (op. cit. pp. 27–8) demonstrates her thesis in an exhaustive analysis of the official statistics of motoring offences in England and Wales for 1955. She shows that over five times as many persons aged 17 and over were convicted in the magistrates' courts for driving dangerously, etc., as were convicted for breaking and entering. She found also that convictions of adults for dangerous driving, drunken driving, speeding, and failing to stop after or to report accidents exceeded the convictions of all adults for crimes of dishonesty and crimes against the person by approximately 50 per cent.

However, although she seems to stigmatize the motoring offender as a criminal, she does so in a rather special sense, since she appears to accept the view that 'the motorist seldom sets out to do mischief'. Hence his criminality lies in his negligence rather than in the kind of antisocial behaviour that is usual in the commission of those offences in which deliberate intent is presupposed. If this is so, it is perhaps rather inconsistent of Wootton to ask why motoring offenders are considered by the public to be less antisocial than housebreakers or 'the shop assistant who fiddles a pound from the till'. She supplies one possible answer by her frequent use of the term 'accident' in connection with motoring offences.

Despite her strong condemnation of the motoring offender, Wootton does not produce any substantial reason to show that the public are wrong in regarding motoring offences as less heinous than those against the person or property, and one gets the impression that the work is an attack on a privileged group as well as a criminological analysis. There is, for example, the author's remark (op. cit. pp. 48, 70) that 'nothing induces so strong an inclination towards the Marxist theory that the law is made and operated in the interests of the well-to-do as the difference in the prevailing attitude towards motoring offences'. This appears to mean that those who make and administer the law are much more tolerant towards motoring offences than they are towards other offences, since they are prone themselves to commit the former; there is also the inference that the typical motoring offender comes from the well-to-do classes or white-collar occupational groups. Indeed this is the historic stereotype of the motoring offender: the well-to-do owner of a private car who sees himself as a privileged person and a law unto himself. Albeit inadvertently, Wootton seems to have done something to harden this 'Mr Toad' stereotype, but this should not detract from the value of her study since it provokes much curiosity about the kind of person the motoring offender is, and about his position in the social and criminal hierarchy. It also emphasizes the incongruity of the ignorance and the lack of interest that are manifest in respect of these offenders, when the size of their contribution to the total number of offences is realized.

Another interesting contribution from British criminological literature is Gibbens's study (1958) of thirty-nine lads convicted of taking and driving away vehicles without the owners' consent. This is not, strictly speaking, a motoring offence since the substance lies in the taking of the vehicle and not in the way in which it is handled; but the central element in the offence is the motor vehicle and the attitudes towards it, so much of what Gibbens has to say is apposite to motoring offenders in general.

It seems that taking and driving away is mostly an offence of the teenager from an 'intact' home in which he is on good terms with his parents, and Gibbens suggests that the attractiveness of the vehicle may stem from its significance to the youngster as a symbol of masculinity and power. Hence it is much sought after by the boy whose ties with his mother have been very close and who wishes to prove himself as a male adult. To support this view Gibbens quotes Parsons's theory that boys from this type of background often associate 'being good' with femininity because the mother is usually the main regulator of morality in the home; thus 'being bad' is to reject femininity and to become more masculine.

Orientation

These ideas are of relevance to the controversies about sex differences in driving behaviour. It may be that male drivers identify driving cautiously at a modest pace with femininity, and so, according to Parsons's theory, are tempted to take risks and to drive more aggressively. And here the writer recalls a remark made by a senior police officer, that 'most men think that criticism of their driving is criticism of their manliness'. It is, indeed, a fact that males far outnumber females among motoring offenders, as they do among offenders of all kinds; hence Wootton's point (1959, p. 32) that 'if men behaved like women the courts would be idle and the prisons empty', an argument that many male drivers might find rather provocative.

From what has been said above, one would expect Gibbens's offenders to have been reckless and aggressive drivers but, on the contrary, he reports that they were quite careful although they were unskilled, and the same is said of similar offenders in Scandinavia. It may be, however, that this kind of offender is careful not to attract the attention of the police by exhibitionistic driving, and contains himself until the chances of being caught are minimal. This could explain why there are only four of these offenders among the 285 drivers in this study who were convicted of dangerous driving (see Chapter 8), and Gibbens has a valid point when he questions the rationality of always disqualifying them. It is this automatic disqualification, to which Gibbens draws attention, that makes his study relevant to other motoring offenders, notably those who drive while disqualified, since this is an offence to which the car thief seems particularly prone.

In discussing 'taking and driving away' Gibbens shows that there is good reason to think that it is a compulsive form of behaviour with a neurotic origin in the family relationships, especially with the mother; so there is a tendency to repeat the offence, despite disqualification and the warning that driving while disqualified must mean a prison sentence. Thus it would seem that there are additional reasons for doubting whether the usual practice of disqualifying the car thief is a wise course to take since it makes a further serious offence more or less inevitable in a compulsively inclined offender.

Another British study that throws light on the characteristics of offenders is that of Clarke (1949), concerning the 'extent to which any broad personality characteristics of army drivers who have accidents might emerge from a study of their personal records'. The subjects were 431 drivers in transport companies of the Royal Army Service Corps, of whom 254 were regulars and the remaining 177 were conscripts; the mean age was 22. A number of contingency tables were set up to see if any particular constellations of the following criteria were clustered about subjects who

15

had traffic accident records, which could distinguish them significantly from drivers who were accident-free:

Age
Rank
Type of army engagement
Length of service
Driving experience
Type of vehicle normally driven
Marital status
Selection grade given when entering service
Education
Number of jobs held in civilian life
Number of military offences during service driving experience

Only two of the criteria were associated significantly with a history of one or more accidents: the number of military offences, and the number of jobs held in civilian life. Of the 168 drivers with one or more accidents, 111, or just over 66 per cent, had been found guilty of one or more military offences ($p < \cdot01$). And of the 139 drivers whose records of pre-service employment were available, and who had one or more accidents, forty-five, or just over 32 per cent, had changed their jobs more than once before joining the army (p between $\cdot02$ and $\cdot01$). Some offences may have been trivial and it is conceivable that a driver whose accident had caused some inconvenience and had possibly marred the unit's accident record might have become so unpopular with NCOs as to find himself on charges more often than others. But the fact remains that offences and driving behaviour appear to be associated in some way.

The association of job-changing with accidents is also of interest in a criminological sense, for Mannheim and Wilkins (1955) held that this factor was a significant indicator of poor prognosis when found in the records of young offenders in Borstal institutions. So there is here a hint that driving behaviour and a tendency to offend against the law, albeit military law in this case, may not be unrelated. It is, however, no more than a hint since there is no indication that the accidents in which the subjects of this study were concerned involved antisocial conduct, or were even their own fault.

Some support for the view that a history of previous convictions might often be found among those who have traffic accidents is given by Bebbington, the chief constable of Cambridgeshire, in two unpublished papers (1954). Two groups of 131 drivers of vehicles other than public-service vehicles were compared: one group were known 'accident-repeaters', having 660 accidents between them; the other group comprised 131 motorists taken at random from licensing records. The latter group included twenty-one who had had accidents, of whom three were among the accident-repeater group; excluding these three, there were only twenty-six accidents to be shared among eighteen drivers – a much lower accident record than found in the repeater group. When previous convictions were considered it was found that seventy-one, or 54 per cent, of the repeaters had previous convictions as compared with twenty-three, or 17·5 per cent, of the random sample; moreover, seventeen of the repeaters had non-traffic offences on their records in contrast to only four of the sample.

There is also some evidence from an analysis of the claim records of an insurance company by Munden (1962), in which he shows that individuals who had been convicted of an offence (the kind of offence is not indicated, but presumably a motoring offence is meant) had a higher claim rate than those not previously convicted, but he points out that it was unknown how long a driver had been driving before taking up the policy with the particular company, and the greater the prior experience the greater the opportunity for committing an offence.

Munden's examination of 2,640 insurance policies yields some further information that is of interest, since knowing something about those who have accidents may provide useful clues about the characteristics of those who commit motoring offences. His analysis showed that the peak ages for claims were about 30 and 60, with low rates among the youngest and the oldest drivers; and it was found that those who claimed in the first three years of their policy's life tended afterwards to make more claims than the average. Indeed it was possible to discern the proportion of policy holders who were more disposed to have accidents than the majority, and to have more accidents than mere chance would lead one to expect. Munden thought that this was attributable to some inherent personal characteristic which he does not define beyond calling it 'accident-proneness'. As might be expected, the drivers who lived in cities had higher claim rates than those living in rural areas, though the former drove fewer miles; and females tended to have lower claim rates than males. Of the various classes of user it was found that the highest claim rates were among commercial travellers and others who used their cars for business; their rates exceeded the rates for 'private use only' drivers by 120 per cent and 66 per cent respectively. None of these findings is surprising, and most of them would be suggested by common sense alone; it is interesting, however, to see to what extent they are supported by the evidence reported in the present study.

Support for the view that drunken drivers are mostly from age groups over 21 is found in an interesting pamphlet by Stack and Walker (1959), aptly titled *Motorized Drunkenness*. The authors analyse for the period 1955–57 the press reports of 700 offences in which there had been a conviction for either driving under the influence of drink or being in charge while under the influence. These show that the highest proportion of the offenders – 33 per cent – were in the age range 40 to 49, with a substantial proportion, 27 per cent, in the range 30 to 39; only 2 per cent were under 20. It seems also that most offenders had been drinking beer (average five pints), and that the peak hours for arrests were on Fridays, Saturdays, and Sundays after the bars closed in the afternoon and evening. A short analysis of sentencing is included, which shows the most frequent fine to have been between £10 and £20; and in the proportion of cases sent to prison (just over 3 per cent) the usual sentence was twelve months. All the offenders were disqualified, usually for twelve months also.

Since this study was sponsored by a religious organization with a special interest in abstinence, most of the discussion, as one might expect, concerns the role played by alcohol in traffic accidents and offences, but there is not much indication of the influence of alcohol in motoring offences other than the specific 'drink' offences. Little information is given about the offenders: distributions of age and sex are presented, but without comment; and there is no analysis of occupations although it is said that these were recorded.

More information about this type of offender is available in two statistical studies of similar sponsorship to that of Stack and Walker: namely, the Christian Economic and Social Research Foundation. The first (1959) analyses the Home Office Returns of *Offences relating to Motor Vehicles* for the years 1953 to 1958 inclusive, and again the focus is on the 'drink' offences. It is shown that they increased by 50 per cent during the period, without, it is noted, the change in the law in 1956 (separating the offence of being in charge, but not driving, while under the influence, from that of driving under the influence) making any appreciable difference to the offence rate. The analysis showed interesting differences in the offence rates between geographical regions: the highest incidence was in the urban industrial areas of the Midlands and Tyneside. It is a measure of the care with which this study was carried out that increases in the numbers of vehicles and licences are taken into account: the possibility that the increase in offences was due to the increase in either vehicles or drivers is negatived by the fact that there was a consistent rise in offence rates in only thirteen of 126 administrative areas; in the others there was either stability or a temporary decrease, despite the countrywide increase in drivers and

18

Orientation

vehicles. It was shown also that the modal age tended to remain high for this group of offenders, despite the considerable annual increase in new licence holders among the young; this conclusion is the same as that of Stack and Walker, i.e. that the drunken driver is well over 21 and is usually middle-aged.

That increases in vehicles and drivers may not be the basic cause for the surge in these offences is demonstrated also by the second report (1960), which is concerned mainly with the publican's role in influencing drunken driving. It suggests that most offenders often move from one public house to another so that no one landlord has much idea of what they have drunk before serving them; as they are 'strangers', there is not the knowledge of character which helps a landlord to keep his customers in bounds, nor are the regular customers prepared to adopt a modifying influence as they would with one of their own number – 'there is often latent antagonism' between the locals and the motorists, who simply go elsewhere if their needs are not met. The report states that the statistics concerning offences in which drink is a factor are 'deficient, unsatisfactory, and even misleading . . . nobody – the police least of all – regards the number of prosecutions and convictions recorded as coming near the totals of incapable motorists on the road'. The incidence grows none the less, and the report's view is that 'the proportion of the motoring public which is most involved in police prosecutions and drink accidents is not growing rapidly but is becoming more prone to drunken driving'. However, such a conclusion is questionable, given the available data; for instance, the inadequacy of the information about the ages of new and existing licence holders makes verification virtually impossible.

As Stack and the CESRF workers had to rely mostly on statistics for their material it is not surprising to find that they make hardly any mention of personality characteristics. Yet, among British studies, those which have concentrated on drunken driving have been to the fore in calling attention to the personality as a major factor in driving behaviour.

The importance of the personality factor emerges clearly from the work of Drew *et al.* (1959) on the effect of small doses of alcohol on skills resembling driving. Increasing doses of alcohol were given to forty drivers, of whom five were women; it was shown that errors in driving tended to increase markedly with the consumption of alcohol (the highest dose was the equivalent of three pints of beer), but there were differences in the extent to which the alcohol affected the accuracy, speed, and control of the individual subjects. Within the limits of this small sample these differences in response could not be attributed significantly to age, sex, drinking habits,

19

or driving experience; however, personality ratings – especially those relating to extraversion-introversion – had a definite relation to changes in driving behaviour. Extraverts did not alter their speed very much, but manifested large increases in error. Introverts showed considerable changes in speed: some increased it, others decreased it.

Considerable caution is shown in the interpretation of the results of this carefully planned study, especially since the subjects were members of the Road Research Laboratory staff and so were not really representative; but it offers more than a mere shred of evidence to suggest that differences in driving behaviour are related to differences in personality. There is a strong possibility, then, that people 'drive as they live', as Tillmann and Hobbs (1949) have suggested.

Nevertheless, apart from the few studies of drunken driving, studies that deal with psychological factors in driving – and especially deviant driving – are much harder to find in Britain than in other countries. This is in spite of the fact that in 1937 there was a special issue of *The Practitioner* devoted to medical aspects of motoring, in which Culpin drew attention to the need for psychological analysis of the desire for speed and the stimulation derived from it. He suggested that the thrill of speed is a 'conative propensity' which does not fulfil any biological need, and has not therefore been brought under control. He stressed the urgent need for the psychological study of serious motoring offenders, and predicted that psychopathological traits might be well marked, such as hypomania, obsessional desire for hurry, and such irrational impulses as to resist being overtaken or to charge oncoming vehicles. (For an actual example of 'charging' of this kind, see p. 231 below.)

Culpin also developed a particularly interesting sociological line of thought in relation to motoring. He drew attention to 'a generation which has grown up side by side with a developing mechanical capacity for speed', which has 'unquestioningly accepted that speed as part of its normal environment. . . . The absence of emotional reaction in the face of a casualty list of killed and injured as great as in a nineteenth-century war suggests that, in spite of the efforts of responsible authorities to lessen the totals, we have now become reconciled to conditions at the thought of which earlier generations would have shuddered. Anthropologists speak of "cultural mosaics", i.e. patterns of belief and usage into which individuals are moulded, so that what appears as ill-advised, foolish or repugnant to the outsider is accepted without question; the desirability of speed, even at the cost of a few thousand lives per annum, has become part of our cultural mosaic.'

Orientation

Culpin's plea for more research into the psychology of speed should be heeded, because the question of whether speed is dangerous is central whenever the control of driving behaviour is discussed; it is also an important factor in the motoring law. There is much naïveté about this matter, as when it is suggested that the imposition of a speed limit of, say, 30 mph causes more accidents through frustration and dawdling than if the judgement of what is a 'safe' speed were left to drivers. The technical editor of *The Motor* put the argument well (in a broadcast programme, 'Matters of Moment', 26 May 1960) in the simple statement that 'speed is a relative term'. Indeed it has been held that 'the faster you drive the fewer accidents you have': a comment quoted by Moynihan (1960) in reporting a survey by the United States Federal Bureau of Public Roads, which showed that cars travelling at 35 mph were involved in 600 accidents per 100 miles travelled compared with those travelling at 65 mph which sustained fewer than 100. At 65 mph the rate began to rise, but even at 80 it was still only one-quarter of what it was at 35. Teenagers, it appeared, had four times as many accidents at 30 mph as at 65, and Moynihan asks – no doubt with irony – if 'this means that we should urge juveniles to drive faster'.

This survey was derived from the roadside questioning of 29,000 drivers, and Moynihan hints that the evidence may be biased. It may well be biased, if the present writer's experience of listening to numerous motoring cases in court is any indication: it was quite incredible how many drivers said in court that they were doing almost exactly 30 mph, and few admitted to faster speeds. Yet perhaps the commonest form of dangerous driving is overtaking blindly at speed, and this happens at speeds well over 30. Observation suggests that many drivers travel considerably faster than 35 mph whenever they can – whatever the law imposes – and the Univision survey quoted above gives some indication of what really goes on.

Moynihan and many others make the point, when discussing speed and driving, that the driver's personality is reflected in his handling of a vehicle. And it is this psychological approach that distinguishes the relatively more numerous American studies of motoring offences and offenders – traffic violations and violators, as they are called – from the British work. In the United States the automobile has been a universal and taken-for-granted mode of transport for rather longer than it has in Britain, and it is possible that the legal and social problems associated with its use have become manifest sooner there. Perhaps that is why a large number of the American studies treat traffic violations and violators as phenomena that are – potentially at least – pathological and delinquent.

This particular approach has derived mostly from the experience of the

21

traffic divisions of the psychopathic clinics that are attached to some American courts, notably in Detroit and Chicago. Since 1930 it has been the practice of the courts in these two cities to refer selected traffic violators to the clinics for psychiatric examination, and in 1936 the work was considered to be sufficiently important to justify the establishment of separate traffic divisions of the clinics to deal exclusively with violators, applicants for driving licences whom the authorities wished to 'vet', and many other kinds of special case in which fitness to drive was an issue.

The work of the Detroit clinic has been comprehensively described by its executive director, Alan Canty (1953), and some valuable studies have been published based on the results of apparently very thorough examinations of offenders by the psychiatrists, psychologists, and physicians on the staff. The commitment is considerable: i.e. nearly 10,000 offenders were examined in the traffic division between 1936 and 1953. These are, however, a selective sample of the violators who appear before the courts, not all of whom are 'referred' to the clinic; for example, in 1953, 854 offenders, or about five in every 1,000 before the court, were examined. The criteria for referral are peculiar or unstable behaviour on arrest or in court, the possibility of alcoholism, previous mental illness, or a remarkable record of previous convictions of any kind. Hence the subjects of Canty's work are a rather special group.

One of Canty's more recent studies (1956) is particularly relevant. It compares the characteristics of 812 traffic violators examined in his clinic in 1953 with 812 convicted offenders selected at random from the files of the separate criminal division of the psychopathic clinic. *Table 1* shows the comparison according to diagnosis.

From Canty's description of the clinic it can be assumed that neither group of offenders is more selective than the other, since, in the case of both groups, offenders were referred to the clinic only when judges found difficulty in deciding disposal. Hence it would seem that there are some meaningful differences between the two groups.

The traffic offenders include a larger proportion of persons of low intelligence, some of whom could become licensed to drive only if there were grave deficiencies in the testing system. It is not surprising, then, that a considerable number of them should be among those referred to the clinic, since they would be sure to attract judicial attention as 'special cases'. Nor is it surprising that the psychoneuroses are more evident among the traffic violators than in the other group: neurotic persons might be inhibited by their characteristic guilt feelings as far as non-traffic crime is concerned, but because they are preoccupied they might commit the kinds

Orientation

Table 1

PSYCHOPATHIC TRAITS AMONG TWO GROUPS OF OFFENDERS

Diagnosis	812 Traffic Violators		812 Other Offenders	
	Number	Per cent	Number	Per cent
Feebleminded and borderline feebleminded	90	11·1	66	8·1
Inferior and borderline inferior intelligence	154	19·0	40	4·9
Psychotic	16	2·0	50	6·1
Psychosis in remission	6	0·7	2	0·2
Psychoneurosis (all types)	22	2·7	5	0·6
Organic brain disorders, etc.	23	2·8	12	1·5
Convulsive states without psychosis	18	2·2	1	0·1
Senile deterioration	7	0·9	1	0·1
Chronic alcoholism	19	2·3	3	0·4
Personality pattern disturbances				
Inadequate	103	12·7	223	27·5
Schizoid	0	—	31	3·8
Cyclothymic	0	—	1	0·1
Paranoid	0	—	1	0·1
Personality trait disturbances				
Emotionally unstable	101	12·4	26	3·2
Passive-aggressive	37	4·6	183	22·5
Egocentric	31	3·8	2	0·2
Immature	93	11·4	28	3·4
Sociopathic personality				
Disturbance	3	0·4	118	14 5
Antisocial reaction	9	1·1	11	1·4
Dyssocial reaction	1	0·1	1	0·1
Sexual deviation	0	—	3	0·4
No major psychopathy	79	9·7	4	0·5
Total	812		812	

Source: Canty (1956)

of offence that are the result of neglect. However, no detailed information is given about the offences committed by either group. There are unstable and immature persons in both groups, as would be expected, but it is perhaps unexpected that they are more often present among the traffic violators; this calls to mind Gibbens's (1958) point that the motor vehicle may appeal to such persons as an instrument and symbol of power.

Alcoholism might have been supposed a predominant factor among the traffic offenders, yet the proportion of cases is very small compared with the 15·2 per cent so diagnosed among the first 500 violators seen in the clinic before 1939.

Turning to similarities, there is a high proportion of the mentally ill in both groups: just over 90 per cent of the traffic violators and 99·5 per cent of the others must have shown some psychopathy. Unfortunately we have no way of knowing what the percentage of such persons is in the population at large, but it is a sobering thought that there were over 700 drivers of severely disturbed personality on the roads of Detroit at some time in 1952–53. Such a reflection prompts the question whether there is an equally disquieting number of mentally afflicted people on our own roads; it would be a serious matter if there were even half the number that were revealed in Detroit. Finally it is interesting to note that the teams could not find one case of 'sexual deviation' among these 812 traffic violators, who could not have been selected in this respect; perhaps homosexuality and other sexual difficulties are not so widespread in the United States as Kinsey led us to suppose.

Unfortunately, Canty does not include case histories in this study, or any indication of the motives for the offences; nor does he disclose the nature of the offences, which would have been a useful basis of comparison between the two groups. However, it is clear from his work that the psychiatric clinic is a necessary adjunct to courts dealing with traffic offenders, of whom some are likely to exhibit mental illness to such a degree that the habitual treatment of their behaviour by fines or imprisonment would appear to be unproductive.

Canty makes this point about treatment in an earlier study (1942) dealing with the young 'problem driver', in which he puts a case for probation, with or without psychotherapy, for these offenders. Here he gives seven case histories, and their content will be familiar to readers of the literature on delinquency: they show the usual pattern of delinquent contacts, broken homes, hostility to the police and to authority in general, and feelings of inferiority for which subjects try to compensate by daring and exhibition-istic behaviour. A typical example is that of an 18-year-old boy who was arrested for dangerous driving while sitting on the back of his car, steering it with his feet. There was a history of polio and a resulting atrophy of the lower left extremity, from which the boy developed 'marked feelings of inferiority'; as he became older he became aggressive and egocentric in his compensatory efforts. His offence so endangered a group of schoolchildren as to cause a demand by the public for severe punishment, and the clinic staff came in for considerable criticism because they recommended one

24

year's probation with disqualification from driving. As Canty says: 'This case illustrates very well the difference in the recommendation that is made following a careful scientific investigation, and the decision that might follow only a consideration of the offence itself . . . we believe that, as in the case of criminal behaviour, the punishment should fit the offender rather than the offence.' This last sentence implies that in 1942 we could have added Canty to the list of those who somehow cannot regard traffic offenders as criminals, even though numerous factors in the environment and make-up of traffic offenders seem to make them almost indistinguishable from juvenile offenders of other kinds.

However, in a later study Canty (1953) clarifies his position in stressing that 'the chronic violator is a social problem child whose traffic mis-behaviour is but a symptom of his personality maladjustment. The same factors which cause marital unhappiness, divorce and separation, frequent job changes, economic distress and unhealthy recreational activities contribute to his contempt for social and legal conventions, as exemplified by his chronic defiance of the traffic laws.' Canty then makes a point that was to be most useful in formulating the hypotheses for the present research: *'It has often been said that a person behaves in a manner totally different from his usual pattern when he is behind the wheel of his car. This is not so. His personality does not change. There is one significant difference: when the driver is in his own car there is more freedom to demonstrate the presence of unsocial, irresponsible and even antisocial traits. The complete clinical study to which these chronic traffic violators are subjected . . . unmasks these people for what they really are, social misfits.'*

These are such strong words that one hesitates to go all the way with them; but it is salutary to remember that they are the result of detailed examinations of nearly 10,000 traffic offenders. However, it must be stressed that the offenders were a selective group, made up of one in 200 of all traffic violators appearing before the Detroit court; hence any extension of Canty's comments to motoring offenders in general can be only tentative.

Lest Canty's evidence be thought too damning, it should be emphasized that his findings are substantially confirmed by the work done in a similar clinic in Chicago, under the direction of Dr E. J. Kelleher since 1956. In his unpublished reports (1959) to the Chief Justice for the City of Chicago, Kelleher deals with just over 100 offenders referred in 1957 and 1958; we find the same depressing picture of low intelligence (11 per cent) and pathological personality states (34 per cent); and although these are also selected subjects, Kelleher echoes Canty's discomfort at the idea of so many individuals who are clearly unfit to drive being loose on the busy roads of an American city.

Kelleher's reports are especially interesting in that they include data on age, sex, education, previous convictions, and – to some extent – occupation. As in the British work, we find the serious offenders concentrated in the age range 21 to 50, with a mode of about 43. Men greatly outnumber women by nearly nine to one. The poorly educated provide about one-third of the subjects, and only 17 per cent are classified as having received advanced education; 67 per cent had been arrested previously for traffic violations, and 22 per cent for non-traffic offences. And Kelleher stressed the 'particularly startling fact' that about 19 per cent of the referrals were 'professional drivers' who, in theory anyhow, are believed to be highly selected in the United States; he does not, however, define the 'professional driver'. ¶

Of the offences for which the subjects were convicted, 51 per cent were cases of drunken driving; only 4 per cent of the offenders were found guilty of dangerous driving, including one who was wearing roller skates when driving his car. A substantial number of offences were relatively trivial, e.g. parking (one offender had seventeen previous parking convictions), and driving without a licence. Kelleher makes a telling point when he remarks on the proportion of offenders who drove without a licence because they would not be granted one if they applied formally, since they would be excluded on physical or mental grounds, e.g. epileptics and the near-sighted. In the United States and Britain this is considered to be a very minor offence with a light penalty (usually a fine of about £1 in Britain), and it may be that these offenders need to be dealt with more firmly in the interests of public safety. If the qualifications for driving licences become more rigorous, then the offence of driving without one would have to be treated more seriously.

As motoring offenders are not apparently a very homogeneous group, it is rather a pity that Kelleher does not break down the information about his subjects according to the particular kind of offence committed; as it is they are dealt with 'in bulk', and it is impossible to see to which offences particular kinds of subject were most prone – though the association of drunken driving and alcoholism is, of course, obvious. However, these are useful and lucid reports.

One of the best-known American studies of traffic violators convicted of a specific offence is that of Lowell S. Selling (1941), a former director of the Detroit traffic clinic, on the 'hit-and-run' driver. In this the characteristics of fifty offenders found guilty of 'leaving the scene of an accident after killing or injuring someone' are discussed, and compared in certain respects with the characteristics of 500 traffic violators taken at random from offenders convicted by the same court for other offences.

Selling found that abnormal traits of personality were well marked among the fifty hit-and-run drivers, whom he classifies as follows:

	Percentage
Unstable psychopaths	40
Egocentric personalities	12
Mental defectives	22
Chronic alcoholics	10
Psychoneurotics	4
Schizoid, etc.	10
Not ill	2
	100

That they constitute a grossly disturbed group seems to be indisputable, and as such they could probably hold their own with any criminal group. But here one must take into account the offence of which they had been convicted, since it is one in which there is usually a flight from the consequences and a guilty mind. This must be so if the offender knows that an incident has occurred.

In this study, as in those of Canty and Kelleher, there is a high incidence of mental defectiveness among the offenders: 22 per cent of the hit-and-run group were classified thus, and 52 per cent of the 500. Indeed it does not seem unreasonable to suppose that limited intelligence is likely to lead to difficulty in handling a vehicle on the congested roads of a city like Detroit. It would be valuable to have information about intelligence levels among British offenders, but the collection of such data would probably require the establishment of traffic clinics similar to those in the United States.

Also like Canty and Kelleher, Selling found that a high proportion (62 per cent) of the hit-and-run offenders admitted to drinking before the offence; 48 per cent showed symptoms of alcoholism; and a further 10 per cent were diagnosed as chronic alcoholics. Hence Selling deduces that 'alcoholism is an important factor in the hit-and-run situation, and it is also said that the psychopathic personality which predominates in this group has a tendency to resort to alcohol'. Among the 500 other violators, 35·8 per cent are classified under alcoholism and a further 12·5 per cent as chronic alcoholics – which suggests that alcoholism of one kind or another may be an important factor in a wide range of serious motoring offences.

There is further evidence to this effect in a more recent monograph by Selzer (1961) on the question of whether it is intoxication *per se*, personality, or an explosive fusion of the two that leads the drunken driver to dangerous behaviour. He quotes an impressive list of authorities to show that alcoholics are found frequently in studies of drunken drivers, thus opposing the belief that it is the slightly squiffy individual, rather than the genuine alcoholic, who is the menace on the roads. Selzer analyses the concept of 'the alcoholic personality' who, he suggests, displays traits of egocentricity, chronic depression with tendencies to self-destruction, and chronic hostility. He suggests further that the egocentricity 'may have the quality of an absolute conviction of omnipotence and invulnerability . . . The depression may be linked with a marked urge to commit suicide', and the hostility may be expressed in a 'passive subtle way that inebriety will change, and chronic rage, coupled with low frustration tolerance, may erupt into violence'. He points out that the automobile appeals to the alcoholic as an instrument of 'almost socially acceptable violence' because it appears to afford him a means of aggressive expression that is otherwise denied him. Selzer quotes one of his alcoholic patients answering the question: 'What effect does drinking have on you as a driver?' The man replied: 'It makes me feel that I can't be outdone in an automobile. I feel this is something I can control completely. I can make it go fast, or I can make it go slow, but I never want to make it go slow. Drinking makes my accelerator foot get heavy.' This man had had five serious accidents in twelve years of driving, and he had been convicted fourteen times for traffic offences.

In all, Selzer quotes only three case histories, and these might have been selected to prove his point, since he seeks to show that accident-prone drivers display the same characteristics as alcoholics by applying the criteria used for the alcoholic subjects to a group of only ten accident-prone drivers. However, it must be said in fairness that the group of ten were said to have been studied independently by another worker, Conger, who reported a close similarity in the characteristics displayed by the two groups.

To return to Selling's work: one of its most significant aspects is the author's analysis of the previous convictions of his subjects. Both groups had a surprisingly large number for traffic and other violations, ranging from one to eighteen traffic violations, and from one to thirteen other offences. Of the hit-and-run group, 80 per cent had two or more previous convictions for traffic offences, and 38 per cent had two or more convictions for non-traffic offences – a possible reason for 'running', as Selling says.

The presence of up to eighteen previous violations on their records suggests that the concept of recidivism may be just as applicable to motoring offenders as it is to others, and it would be interesting to know what proportion of the many serious motoring offenders in Britain would be eligible for such a category. For this purpose it would be necessary to make a definition of recidivism that would be appropriate in motoring cases.

A disturbed and unhappy background was common among the hit-and-run cases, and one case history is quoted in which the situation was 'soon elucidated in an interview'. It is not clear, however, just how many of the disturbed backgrounds were elucidated in this way; if there were many, suspicions are roused, because it seems unlikely in the psychiatry-ridden United States that many offenders accused of such a manifestly blameworthy offence would miss the chance to excuse their misbehaviour on these grounds.

As might be expected, all Selling's offenders but one were males, and women were not found in anywhere near the proportion of between one in six to one in three that was expected. So it seems that the traffic offence is a male prerogative, as is the non-traffic offence also. Age was distributed widely among both groups of offenders, a surprise to Selling who expected the hit-and-run offence to be a teenage phenomenon. Moreover, 50 per cent of the hit-and-runners were experienced drivers who had held licences to drive for over five years, and 22 per cent had fifteen to twenty years' driving experience.

Another rather surprising fact for those who think of motoring offenders as coming from the white-collar classes is Selling's statement that the majority of the offenders studied had occupations that were 'marginal and unskilled', and the group included a higher proportion of Negroes than would be expected from their numbers in the population of Detroit. It may be that the occupational class distribution of motoring offenders in this country is not as we imagine it to be, which would suggest that the sociological and psychological differences between motoring offenders and other offenders may not be so marked as is often supposed.

From a criminological standpoint this work of Selling's is extremely useful because, in addition to describing characteristics, he examines the motivation behind a common motoring offence – a procedure that is not usual except, perhaps, in the drink offences. In his analysis of the motivational factors underlying the hit-and-run offence, Selling produces case-history evidence to suggest that flight from the scene of an accident (he uses this term) results from a panic reaction, followed by a claim that the offender was unaware of hitting anything; there is, according to Selling, a partially unconscious suppression of the event so that the 'lies' of the offender become unusually convincing. On the other hand, there is the reaction of the feebleminded who 'just does not think to stop'; and of the schizoid who is 'quite indifferent to the harm he does', because there is a 'dissociation between appreciation of the occurrence and any sense of responsibility for it'.

It is peculiarly difficult and hazardous for a writer, who is not himself a psychiatrist, to make inferences from psychiatric data, but it is hard to resist the comment here that Selling's analysis might be appropriate to a wide range of unlawful behaviour that unhesitatingly secures the label 'criminal'. Hence, again, there may be a substantial bridge between motoring offences and other kinds of offence.

The same inference can be drawn from a comparison made by Heath (1955) between 763 traffic violators and 195 drivers with no recorded offences; the two groups were matched according to the annual mileage driven. When the Thurstone Temperament Schedule was applied, statistically significant differences were revealed between the two groups: the offenders showing a higher degree of impulsiveness and sociability, and a lower degree of 'reflectiveness', than the non-offenders. There were marked differences also shown with regard to:

Age:	Offenders were younger.
Marital status:	Offenders were more often single.
Education:	For a higher proportion of offenders it was 'not better than grade school'.
Income:	Offenders were much lower earners, and fewer of them had professional or managerial occupations.
Employment record:	There was a higher job-turnover among offenders for reasons other than self-improvement.
Driving knowledge:	Offenders were more experienced and knowledgeable.

Perhaps the only surprising finding is that the offenders were the more experienced and knowledgeable drivers. Moreover, when sixty-three offenders with a high degree of exposure to accident risk were studied in detail, it was found that they had a better accident record than the non-offenders, though their record of offences was not so good. Most of these sixty-three offenders were professional drivers, e.g. chauffeurs or driver-salesmen.

One important feature emerges from Heath's work that is similar to the British studies: that a personality inclined to extraversion is inclined also to be involved in incidents when driving (see Drew *et al.*, 1959).

THE STUDY OF ACCIDENT-PRONENESS

It will be seen that much of the foregoing work was concerned almost entirely with persons involved in 'accidents', and it is from the study of accidents and the liability to have them that the bulk of all information about driving behaviour that is of criminological interest has been derived. The findings of numerous studies of this kind have been reviewed comprehensively by McFarland (1955)[1] whose comments will now be considered.

In Britain and in the United States there has been considerable interest in the concept of accident-proneness, or the propensity of certain individuals to have more accidents than they would be expected to have by chance alone. This concept stemmed from the studies of industrial physicians and psychologists who found that in certain cases a minority of workers appeared to have a higher proportion of accidents at work than would be expected from calculations of normal probability. Accordingly, the hypothesis was put forward that it should be possible to identify a group of drivers as having a greater inherent propensity to accidents than others. Unfortunately, as McFarland has said, there was a tendency in much of this work to be over-zealous in trying to isolate predictable characteristics, and to omit the statistical tests necessary to show that the accidents were *not* due to chance. McFarland has also exposed some of the difficulties in accepting the view that any particular group of subjects can be identified merely because they have more accidents than would be expected by chance: there is, for example, the likelihood that the members of the group would not all have the same liability or exposure to risk, in that the conditions under which they lived and drove would probably be very dissimilar. So we have not progressed far if we find that X has had six accidents when by chance alone he might have been expected to have three, since the explanation may be X's greater exposure to risk; hence a comparison of personal characteristics between X and others, whose accident frequency exceeds chance also, would not be particularly meaningful. To get anywhere it would be necessary to ensure that exposure to risk is taken into account and, as McFarland shows, there is no really satisfactory way of doing this. Mileage covered would certainly not meet the requirement, because conditions vary so much: e.g. 2,000 miles driven in rural areas is a vastly different risk proposition from the same mileage in an industrial urban area – as insurance rates indicate.

Another method is what McFarland has called the 'clinical approach', according to which a number of persons who have had 'several' accidents are intensively examined; whether the number of accidents is greater than would be expected by chance is not regarded as important here. The point is

[1] References are given to the works cited by McFarland (op. cit.), but they have not been read in the original by the present writer, and the descriptions of the studies are McFarland's.

that the subject is an 'accident-repeater' (though McFarland does not say how many accidents would justify this appellation), and in this view the emphasis – to quote McFarland – 'is upon the psychological characteristics of the persons who have the accidents [which] result from the psychological make-up of the individual, and when they occur, they are deemed to serve certain purposes of personal need'. McFarland (1955, p. 26) considers this approach as deriving from the clinical studies of persons sustaining accidental injuries, and he cites Dunbar's work (1944) as typical. In examining patients who were in hospital for fractures sustained in accidents, she noticed marked differences in personality among them as compared with patients admitted for heart and circulatory complaints: 'Psychological conflicts in the area of reaction to authority were focal, and accidents occurred as the result of the impulsive attempts to resolve the tensions'; injuries were envisaged as means by which guilt could be assuaged and attention secured.

To the criminologist there is nothing new in this kind of clinical, albeit speculative, approach, and we are on familiar ground when we consider one of the best examples of it, a study by Tillmann and Hobbs (1949). They carried out in London, Ontario, an intensive analysis of the personal history and characteristics of three groups of twenty taxi drivers, all of whom were known to the workers; the subjects were classified initially into three categories of high, low, and medium accident frequency, and comparisons were made from personal histories and from data compiled from police, juvenile court, and social agency records. *Table 2* presents the results of the comparison between the high and low frequency groups, according to various criteria.

The first two columns show the numbers of subjects in each category, and the third column shows the extent to which the difference between the two groups is greater than it would be if the relationship were one of pure chance only (chi-square = 0). In fact a significant difference at the 5 per cent level is given by a chi-square value exceeding 3·84 (there is, however, some inaccuracy in the chi-squares for $N = 40$, since full information was not available for all the subjects).

The highest values of chi-square are associated with factors that are usually found in case studies of offenders, i.e. histories of excessive aggression, of truancy and poor discipline at school, of absence without leave from the armed forces, and of domestic disharmony; there is also 'bootlegging on the job', whatever that is, but it may be that the low accident group were as guilty of this as the high accident group, but were not prepared to admit it. In fact it might be wise to treat with reserve any criteria that depend on

Table 2

PERSONAL ATTRIBUTES OF 20 HIGH AND 20 LOW ACCIDENT FREQUENCY DRIVERS

	High accident	Low accident	χ^2*
Birthplace			
urban	15	15	0
History of parents			
divorced	6	1	4·63
excess strictness and disharmony	13	5	6·28
Neurotic traits			
excess childhood phobias	11	5	4·48
excess childhood aggression	11	0	23·60
School adjustment			
completed grade school	15	15	0
truancy and disciplinary problems	12	2	10·98
Employment record			
5 or more previous jobs	13	7	3·60
history of being fired	10	4	3·98
Armed service record			
member of armed forces	15	9	
frequent AWOL	11	1	8·60
Marital status			
married	8	11	—
Sex adjustment			
admitted sexual promiscuity	8	2	4·00
Social adjustment			
2 or more hobbies	9	17	8·50
admitting bootlegging on job	14	3	12·20
conscious of physique	11	3	5·40

Source: Tillmann & Hobbs (1949)

* χ^2 = 3·84 significant

personal admissions, e.g. parental history and neurotic traits, since these could easily be used to rationalize a poor record; however, this would not apply to most of the other significant differences between the groups, because the information did not come from the subjects alone.

The employment record is interesting in view of its importance in such studies of criminal offenders as that of Mannheim and Wilkins (1955); a more significant difference might have been expected with regard to this factor, but perhaps taxi drivers are more likely than other workers to change their jobs. Also it is rather surprising to find no item linked to drinking, though presumably alcoholism would be unacceptable in this kind of job.

Legal and Social Background

In another project Tillmann and Hobbs (1949) eliminated objections to the use of personal admissions as evidence by obtaining their information *solely* from sources other than the subjects, i.e. courts, social agencies, and credit bureaux. In this study they matched ninety-six accident-repeaters with two control groups of a hundred drivers, one taken from the claim-free records of an insurance company or companies, and the other from official licensing records. Their findings are presented in *Table 3*.

Table 3

PERCENTAGES OF ACCIDENT-FREE AND ACCIDENT-REPEATER
DRIVERS KNOWN TO VARIOUS AGENCIES

Criteria	Accident-repeater	Accident-free Group A	Group B
	%	%	%
Known to one or more agencies	66	9	9
Known to more than one agency	32	0	0
Credit bureau had contacted	34	6	6
Social service agencies	18	1	1
Public health venereal disease clinic	14	0	0
Adult court (exclusive of traffic charges)	34	1	1
Juvenile court	17	1	2

Source: Tillmann & Hobbs (1949)

The comparative percentages reveal marked distinctions between those who have repeated accidents and those who are more or less free from accidents. Of most relevance to this particular study is the proportion of repeaters who have been before courts on charges other than traffic violations: 34 per cent had been before adult courts, as against only 1 per cent in each of the accident-free control groups; and 17 per cent had been before juvenile courts in contrast with 1 and 2 per cent in the two control groups of the accident-free. It would obviously be unsound to add the two percentages referring to the accident-repeaters and say that 51 per cent of them had been before the courts, since it is not clear whether the 34 per cent includes some who had earlier appeared before juvenile courts; however, 34 per cent is a larger proportion than would be expected if it were true that the motoring offender is normally an upright law-abiding citizen away from his vehicle. The other criteria suggest personality disturbance, worry, and preoccupation, or all three combined, and indicate that at least one-third of the repeaters had backgrounds that might be unstable.

34

Orientation

From these two studies Tillmann and Hobbs concluded that a person 'drives as he lives', and so put forward a concept of driving as just one of the manifestations of personality. There seems to be ample support for their conclusion in *Tables 2* and *3*, and the idea is of such importance that it is one of the aims of this study to test it.

A confirmatory study was, in fact, done by McFarland and Moseley (1954), in which fifty-seven accident-free drivers were compared with a control group of fifty-seven accident-repeaters. The results are presented in *Table 4*. There is here an interesting contrast with the Tillmann findings:

Table 4

RELATIVE VALUES OF SELECTED ITEMS TO DISCRIMINATE
BETWEEN DRIVERS WHO ARE ACCIDENT-FREE AND
DRIVERS WHO ARE ACCIDENT-REPEATERS

Criteria	χ^2
Court record of automotive offences	7·48
Minor violation, in motor-vehicle records	6·76
Court record of offences against persons	6·43
Unfavourable business inspection report	3·84
Court record of offences against self	2·55
Court record of offences against property	2·01
Accident, in motor-vehicle records	0·61
Licence suspension, in motor-vehicle records	0·60
Serious violation, in motor-vehicle records	0·03

Source: McFarland and Moseley (1954)

McFarland and Moseley give the existence of previous motoring convictions the highest priority in their table, which consists largely of criteria concerning previous offences of various kinds. Using this particular table in later research these workers were able to identify 85 per cent of the accident-repeaters in a random sample of drivers.

Still more support is available for the view that a driver is influenced by his social conditioning as well as by his innate characteristics. McFarland and Moore (1957, para. 20) report on an investigation of personal and interpersonal factors in motor accidents, made at the University of Colorado and the Fitzsimons Army Hospital; in this study the most powerful item in discriminating between the accident-repeater and the accident-free is the response to a modified version of the Allport-Vernon scale of values: 'Subjects who have had accidents score consistently high on the aesthetic

35

and theoretical scale but consistently low on the religious scale. . . . Analysis of the emotional projection tests used in the study suggests that the accident-free subject is relatively more likely to identify with the father and have a positive self-picture than is the accident-repeater.' The latter is 'less likely to identify with his parents and is more likely to show regressive masochistic phantasy'; he is also 'more likely to consider authority figures as unpleasant'. Furthermore, 'the accident-repeater appears to feel that his social environment is unsatisfactory and barren in relation to his strong needs for affection and for recognition'.

It is tempting to criticize the Colorado study as over-speculative and unrealistic in making many inferences from data that cannot be checked; McFarland (1955, p. 27) remarks that 'it would be an unimaginative psychologist or psychiatrist who could not, after an accident has occurred, find some indication of conflicts and repressed feelings consistent with his theory'. However, it does not mean that caution is discarded by concluding that substantial support is given to Tillmann and Hobbs's view that an individual 'drives as he lives'.

Other American studies which deal with personality factors in accidents and to which McFarland (1955) refers include that of Brody (1941), who found accident-repeaters to be more frequently maladjusted than the accident-free; and a study by the Eno Foundation (1948), in which a group of accident-repeaters were compared with a matched group of accident-free drivers – the latter were found to be more stable emotionally than the repeaters. A similar finding is attributed to Parker (1953) who compared two groups of thirty tractor drivers, one of which had accident records and the other was accident-free. It was found that the accident-free drivers were less dominant, less self-sufficient, and more tense than the accident group, according to results derived from the administration of the Bernreuter Personality Inventory.

In considering specific factors in driving behaviour that might be especially associated with high accident propensity, McFarland stresses four: intelligence, sex, age, and personality. And here it should be noted that the focus is upon *accidents and not offences*, since not all accidents involve offences, and vice versa; there may, however, be a strong enough relationship between the two for McFarland's discussion to be useful.

McFarland (1955, p. 35) does not appear to give intelligence the importance accorded to it by Canty, Kelleher, and Selling in discussing offenders, but he does suggest that the better-endowed are safer drivers than the less intelligent. Clarke found this to be indicated in his study of drivers in the British army, since his subjects with low selection grades had a fairly high accident rate in proportion to their small numbers. In a study of American army motor transport units, Edgerton (1951) compared a unit 'rated highly for safety with another rated low'; he found that the average scores on intelligence tests by the drivers in the highly rated units were significantly better than those by the drivers in the low-rated units. But, as McFarland emphasized, 'superior intelligence by itself is no guarantor of freedom from accidents'; and there is evidence from a study by Laur (1939) that high intelligence can be associated with dangerous driving when the IQ is between 110 and 125. On the other hand, Brody (1941) considers that intelligence has very little to do with the propensity to have accidents. So the evidence is equivocal on this point.

It may surprise those who so readily castigate women drivers to learn that there is no evidence at all to suggest that they are more prone to accidents than men. There have been several studies on this issue in the United States, where the proportion of women drivers is higher than in Britain, and they have found nothing manifestly unfavourable to women (see McFarland, 1955). This has been demonstrated also by an analysis of insurance company records, although men outnumbered women drivers by five or six to one (Munden, 1962). The same is true of motoring offenders, among whom women are rarely principals: Selling produced only one female offender; in Kelleher's highly selected group 11 per cent were women; and it would appear from the available data that the ratio of motoring offenders in Britain in 1959 was about twenty-one men to every woman (the ratio for non-motoring offenders was about eight men to every woman).

Where age is concerned it seems that high accident rates are found more often in the age groups under 30, and there is another high point in the range over 55; the best records appear among those aged 30–50. Yet it has been shown by Stack and Walker (1959) that the age range 30–50 is likely to produce a disproportionate number of offenders in the 'driving under the influence' group. Little evidence is available concerning the typical ages of motoring offenders, though Canty (1940) has mentioned a tendency for higher concentrations of offenders in the age group 20–29 than would be expected from the proportion of licence holders in this group. The evidence is, therefore, inconclusive as yet. One thing is clear, however: since it has been found that the best scores in tests of physiological, sensory psychomotor, and mental ability are made by young people, their propensity to accidents, and perhaps to offences, may be due to what McFarland (1955, p. 40) has called 'youthfulness and the particular kind of immaturity, inexperience, and temperament that go with it'.

So here again we begin to overlap the psychological field and to find substance for Moore's (1956) view that 'something other than pure skill or physical fitness must be of great importance in determining accident liability . . . and recent work suggests that the missing factor is what psychologists call "temperament"' (defined by Moore as an individual's mental and emotional outlook).

There is confirmation of the significance of the temperamental factor in the work by Dr Russell Davis (1948) on the classification of pilots in the Royal Air Force. In a number of tests of pilots flying under instrument conditions he designated three apparent groups: those showing normal reactions to the complex (instrument-flying) situation; those showing over-activity, tenseness, and irritability; and a third group showing inertia characterized by lack of attention, lowering of standards, tiredness, and emotional difficulty. In a follow-up study of these subjects, pilots in the second and third groups were found to be suspended from flying duties more frequently and were involved in proportionately more fatal accidents, than those in the first group. Similarly, Bieshevel and White, in a study reported by Moore (1956), found that tests for coordination, mechanical aptitude, emotionality, and parental relationships discriminated between 200 pilots who had blameworthy accidents and 400 who had none; they claimed to predict accident-proneness in thirteen out of seventeen pilots who had blameworthy accidents while flying.

It may be held that studies concerned with flying are somewhat out of place in this context, but it is suggested that the whole problem of what used to be called 'flying discipline' has many things in common with traffic discipline and its breach – the traffic offence. In the second world war the air staff were much disturbed by the incidence of flying accidents that were thought to be due to carelessness and to breaches of flying regulations concerning, for example, low flying and aerobatics. An intensive campaign against such occurrences was carried out through films, magazines, and posters to supplement the increased severity with which authorities were ordered to deal with offenders. The campaign aimed to convince pilots that careless damage to aircraft was severely detrimental to the war effort, and that most behaviour of this kind was, in any case, stupid. The stereotype of the careless pilot was developed through the striking personality of 'Pilot Officer Prune', whose inanities were featured in an attractive and widely circulated training magazine called *Tee Emm*. It was by these means, and with the support of enthusiastic and responsible aircrew, that the slapdash pilot became stigmatized mercilessly as a 'clot' (i.e. an incompetent or stupid person), and since none liked to be labelled in

38

Orientation

this way the standards of behaviour improved markedly and quickly. This was the ancient device of group ridicule at its most effective, and the results were good. It is possible that equal success could be achieved if road users were to treat bad or exhibitionist driving behaviour in a similar way.

CRIMINOLOGICAL APPROACHES

Perhaps the most striking feature of the available literature is the absence of a comprehensive study that attempts to discuss the motoring offence and offender within the framework of existing criminological theory. Wootton, admittedly, touches on this broader problem, but only very sparingly, so that she is unable to analyse the offences or the motives and characteristics of offenders at any depth. Middendorff (1959) makes some provocative and stimulating remarks about the way in which motoring behaviour reflects national characteristics, but he does not found these on any detailed and specific research data.

It is perhaps surprising that no attempt has been made – as far as is known – to treat the subject in relation to criminological theory, but the reason is probably that we do not yet know enough about motoring offences or offenders to be able to do this. Such information as we have is essentially monographic and 'bitty'; so much so that it is hard to draw the strings together in a summary. Accordingly, it will be left until the end of this study to see how far our body of theory can be applied to motoring offences. To take up the question now would be premature.

The relatively sparse British literature seems mainly concerned with telling us that the incidence of motoring offences is a serious matter, and that a high proportion of offences which involve the handling of vehicles are due to the 'demon drink'. Almost the only attempt to go into any detail is Stack and Walker's (1959) study (see above, p. 18), and that deals with only one kind of offence. Even here the evidence is slender, and all we know about the offenders is that they are mostly over 30 and live in towns. Of the offences we are told next to nothing, and the mild case of the inebriated but safe slow driver is one with the headlong dash of the drunken exhibitionist.

The most significant British work may be that which deals with people who have accidents, and with the influence of alcohol on driving. The studies mentioned, those of Clarke and of Drew *et al.* for example, leave little doubt that the personality factor looms large in driving behaviour – and in driving misbehaviour too. Yet we have to rely almost entirely on American work to examine this approach. And in all the studies reviewed from American sources the thesis that one 'drives as one lives' seems to

39

find support; or it may be more accurate to suggest that 'one drives as the kind of personality one is'!

In the work of Canty, Kelleher, and Selling there is evidence to indicate that among serious motoring offenders there may be a proportion of the maladjusted, the delinquent, and the inadequate that is large enough to be worth worrying about. From the facts presented in any of these studies it seems *possible* that a higher proportion of motoring offenders than might have been expected are not readily distinguishable from 'criminals'. Although it must be stressed again that the subjects of these studies were highly selected, it is suggestive that between 86 and 90 per cent of them were found to be psychopathic in some way.

Even though the treatment of motoring offences has been more thorough in the United States than in Britain, it is necessary to use many data from the study of accidents in order to build up a mutually supporting body of knowledge. And here again the importance of personality is inescapable, particularly in Tillmann and Hobbs's work, where the association of social maladjustment with a record of accidents and traffic offences is manifest. Otherwise much of the evidence in the literature is equivocal. The age, intelligence, and social background of persons who are or might be offenders are by no means clear cut.

On balance it seems that offenders come mostly from the age groups under 30, as is the trend in other kinds of crime, except for the 'drunken driver' who tends to be older.

The evidence about intelligence is slight, and somewhat biased by reliance on such highly selected groups as Canty's and Selling's, in which about one-third of the individuals were rated borderline or below in this respect. But a number of studies of the accident-prone lend support to the view that below-average intelligence is a significant factor in many accidents. The findings are not unanimous, but there is no reason to suppose that the distribution of intelligence among motoring offenders is much different from that found among offenders of other kinds.

About social class and occupation there seems to be enough information to suggest that any assumption that motoring offenders are mainly from white-collar groups should be challenged. In no study has the social status of motoring offenders been dealt with adequately, but there are inferences that their class distribution may correspond more closely to that of offenders in general than is often thought to be the case.

When the sex ratio is considered the ground becomes firmer, and it is no surprise to find that the female is less active as a detected law-breaker than the male. The literature mentions females but rarely, and even if we can assume that male drivers exceed females by between five and eight to one, it is indisputable that the motoring offender is nearly always a male.

On motivation there is little in the scientific literature to supplement Selling's work on the hit-and-run offender and Gibbens's study of car thieves. Here again it is striking that there has been so little interest in diagnosing the motives for motoring misbehaviour, in contrast to the intense interest shown in the motives for 'criminal' offences against property and against the person.

So perhaps a criminologist might be excused for turning to a theologian for the postcript to this chapter, and asking, with Waterson (1961), the Vicar of Stoke D'Abernon: 'What is it that happens to many an ordinary, quiet, good-natured husband and father, for instance, which often so oddly debases him when he takes charge of a motor car in, say, the rush hour? On foot he may be continually jostled without irritation, or wait patiently in queues and be courteous to women; but driving he turns to cursing everyone who gets in his way, feels that pedestrians and cyclists are provocative menaces, finds it degrading to be overtaken, adopts a dangerously competitive attitude to other cars and expatiates on the inferiority of women.' Waterson comments also on the remarkable lack of objectivity of drivers towards their driving skill, which he suggests implies a deep-seated deficiency in insight; on the appeal of different designs of vehicle to specific personality types (the car as a 'personalizer'); on the regression to 'atavistic and primitive' behaviour in motoring situations, even to the use of ritual superstitions such as the carrying of 'lucky' charms (Roche is quoted as reporting that 90 per cent of a sample of drivers touched wood when asked if they had ever been in an accident!). He also shares some of Middendorff's (1959) views concerning the expression of national characteristics in motoring behaviour.

Some of Waterson's ideas are too general to be more than stimulating provocations to focused research, but he is more than just suggestive when he points out that 'the motor car puts at human disposal a phenomenal increase in personal power in response to an extremely small effort. The slight movement of one foot can transform every little Charlie into an astronaut.' An unconscious sexual element is inferred when 'the vast virility of the machine is transferred to its master', yet the machine is 'personalized' in that the driver's personality is projected onto it. . . . 'It thus becomes his *own* power and will which are so vastly multiplied and projected that both time and space alter their characteristics to suit his every whim' (op. cit. p. 229).

2

Design of the Study

During discussions with the supervisor of this research, with police officers, lawyers, and members of the public when planning the study, it became evident that a fairly definite stereotype of the motoring offender seems to exist. Generally speaking it is that he – the offender is typically a male – is a thoroughly respectable law-abiding person when he is not behind a steering wheel, and that he usually drives a private car. He is seen to take his offence and punishment in his stride and not to suffer any social ostracism as a result. And as an 'upright' citizen he learns his lesson from his prosecution and does not tend to repeat his offence. Overall the picture is of a technical offence, and of an offender with whom we can identify easily, and about whom jurymen tend to think 'there but for the grace of God go I'.

But the review of the literature in the preceding chapter casts doubt on this stereotype, which, on balance, it does not substantiate. Indeed, it is pertinent to ask whether the motoring offender, and in particular the serious motoring offender, *can* properly be classed with those who forget to renew their wireless licence or dog licence. Perhaps we would not say 'there but for the grace . . . etc.' if we knew more about these people. To what extent *do* they differ from those whom we somewhat arbitrarily call 'criminals'? Do they really exhibit so few of the traits that we have come to call 'psychopathic' that they cannot be compared with the burglar, the embezzler, and the sex offender? By objective standards there does not seem to be any answer to these questions: we just do not know, and we give the motoring offender – even the serious one – the benefit of the doubt and tend to put him in a non-criminal category.

It is a central part of this research to find out whether this comparatively lenient view of these offenders is justified, and the problem was to find an effective way of doing this.

DEVELOPMENT OF HYPOTHESES

The first step was to devise some hypotheses that could be tested in a one-man research for which time and means were strictly limited. Also it was felt that these hypotheses should reflect 'public opinion' about the serious motoring offender; they could then be exposed to the usual scientific procedure whereby one tries to adduce facts to disprove them. Failure to disprove a hypothesis leaves it in a state of at least tentative validity.

It seemed, in the planning stages, that the following hypotheses constituted the minimum that would have to be examined in order to present a picture of the serious motoring offender that was to have much meaning:

(*a*) *The serious motoring offender, unlike the majority of other offenders found guilty of criminal offences, e.g. offenders against property, is a respectable citizen whose behaviour apart from his offence is reasonably in accord with the requirements of law and order.*

This hypothesis was suggested by attitudes noticed among friends, and among students of criminology, whenever motoring offences were mentioned in discussions. Its usefulness was confirmed also in conversations with police officers, whose first reaction to the research proposals was that they saw no point in looking for 'criminals' among motoring offenders *per se* – they were, they said, an essentially different group from the criminals.

(*b*) *The majority of serious motoring offences are derived from accidents, and there is nothing in the offender's personality or background that predisposes him to break the law.*

This seems to be believed widely, and it is linked with the conviction that the *mens rea* does not arise in motoring offences. Hence, perhaps, the ease with which juries are said to identify with the offender in saying 'there but for the grace of God go I', because the offence is thought to be derived from accidental circumstances that were not premeditated or intended. Moreover, it is inferred that dishonesty and malice do not come into these cases, which puts them at once into a different category from offences against property or the person.

(*c*) *The offender convicted of a serious motoring offence does not regard himself as a criminal, nor does he think himself to be regarded as such by the rest of society.*

It seems reasonable to suppose that the motoring offender has no 'professional pride' as a criminal, as those who live by the proceeds of crime are believed to have. He does not, therefore, identify with the 'criminal classes', and does not suffer any social ostracism as a result of his conviction – an incident that makes little difference to his social status.

43

Legal and Social Background

(d) *If the Registrar-General's classification of occupational groups is taken as a criterion of social class, serious motoring offenders will be distributed widely over the range of occupations, in contrast to the majority of other offenders convicted of indictable offences (or those akin thereto), who tend to come from the manual groups.*

This hypothesis was developed to examine the view that most serious motoring offenders come from the white-collar occupational classes. To test the hypothesis it was intended to classify the offenders according to the Registrar-General's five occupational classes, and to compare the distribution with that given in the latest census for the population as a whole. But this proved unsatisfactory since the Registrar-General's classification does not discriminate adequately between the white-collar and the skilled manual groups: as everyone has to be compressed into five classes, the skilled manual class includes a great many people who might properly be regarded as white-collar workers. Hence, if the offender population *did* show a concentration in the manual groups, this would not appear at all significant when it was compared with the census which would show these classes in an unrealistically inflated form. So it was necessary to modify the hypothesis to read:

If occupation is taken as a criterion of social class, the majority of serious motoring offenders will be found to come from non-manual occupations, in contrast to the majority of other offenders convicted of indictable offences (or those akin thereto), who tend to come mostly from manual occupations.

This, so far as motoring offenders are concerned, is a hypothesis that can be proved or disproved, but to do so it was necessary to use an occupational classification that distinguished fairly well between white-collar and manual working-class groups. The choice of a classification was peculiarly difficult since no classification is without shortcomings; but eventually it was decided to use a form derived from Hall and Moser (1954), as follows:

White-collar :   Professional and higher administrative
                 Managerial and executive
                 Lower non-manual grades

Manual :   Skilled manual
                 Semi-skilled manual
                 Unskilled manual

This seemed to offer an adequate range, and where there was doubt – as in cases like members of the armed forces and housewives – allotment could be made to a higher, rather than a lower, group. Hence the distribution would be biased towards the white-collar groups; but this would not be unrealistic, having regard to the reduction nowadays of the distinctions between manual and minor white-collar occupations.

However there still remained the problem of showing whether any occupational/class group in the population was under- or over-represented among the offenders, or whether the distributions were reasonably coincident. Unfortunately no satisfactory solution was found, but rather than admit defeat it was decided to use for comparison a classification devised by Cole (1955, p. 153), based on the 1951 census; this shows the estimated distribution of occupied heads of households in Great Britain. It was attractive because the breakdown by occupational groups is very similar to that of Hall and Moser, and its population would be predominantly male, with probably a high proportion of licence holders; but, on the other hand, it would exclude most of those under 21 of whom there is a substantial minority among the offenders. The method of comparison is, therefore, very imperfect, but perhaps it does give a more accurate idea of the position than has been available hitherto.

(e) *The typical serious motoring offender is 'the motorist' – the driver of a private car. These drivers form the majority, in contrast to drivers of public-service vehicles, drivers of goods vehicles, and motor cyclists.*

The correspondence columns of the press leave an impression that this is a generally held view; moreover, when motoring offenders are being discussed, the hypothetical offender is usually referred to as a 'motorist': a term that is not normally applied to anyone but the driver of a private car. For instance, *The Times* ran a descriptive heading 'Motorists in Court' for a correspondence series in October 1959; and the *Daily Telegraph* for 18 January 1960 devoted a leading article to discussing the reaction of 'motorists' to the proposed changes in the law dealing with drunken drivers; no mention was made of other drivers or riders who might be equally concerned. Indeed the term 'motorist' has been used in aspersion so extensively that the Automobile Association was moved to stimulate a correspondence in *The Times* (20 October 1961) to get ideas for another generic term for those in charge of mechanical vehicles; the suggestions ranged from 'martyrists' to 'maniacs'. Yet if the proportions of the different classes of vehicle on the roads are taken into account, it may be found that the driver of the private car is not the most frequent transgressor of the law, especially where the more serious offences are concerned.

45

(*f*) *Serious motoring offenders are not concentrated in any particular age group.*

According to the *Criminal Statistics* for the years 1950 to 1960, the majority of offenders convicted of indictable offences are in the group aged 21 and under. In view of the equivocal evidence about the age of motoring offenders presented in Chapter 1, it is interesting to inquire whether serious motoring offenders differ from other offenders in being older as a group, or in being distributed over a wider range of ages.

(*g*) *Having been found guilty and punished for one offence of a serious nature, the motoring offender does not repeat the offence.*

This is another hypothesis that supports the belief that motoring offenders are usually respecters of the law, who take their punishment in the spirit of a lesson and do not offend again in the same or similar ways. Hence one seldom, if ever, hears the term 'recidivist' applied to motoring offenders with several convictions.

(*h*) *Given the opportunity to do so, the serious motoring offender will usually elect to be tried before a jury.*

Discussions with motorists and solicitors prior to starting on this research made it clear that it is believed that juries are likely to be more lenient and sympathetic towards the motoring offender than are magistrates. An example of this belief can be seen in a speech by Lord Goddard in a House of Lords debate, during which the leniency of magistrates towards motoring offenders was held to be partly responsible for their high incidence. Lord Goddard said: 'There have been a good many hard things said about magistrates, but they are not the only people who have to take responsibility. Of all the people concerned I would put at the head the quarter sessions' juries, remembering that in all cases of dangerous or drunken driving the defendant has the right to trial by jury, and many of them exercise it because they know that their chances of acquittal are much greater. No one has yet found a way of preventing a jury from returning a perverse verdict' (*The Times*, 11 June 1959).

(*i*) *The treatment of serious motoring offenders by the courts is much more lenient than the treatment of offenders charged with offences against the person or against property, or with sex offences.*

Despite the belief that underlies the preceding hypothesis, this statement also expresses a view that seems to be quite firmly established, and Wootton

(1959, pp. 26–9) makes this point the burden of her references to motoring offenders. There is evidence that the belief exists in the Magistrates' Association too, since its Annual General Meeting for 1959 heard a motion proposed that 'in general, magistrates' courts had failed to impose adequate penalties for road traffic offences' (*The Magistrate*, December 1959, p. 134). Wootton (op. cit. p. 49) comments that the proportion of motoring defendants convicted of driving under the influence of drink or drugs, or of dangerous driving, is negligible in contrast to the proportion of defendants convicted of larceny, breaking and entering, and even of begging. Further, if more sensational, support is provided by the middle-page spread in the *Daily Sketch* of 3 June 1960 under the headline 'An Hour Apart in the Same Court', reporting the sentence of fifteen months' imprisonment with three years' disqualification imposed on a lorry driver for causing the deaths by dangerous driving of two persons (it was shown also that he was drunk at the time), and the two-year prison sentence passed on a 'foolish woman of 43 for obtaining £1,490 from a finance company by false pretences'. Both sentences were said to have been passed by the same judge in the same court with no more than an hour between the two cases.

(*j*) *The courts rarely use their power to order a serious motoring offender to take another driving test.*

This supplements the preceding hypothesis, and if it is proved it suggests a sympathy with the offender's difficulties that may not be shown when non-motoring cases are dealt with. A reluctance to order re-tests has been criticized often; for example by Lord Selkirk, who said in the same debate as that from which Lord Goddard's speech was quoted (hypothesis (*h*) above): 'It is beyond my understanding why the penalty of disqualification is not more widely invoked; I feel it is a great pity that it is not sufficiently used. I think that the power to order an additional driving test should be invoked more often.'

The following three hypotheses were not proceeded with after consideration:

(*k*) *The serious motoring offender who is sentenced to imprisonment does not regard his punishment as having as severe a social stigma as it would have, had he been convicted of an offence against property or the person.*

For reasons which will be explained, it was decided not to use offenders in prison as subjects, and consequently it would have been impossible to test

47

this hypothesis. A slender piece of evidence came, however, from an article in a popular magazine by G. Taylor (1961), a 20-year-old man convicted for driving while disqualified, and imprisoned; of his experiences he wrote: 'The other men always know what you're in for, you can't hide the truth. I had a good time because I hadn't done nothing that put me in one social scale or another.' So it would seem that the motoring offender is as unplaced in the prisoner's frame of reference as he is outside prison.

(*l*) *Because serious motoring offenders are distributed over the whole social hierarchy, they will not include an undue proportion of those with the minimum standard of education.*

This was abandoned because hypothesis (*d*), about social class, seemed to deal with it to a point. To test it would have meant asking direct questions about educational background, to which the answers might have been both unreliable and difficult to verify.

(*m*) *The serious motoring offender is likely to be accident-prone; i.e. he is likely to have a history of accidents at home and/or at work.*

On reflection this seemed to be a peculiarly difficult hypothesis to test. It could have been dealt with only by interviews, and it was felt to be unlikely that truthful answers would be given to such questions as 'Are you unlucky?' or 'Have you had many accidents at home or at work?' There might be a tendency to play down a record of previous accidents, since a respondent would scarcely wish to be thought one of those who are always having accidents or – put in another way, as he might see it – are always in trouble. However, this would have been an interesting and perhaps useful hypothesis to test, and it is a pity that it was not included among the matters discussed in the interview phase of the research.

So much for the hypotheses. Now came the problem of deciding how the job could best be done.

THE BASIC CONCEPT: THE SERIOUS MOTORING OFFENCE

First it was necessary to establish working concepts of 'the serious motoring offence' and 'the serious motoring offender'. This had to be done to make the research at all credible as other than a study of the trivial and the mundane.

It was not easy to select the offences, for the obvious reason that it is a matter of opinion as to what is, or is not, 'serious'. Moreover, many motoring offences – such as failing to stop after, or to report, an accident; or failing to stop at a police signal – embrace a wide range of circumstances, from those where there was a deliberate refusal to obey the law to those where the omission was no more than mere forgetfulness or lack of concentration on what one was doing.

However, the choice was made easier by the specification by the law of the maximum sentences for particular offences. This is often as good a criterion as any of the gravity with which the legislature regards the offence. For example, it could be said that causing death by dangerous driving stands out, since it is the one motoring offence for which an offender can be sent to prison for more than two years in the first instance.

Only two other offences carried maximum sentences of longer than six months' imprisonment under the acts current at the time this research was being planned: driving under the influence of drink or drugs, and driving in a manner, or at a speed, dangerous to the public. And, since these are offences that can be dealt with on indictment, they might be regarded as 'serious' among motoring offences. As such they stand, with causing death, rather on their own as obviously serious; but the selection of other offences from a fairly long list of motoring offences for which lesser terms of imprisonment can be given was still a problem.

Perhaps the outstanding offence that comes to the attention in addition to those already mentioned is that of driving while disqualified. This offence is unique in that a sentence of imprisonment is mandatory unless the circumstances are such that they can be regarded as 'special to the offence' rather than to the offender; in other words, there must be some facts that mitigate the offence other than reasons for not sending the offender to prison (see Wilkinson, 1960, pp. 247–8).[1] Clearly this offence is treated in a class of its own, and consideration of the elements involved justifies a serious view since it is usually a deliberate defiance of a court order; it also amounts to driving without insurance since a driver is excluded from cover unless he holds a valid driving licence. So the consequences for the victim are likely to be serious if the offender does damage and is unable to pay anything in compensation. It will be seen that this offence contains two of the three elements considered to merit the label of 'criminal'; i.e. it is usually deliberate, and there is dishonesty in that the defendant is falsely representing himself to be a licensed driver when he knows that he is not. These were considered to be adequate reasons for including this offence in the serious group.

[1] Under the Road Traffic Act, 1962, circumstances special to the offender can be considered as mitigating the offence.

49

Two more offences were chosen after careful thought, and discussion with lawyers and police officers: failing to insure against third-party risks; and failing to stop after, or to report, an accident.

Although failing to insure can sometimes be technical – as when the charge is aiding and abetting, or when the buyer of a vehicle thinks that he is covered by the previous owner's policy – some of these offences could be as intentional and irresponsible as driving while disqualified. Whenever the offender does not think he is insured some measure of deliberate intent and of dishonesty can be assumed, since, as in driving while disqualified, the defendant is riding 'under false colours', and someone may be injured without a hope of protection or recompense. Indeed, some idea of the attitude of mind that can attend this offence can be formed from the view expressed by one of the divisional police superintendents interviewed in the course of this work: that some of those who commit this offence do so because it is cheaper to pay a fine, if caught, than it is to pay an insurance premium. And, of course, the consequences of this offence can be anti-social in the extreme; for example, an offender with no means may kill or injure a breadwinner, with the result that a family may be reduced to living at subsistence level for many years.

Seen thus, failing to insure becomes a serious offence by any standards that are at all responsible, and one might say the same of the hit-and-run offence of failing to stop after, or to report, an accident. For here again we find the elements of deliberate intent and dishonesty; on some of the worst occasions it could also be said that malice is present, in that an injured person is left lying unaided, without regard to his fate, or damage is inflicted to someone else's property, which cannot be recovered or com-pensated in any way without loss. It may be that an offender has some idea that the injured party is insured, or that he runs away in a panic; but consideration of Selling's (1941) group of these offenders shows that the offence is justifiably included in the serious category by its very nature.

Looking back over these offences it would seem that they have the following criteria in common: first, they are offences that tend often to involve behaviour that is manifestly wrong, not only because it is a breach of the law but also because it is clearly to the disadvantage, and sometimes even the peril, of other users of the road. Second, they are offences in which, when there are no specially mitigating circumstances, the offender has selfishly put his own interests and convenience before those of others or, put more bluntly, he has deliberately disregarded that consideration for others which is fundamental to any society that upholds the rule of law. Finally, there is the strictly functional aspect mentioned already: that the law itself regards them as more serious than other motoring offences, as shown by the maximum sentencing provisions.

Having regard to these factors, it may be wondered why the offence of taking and driving away a vehicle without the owner's consent was not included also. Much thought was, in fact, given to this point, especially as it is likely that such offenders would have criminal records for non-motoring offences, and thus would help to disprove the hypothesis that the motoring offender is a law-abiding person. But is was eventually decided not to include the offence on the grounds that it is not, strictly speaking, a motoring offence at all, since it is not the driving behaviour or the manner of use that is the subject of the offence: rather, it is a straightforward mis-appropriation or unauthorized use of someone else's property – and no more than that, unless another motoring offence is committed after the taking of the vehicle. In that event, if the other offence were one of those with which this research is concerned, the case would be included.

Logically, then, the serious motoring offender, for the purpose of this research, must be anyone convicted of one or more of the six offences selected for study. It is evident, of course, that this means a considerable stretching of practical limits in many cases in which the offence was, to say the least, a mishap; for example, the frequent cases in which the 'dangerous' driving was due to forgetting to act in time in circumstances that could equally have been regarded as failure to exercise due care or attention – a theoretically 'less serious' offence that is not usually thought of as serious by anyone. There are also the 'technical' cases of failure to insure against third-party risks, and some of the doubtful cases where there was failure to stop after, or report, an accident. It may not, therefore, be very realistic to expect others to agree with the description of *all* offenders convicted of any one of the six offences as 'serious' motoring offenders. However they *will* be so regarded for research purposes, with the limitations continually in the worker's mind.

A POSSIBLE APPROACH

It was obvious at once that the heart of the study must be a thorough analysis of *actual* cases, and that these must be sufficiently numerous and be taken over a long enough period for the result to be representative and meaningful. Then it was necessary to consider how to assemble the cases, and how they should be studied: by interview, from documents alone, or by both means.

One possible approach was to use a sample of serious motoring offenders in prison, compiling the data from the administration of a suitable personality inventory supplemented by interview material and from prison records. By comparing the results derived from a group of motoring offenders with the results of the same procedures applied to a group of other prisoners it could perhaps be shown to what extent the groups differed. Then the significance of any similarity or difference between the two groups could be tested by applying the same measures to a group of drivers with no record of offences. Moreover, there was a very suitable and validated personality inventory ready to hand in Grygier's *Dynamic Personality Inventory* (1956), a method that is especially useful for the diagnosis of excessive aggression, fears, and other symptoms of neurosis.

There were, however, a number of difficulties. The first was the problem of persuading the subjects to do the Dynamic Personality Inventory, which takes over thirty minutes and contains many personal questions. Though a captive population might agree, it is unlikely that a group of non-offenders would do so.

Even if the groups consented to do the inventory, and a clear-cut situation emerged, it would not establish anything very useful. For example, suppose that the results from the two groups of offenders in prison were very similar, and that they differed significantly from the results derived from the group of non-offenders. This would not indicate that the personalities of serious motoring offenders approximated more closely to the personalities of other offenders than to those of ordinary non-offending motorists, for the similarity between the groups of offenders could be the result of an influence common to both – the prison environment itself.

Another difficulty of this approach was that it was most unlikely that any one prison would contain more than a few motoring offenders at any one time. To have access to a sufficient number of offenders for a sample, therefore, would have meant either visiting numerous prisons all over England, or taking several years to gather data from one prison. Neither course was feasible with the resources available for this research.

It was decided, then, to give up the idea of using a captive population as the basis for the research, and in the event it would have been unsatisfactory for other reasons also. For it became apparent later that the vast majority of motoring offenders in prison had been committed for driving while disqualified, and that these were a distinctive group in many respects – for example, they included an unusually high proportion of offenders with criminal records. A captive population, therefore, would not have been representative of serious motoring offenders in general, and might have led to grossly misleading conclusions.

Design of the Study

There remained the alternative of basing the work primarily on a documentary study of cases from reliable records. Police files were indicated as the only source that would provide sufficient information for the testing of the hypotheses – and the next step was to gain access to these records.

THE CHOICE OF A POLICE AREA

Since a nationwide survey was impossible in this instance, it was necessary to choose a homogeneous police area in which documentation and reporting methods were similar; thus a Police District was indicated. Moreover, it was important that the District chosen should be representative of the country as a whole. It should not, therefore, be mostly urban or mostly rural, nor should the occupational distribution of its population be biased towards particular occupational groups, e.g. white-collar workers on the one hand or manual workers on the other. Also the users of its roads should not be disproportionately of one type, e.g. goods vehicles or holiday traffic. 'Balance' was necessary in this respect, and it was not easy to achieve, but in the end a Police District was found in the home counties which seemed to satisfy most of these requirements, and in which the police and the justices were interested and prepared to cooperate. The District is described in Chapter 6 below.

Once permission to do the research had been secured, visits were made to each of the eight police divisions in the District, where the files of cases are kept. These visits involved much travelling, but enabled the writer to see the whole area 'on the ground', and to meet a considerable number of police officers of all ranks.

THE DOCUMENTARY SOURCES

The files for each case usually contained the following:

(a) An Accident Report Book – if the offence had been derived from an accident – completed by the police officer on the spot and containing the following information:

(i) *Details of the accident:* Date, time, place, conditions of light and weather.

(ii) *Particulars of injured persons:* Injuries, personal particulars; statement; friends/relatives to be informed.

(iii) *Position of vehicles involved:* Measurements; whether vehicle had apparently been moved since the occurrence.

53

(iv) *Details of drivers and vehicles:* Index number, make, model, type, direction of travel; owner's name and address; driver's name and address and estimated age; details of driving licence, insurance, and excise licence; driver's statement; details of badge and licences if public-service vehicle or goods vehicle driver; details of passengers carried.

(v) *Other property damaged:* Fences, trees, etc., owner's name, etc.

(vi) *Witnesses and statements:* Names, addresses, and estimated ages; whether independent.

(vii) *Actions of persons involved:* E.g. 'lost control of vehicle'.

(viii) *State of the road:* Speed limits, surface, etc.

(ix) *Sketch of scene*

(x) *Additional particulars:* If motor cyclist, was he wearing crash-helmet, etc; particulars of persons assisting the police.

(xi) *Officer's own report:* Whether names and addresses were exchanged; vehicle to which accident was attributable; description of how accident probably happened and any arrests for drunkenness; opinion as to whether there was any evidence of an offence.

(xii) *Section officer's report*

(xiii) *Subdivisional officer's report*

(xiv) *Result of process (prosecution) or inquest*

(*b*) A Minute Sheet on which the officers concerned wrote their comments as the paper passed through the hierarchy from section to division, and sometimes to the chief constable.

(*c*) A copy of the Notice of Intended Prosecution sent to the defendant.

(*d*) A form from the offender's local police (if he lived outside the District) giving the date, offence, and penalty for previous motoring offences.

(*e*) Statements of prosecution witnesses and of the defendant if he made one.

(*f*) Plans and photographs of the scene.

(*g*) Correspondence with counsel and with the Director of Public Prosecutions.

(*h*) A form used in court summarizing the personal details (name, address, occupation, and estimated age) of the defendant, offences charged, and details of the police case. The penalty was recorded on this form also, and often there were further minuted observations on the outcome of the case by officers.

Design of the Study

It will be observed that this was a very comprehensive list of details, and it was possible to build up a satisfactory scheme for coding onto Cope-Chat cards. The scheme is shown in Appendix A.

However, gaps in the information caused problems, especially when they occurred in connection with matters relevant to the hypotheses. For example, it was not usual to insist on occupation or date of birth being recorded in traffic cases, and there were a number in which these details were missing. Also it was not usual for previous offences other than motoring offences to be recorded, and when the offender lived outside the division, only details of his traffic offences would be supplied to the prosecuting division.

Checks of offenders' records for previous convictions were, therefore, carried out in the division in which offenders lived, and at the Criminal Record Office (CRO). The CRO covered offenders who lived outside the District, but it supplied records of 'fingerprintable' offences only, and it may be that a number of minor non-motoring offences were omitted. The result of the checks is thus likely to be an underestimate of additional convictions: it is certainly not an overestimate.

Although the police files were more informative than expected, they had shortcomings as sources for research data. For instance, some cases were more complete than others, according to the reporting officer's lucidity and thoroughness in writing up the case. Also, it was likely that the material would be one-sided, since it contained almost exclusively the prosecution's case; in most cases nothing was evident about the defendant's side, except on the rare occasions when defendants made statements. This bias was perhaps the greatest drawback to using the files as the main source, since it could be said that only the police case was being presented.

THE DOCUMENTARY STUDY

The scope of the work could now be considered in more exact terms. It looked as though the main documentary study must embrace at least three complete years' worth of offences in order to allow any trends to show, and to be sure that the picture was a representative one. Moreover, from the Home Office Returns of *Offences relating to Motor Vehicles* it was judged unlikely that there would be a sufficient number of cases of causing death by dangerous driving, driving under the influence, driving while disqualified, and – up to a point – of dangerous driving, if the work covered less than three years. Of the remaining two offences – failing to insure, and failing to stop, etc. – there was no such shortage, and it was clear that the

55

study might be overburdened by these much more numerous offences if each case were included. So some form of sampling was needed for these offences if not for the others.

Eventually it was decided to take for analysis every case of causing death by dangerous driving, of driving under the influence, of driving while disqualified, and of dangerous driving, in which there had been a conviction during the years 1957, 1958, and 1959. For the other two offences a form of sampling was devised to cover the same period: this confined the offenders to those who were resident in the Police District, and, out of these cases, every conviction for failing to stop or to report an accident, and every tenth conviction for failing to insure, were selected for analysis. It was decided to exclude convictions for aiding and abetting in insurance cases, since these offences appeared to be mostly without any intent, and were apparently 'technical' in almost every instance seen. Cases were also excluded when the insurance offence was an automatic consequence of some other offence: e.g. it follows automatically that an offender charged with taking and driving away must also be convicted for failure to insure, and similarly a person driving while disqualified must also be committing the offence of failing to insure since disqualification nullifies insurance cover. To have included such automatic charges and convictions would have led to double-counting and a misleadingly false inflation of the data, although, strictly speaking, these convictions are instances of the commission of offences, and they are included in the official statistics without distinctions being made.

It was now possible to predict the probable number of cases that would be available for the documentary study. It looked like being between 600 and 700: a number sufficient to give a representative picture, and perhaps to avoid the criticism of using too small a population.

BACKGROUND AND FRAMEWORK

As the central part of the study had taken shape first, the next step was to design a framework.

The first requirement was the provision of a background or build-up for the major hypotheses. This had to include some analysis of the incidence of motoring offences and their treatment over a relatively long period. But statistics tend to express only the social responses to the law and other kinds of constraint. Hence it was necessary to show something of the development of the law, and of the social attitudes influencing it, if the picture was to have real meaning and perspective.

Design of the Study

Not much will be said about the statistical analysis at this stage, except to explain the factors affecting its scope. It was decided to include motoring offences of all kinds in order to show how the six classes of serious offence fitted into the general picture. Moreover it was thought necessary to show, as Wootton (1959) had done already, the relationship between motoring offences and other offences so that their respective contributions to the general pattern of crime in Britain could be seen.

Since the time span of the main study was only three years, the statistical analysis had to cover a longer period if trends were to be manifest, and if the effects of changes in the law, such as the major change in 1956, were to be evident. The year 1954 was, therefore, chosen as the earlier point because, by this time, the abnormalities due to petrol rationing and the pre-war shortage of cars were beginning to disappear; it also allowed two full years before the Road Traffic Act, 1956, became operative, although the petrol rationing of the Suez period intervened. The remainder of the period was chosen to correspond with the documentary study, i.e. 1957, 1958, and 1959.

The section dealing with the law posed more difficult problems. It had to be quasi-historical to be of interest, and, since the law does not go back much beyond 1908, there was not a very long period to deal with. The evidence, however, was very scattered, since few aspects of the law could have been more subject to the pressures of interest groups in their development. So debates in parliament and famous cases were not very helpful by themselves. Some research into contemporary newspapers and into the annals of interest groups, such as the Automobile Association and the Pedestrians' Association, was necessary. Yet another problem was the writer's lack of legal training and experience, for it soon became evident that the layman is at a considerable disadvantage when it comes to the deeper understanding of the law and its intricacies. Because of limitations in this respect, this section of the work has been restricted to the bare essentials; but it is shown that in this area alone there is scope for a great deal of useful research.

SOME INTERVIEWS

When the plan was reviewed, however, it still seemed to be defective in one major sense: it was focused entirely on documentary evidence and contained no first-hand impression of offenders or their views. Without some actual contact with offenders and some account of their attitudes the study would be one-sided, and it would lack human interest. Hence it was

57

decided to include a small-scale interview study of offenders convicted of one of the serious offences referred to above. Its aims were:

(a) To provide supplementary evidence to test the hypotheses concerning the attitudes of offenders, and of the public towards them;

(b) To see what offenders thought about their treatment by the law;

(c) To get an impression of them 'as people', e.g. personality, driving experience, education, and occupational/class membership;

(d) To get impressions about the antecedents to these offences;

(e) To find out what the actual implications are, for the offender and his family, of such orders as disqualification.

Accordingly, a structure for an interview was devised as shown in Appendix B. The intention was to undertake interviews lasting about thirty minutes, using a guide to ensure that all questions were covered, but not insisting on dealing with them in any rigid order. It will be seen that the structure avoids overtly personal questions; perhaps the nearest thing to a personal question was concerned with education, and this was left out unless it arose naturally. However, the absence of probing or personal questions does not mean that the interview was useless for making some assessment of personality, since attitudes to the law and to other people in general are soon revealed in the discussion of controversial issues in which the subject has some stake.

It was, however, very difficult to decide whom to interview. For reasons given already (p. 52 above), it could not be a group of offenders in prison. Nor was it desirable to interview a sample of the offenders from the documentary study; the police did not like that idea because they thought it would be a misuse of their records if information were used in order to approach offenders. And, indeed, it is possible that it would not invite cooperation if offenders thought that the interviewer had privileged access to the police side of their case; they would almost certainly identify him and his research with 'seeking information for the police' unless he misled them, which would be out of the question, and very unwise.

Eventually it was decided to use an entirely separate group of offenders, though preferably containing similar proportions of persons convicted of each of the 'serious motoring offences' to those found in the documentary study.

At first it was proposed to approach subjects at court, ask for their cooperation before the hearing, and interview them afterwards. To this end four conveniently placed courts were selected, and it was intended to approach all persons charged with any of the classes of offence with which the study was concerned, who appeared within a three-month period. This did not work for a variety of reasons. One was the waste of time: hearing that a case would be 'coming up' at a particular court, the writer would attend only to find that the case was late or, much worse, adjourned. And even if the hearing did take place, it often meant sitting for a long time in court to hear a case which, if it resulted in acquittal, had to be discarded. Another reason was uneasiness about approaching accused people at such a time, and tackling an offender for interview so soon after the double blow of conviction and punishment; quite apart from the fact that the offender would not be in a very objective frame of mind, and would have no idea of anyone else's reaction to his case or punishment – information which it was hoped to include in the study – it did not seem right to intrude on anyone's privacy at such a time. In the event, this approach was tried in four cases: two refused very politely, and the others agreed to interviews in return for the offer of a lift home which, since both had been disqualified, was useful payment. But, despite success in these two cases, the method was rejected on account of the time factor.

So something else had to be thought of, and it was decided to obtain the names of possible subjects for interview from the columns of two local newspapers which covered a large part of the Police District. When a conviction was reported for one of the offences with which this research was concerned, a call was to be made on the offender requesting an interview. It was to be explained, without subterfuge, that the aim of the interview was to get the offender's point of view about the offence and the manner in which it had been dealt with by all concerned, and also to ask about opinions and attitudes on the subject of motoring. It was at once evident that such a plan would be expensive in time and petrol, since it seemed that only a sudden face-to-face call would avoid rejection. To have preceded the visit with a letter or telephone call would have made it easy for respondents to ignore or put off the request, and in this kind of situation it is easier to explain one's purpose in an interview than in writing or by telephone.

Fortunately, in the pilot study of six cases, the plan worked well; but so much time and travel were involved that the number of interviews had to be reduced to the minimum, and this was set – quite arbitrarily – at fifty. A higher figure would obviously have been better, but resources did not permit; moreover, in the planning stage it had not been thought that this phase of the research would produce enough reliable and useful information to warrant a lot of time and effort.

For the same reasons, the idea of using a control group of non-offending

59

drivers, which would have more than doubled the interviewing commitment, was reconsidered. In any case, the selection of a control group posed almost insoluble problems. For example, how could one be certain that any one subject had never been convicted? To find out would have meant contacting the police authority in every place in which he admitted to residence, and in some of the more mobile cases omissions might have been frequent. The only practicable answer was to ask the licensing authority in the Police District for a random sample of licence holders who had always been licensed by them; it would then be possible to check their convictions with their local police and with the Criminal Record Office. But, in the event, the licensing authority refused to supply any names because they thought it improper to divulge confidential information – that a person held a driving licence, and his name and address – to a research worker. Apart from the offenders who refused interview, this was the only refusal to cooperate that was encountered from official and lay sources during the entire research.

Obtaining subjects for research as their names appeared in the local newspapers can hardly be called scientific sampling, and it would be presumptuous to claim that they constituted a representative sample of serious motoring offenders. Indeed it may be that reporters and editors of local newspapers are inclined to print accounts of certain kinds of case rather than others. But it must be said that it seemed to be purely a matter of chance whether reporters happened to be in court for motoring cases; if there was a case of larceny or violence in another court, they were far more likely to be listening to that. Some of the more newsworthy motoring cases did not seem to be reported at all – presumably because the reporters did not hear them; but other factors may have been involved, for instance when the press appeared to play down a story, or when the occupation of the defendant was not mentioned (this happened twice in the same court when professional men pleaded guilty and received the maximum sentence short of imprisonment). It may also be said with good reason that offenders whose cases are reported are likely to feel the repercussions more than those whose cases do not appear in the press.

Eventually, only seven of the fifty persons approached refused to be interviewed, a proportion of 14 per cent which, though large for a random sample, would not be considered high for a selective sample of this kind, in which the material has marked significance for the respondent.

The interviews were not exactly the same in each case, since the order and wording of the questions were not stereotyped; they were what Moser (1958) has called the 'least formal' kind of interview, in which the interviewer varied the order of the questions, explained their meaning when necessary, and asked for all the elaboration that the respondent could give. But, on the other hand, all the interviewing was done by the writer so that the influence of the interviewer was reasonably consistent.

Calls were made on informants not more than seven and not less than two days after their cases were published; this timing was necessary because of the questions concerning the social repercussions of conviction on the offender. It was thought that at least two days were needed for any reaction to show itself, and the limit of seven days was set to ensure that conditions affecting this issue were reasonably the same for all informants. In actuality the visits were made usually between five and seven days after publication.

The approach technique was to present a visiting card, which always seemed to reassure the informant and bring him to the door if someone else had answered it. The card seemed to have a quite amazing effect sometimes: after it had been stated that an informant was out, the production of the card would often flush him from some back room – perhaps his curiosity was too much for him.

There then followed a short explanation that this was research into the law relating to motoring, undertaken for a higher degree. It was stressed that it was a 'pioneer' research in that it sought to discover an offender's views about the law and the manner in which he had been treated under it; and it was pointed out that, although much was known of the views of the bench and the police on these matters, all too little was known about those of defendants. Finally it was emphasized that the researcher had no connection whatsoever with the police or the courts, and that the anonymity of informants would be guaranteed.

The interviews were approached with some trepidation, in the expectation of abrupt rejection. It was therefore a surprise to find nearly all the contacts both pleasant and stimulating, and it was usual to be asked into the house and offered a cup of tea or coffee while the interview proceeded. This invitation was, of course, invaluable because it made available some idea of the informant's background and way of life; but it did seem to be rather an abuse of hospitality to use it thus.

When the purpose of the interview had been explained, most informants were prepared to talk about their cases, and seemed to enjoy doing so. Hesitation was noticeable only when others were present, or when there were interruptions, which occurred frequently because interviews took place not only in sitting-rooms, but in the garden while the informant did his weeding, on doorsteps, in bed-sitting-rooms against the competition of

61

all-in-wrestling on television, in the writer's own car, in bars, in a caravan, and in a doctor's surgery. There was no lack of variety in people or in the circumstances in which they were seen.

It should perhaps be mentioned that no notes were taken during the interviews, since this often seems to put off respondents; interviews were written up from memory afterwards, for which task the writer's considerable experience in interviewing prior to this research proved useful. The written-up material was then codified on Cope-Chat cards, applying a code similar to that used for the documentary cases; certain data could then be compared.

It must be admitted, however, that the assessment of the data obtained at these interviews was highly subjective, depending as it did on a single interviewer's interpretation. Hence this final phase of the research cannot produce results capable of standing up to either analysis or scientific criticism. It is essentially an impressionistic study that can do no more than fill in some of the gaps in the picture presented by the main study, and give life to the rather dry facts and figures which form the greater part of it. Even so, it may be a more realistic account of what offenders think than could have been obtained from interviews with captive offenders only – but it is hard to say without having attempted the latter.

ADDITIONAL SOURCES OF INFORMATION

In order to test the design of the research and the basic ideas behind it – especially that one drives as one lives – interviews were sought with a number of people who, without having any particular axe to grind, might be able to help to keep the hypotheses and analysis within the bounds of good sense. These included magistrates, clerks of courts, lawyers, police officers, officials of insurance companies handling motoring business, and executives of organizations employing large numbers of drivers. Much use was made also of the expert staff of the Road Research Laboratory, whose advice was invaluable.

Generally speaking the interviews were unstructured, and they differed according to the informant's relationship to the research. For example, interviews with magistrates and court officers were concerned mostly with difficulties in interpreting and administering the law, and with factors influencing sentencing; in talking to the police the main interest was in their attitude to the motoring offender as a criminal and in their method of handling these cases. Insurance companies came into the picture because their attitudes and policies seemed to be a major factor in the real effect of conviction on the offender, as when insurance premiums are increased, or insurance is refused, after a serious offence has been proved. And the aim of interviewing employers or transport managers was to find out their reaction to the idea that men drive as they live, and also to get impressions of their attitudes towards convicted employees.

The details of these interviews are referred to in the parts of the study to which they are appropriate, but there are a few points which might usefully be mentioned now.

Among these informants with some special interest in the subject-matter of the research there was almost unanimous acceptance of the idea that one drives as one lives, and many anecdotal examples were given to illustrate it. But there was nowhere the same measure of agreement about the questions, 'Could any motoring offence be considered a crime?' and 'Could any motoring offender be considered a criminal?' In fact just the same confusion and qualification were revealed among these respondents as among those who were not 'professionally involved'. Only causing someone's death by a deliberate act, or by 'couldn't care less' gross negligence, seemed to be regarded as 'real crime', for which the perpetrator could be stigmatized as criminal. Again, there was just the same emphasis on intent, hurt, and dishonesty as criteria essential to crime.

Regarding the basic design of the research, none of these expert informants had much criticism, except to express some doubt as to whether the interviewing of offenders would be worth while, and whether it would be possible to disprove the hypothesis that the serious motoring offender is an upright, respectable, law-abiding citizen apart from his motoring misbehaviour.

These discussions, then, were encouraging, and it was possible to begin the research with confidence that questions were being pursued that other people considered important and sought to answer. There was some disappointment at having to dispense with so much of the original plan for carrying out a tightly organized and controlled study that would stand up well to scientific criticism; but at least some relatively unmapped criminological territory could be explored.

3

The Law and the Motorist

1832–1903

'If the Driver or Conductor of any Stage Carriage, or any other Person having the care thereof . . shall through Intoxication or Negligence, or by Wanton and Furious Driving, or by or through any other Misconduct, endanger the Safety of any Passenger or Person . . . every such Person so offending shall forfeit Five Pounds.'

So runs the principal offence set up by the Stage Carriage Act, 1832, the first time that we find the law of England concerning itself specifically with the manner in which vehicles were driven on the roads.

Though £5 was a lot of money at the time, and may have meant several weeks' wages for one of the working class, it was not a very severe imposition on the subject by nineteenth-century standards. And, in any case, it was felt only by a minority since it was directed at the professional drivers of horse-drawn vehicles whose maximum possible speed could not have been much more than 20 mph.

A similar provision was contained in the Highways Act, 1835, section 78, which required all drivers of 'carriages' to have attendants, and forbade 'furious driving' which, on the evidence of a single witness, could result in a fine not exceeding £5, or up to six weeks' hard labour. The Town Police Clauses Act, 1847, also exacted a penalty of a £2 fine or 14 days' imprisonment for 'riding or driving furiously any horse or carriage in any street'. Both Acts are still in force and the former was used against a cyclist as recently as 1953.

Yet it should not be thought that the legislature of the time had no interest in the development of the revolutionary 'horseless carriage'. A Select Committee had been appointed in 1831 to investigate and report on 'the present state and future prospects of land carriage by wheeled vehicles propelled by steam or gas upon common roads'.

The Select Committee reported that the development of mechanical power for road vehicles was one of the most important improvements ever introduced in internal communication. They considered that its practicability was 'fully established', and that its development should be protected

64

and encouraged by legislation without delay. They were referring, of course, to the steam carriages and 'road locomotives' which, since Cugnot introduced them onto the roads of Paris in 1770, had been appearing in England with increasing frequency and by 1831 were providing a regular road service four times a day between Gloucester and Cheltenham. Only three years after Shillibeer introduced the first horse buses on the London streets in 1829, there was a fleet of steam buses operated by the inventor Hancock plying between the capital, Reading, and Brighton.

The Committee's recommendations were, however, ignored by parliament which rejected a Bill to give effect to them. For the 'horseless carriage' was seen not as a blessing, but as a threat to life, limb, and tranquillity, as well as to the financial interests of farmers and horse-breeders. This was a taste of things to come, and the opening phase of a vigorous contest between the enthusiastic believers in the new invention and the majority who thought it to be an invention of the devil that should be resisted and restricted by every possible means. Typical of the early weapons used against the new vehicles were the closure of roads and bridges to them, and the imposition of heavy tolls for the use of those that were left open. Coming at this time, such restrictions had a most unfortunate technological repercussion in Britain, since inventors in Europe were able to forge ahead with the development of electric and petrol-driven vehicles, relatively unrestricted by their governments.

In 1884 Daimler built his first vehicle driven by a petrol internal combustion engine, and Benz followed a year or so later with the invention of the motor tricycle. So the 'motorist' or 'automobilist' came into the picture for the first time, soon to be followed by his rival for the attentions of a vocal and irate opposition – the 'motor cyclist'. And within fifty years there were to be some two million motor vehicles on British roads, produced and supported by associated industries employing over 350,000 people.

Such a rapid growth bore little witness to the struggles with which it had been attended, and the accounts of parliamentary proceedings since 1896 leave no doubt that this was a cold war of no mean intensity. During the 1890s social antagonism towards the motor vehicle became noticeable. It was expressed mostly in letters to the papers as it is today, and it mounted as pressure began to build up from the champions of motoring for the repeal of the ultra-repressive legislation affecting its movements on British roads.

A typical example of restrictive legislation was the Locomotive Act, 1861, which limited the speed of all horseless vehicles to 10 mph outside towns and 4 mph within them; its main purpose was to control the movement of the fearsome steam traction engines which not only alarmed horses, but also played havoc with roads and bridges. The damage continued, however, and the Act was amended in 1865 to reduce maximum speeds still further to 4 mph outside towns and 2 mph inside them; the amendment also required all horseless vehicles to be accompanied by three persons, one of whom had to walk in front holding a red flag.

The intrepid motorist who would exceed these limits laid himself open to a charge under section 35 of the Offences against the Person Act, 1861, which specified that: 'Whoever, having the charge of any Carriage or Vehicle shall, by wanton or furious Driving, or Racing, or other wilful Misconduct, or by wilful Neglect, do or cause to be done any Bodily Harm to any Person whatsoever, shall be guilty of a Misdemeanour . . . and on conviction shall be liable to be imprisoned for a term not exceeding Two Years with or without Hard Labour' – an Act that is still in force.

Such was the unsympathetic environment for the first British motor cars and it is not surprising that their 'operators' found it irksome and even intolerable. Their views, and those of the motor manufacturers, were forcibly and effectively expressed by the newly formed Motor Car Club and the Self-propelled Traffic Association; sympathetic motorist MPs also pressed hard in parliament. The result was what has been called 'the Motorist's Magna Carta' – the Locomotives on Highways Act, 1896 – which increased maximum permissible speeds to 14 mph for prime movers under three tons unladen, except in areas in which the Local Government Board agreed to local requests for lower limits. The Act was also significant because its first section set the fashion for later legislation, since it stipulated that 'no person shall drive at a speed that is greater than is reasonable and proper having regard to the traffic on the highways'.

The 1896 Act passed through parliament with surprisingly little trouble by comparison with later motoring legislation. Possibly this was because the ground was so well prepared by the two fledgling motoring organizations, the Self-propelled Traffic Association and the Motor Car Club, which were to merge in 1897 and become the Royal Automobile Club of Great Britain. But, in this connection, it is interesting to find a pioneer motorist, Sir David Salomans, writing to *The Times* on 19 February 1896 to dissociate himself from the Club and from the Daimler Company, 'the two concerns being closely related to each other, so many names being common to both'.

This lack of trouble suggested that the anti-motorists were not fully awake, but there can be no doubt about their wakefulness thereafter. Letters bombarded *The Times*, complaining about the 'motoring pest', and the paper was moved to publish a leader on 15 December 1900, wherein it was said that 'it is a fact that in some parts of the country the motor car is an object of hatred. . . . It is not surprising, because there are a number of drivers who are a curse to the neighbourhood in which they drive . . . drivers who seem, when they mount their cars, to put from them altogether the instincts of gentlemen.' The words might have been taken straight from Kenneth Grahame's *The Wind in the Willows*, in which the redoubtable Mr Toad of Toad Hall seemed certainly to have driven as he lived!

After 1900 there were few issues of *The Times* without at least one letter to the editor on 'the motoring problem', and it is fascinating to watch the battle developing as the motorists' supporters pressed for relaxations in the repressive law, especially of speed limits, which were particularly disliked because of the 'speed traps' in which hidden policemen timed unsuspecting motorists over a measured distance, prosecuting offenders for speeding, or 'scorching' as it was then called. An idea of the motorist's unpopularity in some quarters can be formed from a letter to the editor of *The Times* (27 September 1902) from one Mr C. G. Edwards, JP, who wrote that readers would be shocked if they could have overheard the comments at a farmers' hunt luncheon he had attended recently, after the guests had been passed on their way to the venue by one of these 'cads on castors, upsetting their horses and insulting them as he went by'. Another correspondent wrote that 'their manners are so bad that justices should have a free hand with them', and another that 'it is common sense that it is to the public danger to travel on a public highway faster than 12 mph' (*The Times*, 25 September 1902).

But it was not only the behaviour of the drivers that gave offence; their carriages also irritated. For example a letter to *The Times* of 9 October 1902 complained of 'the excessive splendour of the car at night with four acetylene lamps giving out enough light to illuminate St Paul's and frighten any Socialist gas manager'.

However the Automobile Club, and the Association of Motor Manufacturers and Traders (formed in 1902) were not deterred from campaigning for the abolition of speed limits and other restraints, and in 1902 the former organization sent to over 4,000 members of county councils a set of proposed regulations for motor vehicles. They also sent copies of a *Times* leader of 23 September 1902 urging changes in the motoring law since it was founded on legislation 'passed hastily and inconsiderately on the assumption that nobody would ever want to travel faster than he would in a fast horse-drawn carriage'. The leader criticized the law's conception of the motor car as 'just another carriage' rather than as an entirely new phenomenon, and it castigated the 14 mph speed limit as 'absurd' and founded on a complete misappreciation of the capabilities of motor vehicles: 'It is seldom observed by even the most law-abiding citizens, and it is habitually disregarded by persons of high station and authority whose normal respect for the law is instinctive and unimpeachable.'

Motorists had much less sympathy from their parliamentary adversaries, of whom Mr Wason was typical, when he spoke in a debate during 1903 of 'those stinking engines of iniquity from which harmless men, women and children have to fly for their lives at the bidding of one of these slaughterers'. He then moved a resolution for a reduction in the president of the Local Government Board's salary for his inaction in not enforcing lower speed limits. And it was in this debate also that a theme appeared that was to recur throughout the development of the motoring law: a tendency to phrase the problems in class terms. For example, the speech of Mr Harwood that the motor car was 'the luxury of the few, and the time had come when the rich ought to be pulled up from using the roads for sport and endangering the public' (*The Times*, 11 June 1903). Some help in building up the stereotype of the motorist as wealthy, reckless, and inconsiderate was given by leaders in *The Times*, one of which described automobilists as being 'supplied in the majority of instances mostly from a class that possesses money in excess of brains or culture' (*The Times*, 1 August 1903).

It was evidently this kind of thing which stimulated the president of the Local Government Board, Mr Long, to say when introducing the Motor Car Bill, 1903, that he 'noticed with some regret that an attempt had been made to turn this into a class question, and to suggest that motor cars are a privilege of the rich, and that the poor were the sufferers. There was a large increase in motoring by professional men of the smaller grade, such as medical men and those who did work for local authorities. The breaking of the law was by no means confined to those who were termed "gentlefolk", but it was often by people who hired cars to get out into the country' (*The Times*, 5 August 1903).

The Motor Car Act, 1903

The Bill of 1903 was thought to be even more 'the motorist's charter' than the Act of 1896. Its principal authors were the officials of the motoring organizations, and they had powerful parliamentary support from the Prime Minister, A. J. Balfour, who was himself a keen enough motorist to inspire a wag to move in the Commons that 'nothing in this Act shall apply to the present Prime Minister' (*The Times*, 8 August 1903). The Bill proposed a total abolition of speed limits, and the substitution for them of a clause making it an offence 'to drive a motor car recklessly, or negligently, or at a speed or in a manner which is dangerous to the public, having regard to all the circumstances of the case, including the nature, condition and use of the highway, and to the amount of traffic which actually is at the time, or which might reasonably be expected to be, on the highway'. A first conviction was to be punished by a fine not exceeding £20, and a second or subsequent conviction by a fine not exceeding £50 or, at the court's discretion, by three months' imprisonment.

These two proposals are important because they crystallize the attitudes of the two opposing factions: those who were for the motor vehicle and those who were against it; and the two factions persist to this day though a large segment of opinion is uncommitted to either extreme. The motorists and their supporters took the view that the principal criterion of motoring misbehaviour while in motion must be whether the driving was dangerous in the particular circumstances; they held that speed was often irrelevant on this point, since it was possible to drive dangerously while well inside the lowest speed limit, yet it need not be dangerous to drive fast if conditions permitted. Indeed, speed limits were said to be dangerous in themselves since they encouraged the belief that one could not be driving dangerously as long as one were within the speed limit. Moreover, it was held that speed limits were unenforceable – and the more so if they were unrealistic – unless the police used traps. The motoring organizations were opposed also to the clauses in the Bill requiring motor vehicles to carry number plates, and giving police officers power to arrest without warrant: the former were said to be 'degrading', and the latter was objectionable because ambitious policemen 'would find it very easy to sally out from the police station, stopwatch in hand, and shortly find two stripes blossoming on the shoulder' (*The Times*, 8 August 1903). Such was the belief of Mr Healy, MP, speaking on the motorists' behalf in parliament, and it would seem that there are many who would echo it today, since the view is widespread that convictions help promotion in the police force.

The anti-motoring faction was militant and conservative, founding its opposition on such diverse issues as the threat to the Irish horse trade; the threat to the railways; noise, dust, and fumes; and also the perennial class question. Hence Mr Soares, MP, berating the Minister for always 'giving in to the motorist's passive resistance . . . for this is a government by the rich for the rich. When there is passive resistance against the Education Bill you will not give in, but when the motorists resist you give in at once. What's the use of power to arrest without warrant if policemen are open to

69

prosecution for false imprisonment or wrongful arrest by all the power and wealth of the motorists' (*The Times*, 5 August 1903).

The anti-motorist's main argument was, however, an insistence on speed limits since they provided a cut-and-dried rule; whether they were exceeded would be a matter of fact. They considered clauses dealing with dangerous driving to be useless, since their interpretation rested exclusively on opinion. For example, Lord Kelvin said that 'it is easier to say at what speed a car is travelling than to give a definition of reckless driving' (*The Times*, 23 July 1903). Moreover, threats were made that unless limits were imposed the irate public might take the law into their own hands against 'the pest'; and Lord Camperdown, speaking in the House of Lords, offered evidence of people taking 'reprisals' against motorists by throwing bottles, putting nails on the roads, and shooting at the rear wheels of their cars. Harrowing tales were told in parliament of the alarm and indignity suffered by friends and constituents at the hands of motorists, and a speed limit of 20 mph was secured with the proviso that lower limits could be imposed by local authorities subject to ministerial approval.

In the event, therefore, the Motor Car Act, 1903, contained both a speed limit and a clause dealing with dangerous driving. It also made it an offence to fail to stop after, or to report, an accident, and it enabled courts to endorse and to suspend driving licences. In addition, it extended the law to motor cyclists, whose activities inspired Mr Redmond to say during the debates on the Bill 'that it would be an evil day when every artisan went to work on that most detestable form of locomotion, a motor bicycle' (*The Times*, 5 August 1903).

The motorists and their powerful organizations considered this Act to be a penal measure and little more, and they never ceased to fight against it for the next twenty-seven years. They feared that justices would be prejudiced against them, and that maximum sentences would be imposed without hesitation. Feelings ran high in parliamentary debates, and a motorist member, Major Jameson, is typical in saying: 'It is scandalous that these high penalties should be fixed . . . a wife beater was treated no worse than a motorist who exceeded the speed limit by half a mile an hour. Penalties ought not to be left to magistrates' discretion: I have never known a magistrate who had any . . . The interpretation of speed cannot be left to magistrates and half-educated barristers.' There was also some acid comment on the decisions of 'greengrocer juries' (*The Times*, 8 August 1903).

Such views did not endear the motorists to their opponents, and matters were not improved by the Automobile Club's action in circularizing all highway authorities, asking that they should inform the Club as to their

The Law and the Motorist

attitude towards motoring; the Club could then advise members which authority they should approach for their licences. The Club pointed out that members could register for licences anywhere, but would no doubt prefer to do so with authorities who were sympathetic to motoring, and it was intended to issue a Club list of these; authorities were reminded that 'the twenty-shilling fees would be a useful source of revenue', and the clear inference was that it would be profitable to support the cause. This was not very tactful, and it is not surprising to find the chairman of the Lancashire County Council Highways Committee writing to *The Times* that the circular was 'objectionable and unprecedented in tone, and neither the bribe nor the threat therein will influence this Committee in the careful administration of the Motor Car Act' (*The Times*, 16 December 1903).

Because the Motor Car Act, 1903, really pleased nobody, it contained a clause limiting its life to three years. This was inserted to get the Bill passed; without it the arguments, especially about speed limits, would have been interminable. Thus, in 1906, a Royal Commission was set up under Viscount Selby to study the practical working of the Act and its predecessor and to suggest amendments. The Commission's report contained substantial evidence, including an interesting account of what was being done in other countries; it decided against speed limits in open country for light motor vehicles, but it recommended that the speed of heavier vehicles should be further restricted. A more stringent law was recommended for dealing with drunken drivers and with those motorists who would not stop after accidents, but the commissioners stressed that 'the guiding principle in dealing with . . . motoring offences should be to treat the motorist as a person lawfully using the highway, and only create special offences where the great speed of motor cars and their exceptional powers of escape render such provisions absolutely necessary' (*Royal Commission on Motor Cars*, 1906, p. 36).

The government, however, had too many other problems to deal with, and the 1903 Act continued in force – with a number of continuation acts to keep it going – until 1930. The only action taken before then was to embody some of the recommendations of the Royal Commission, principally that concerning drunken driving, in the Criminal Justice Act, 1925, in which section 40 made it an offence to be 'drunk in charge of any mechanically propelled vehicle on any highway'; the maximum punishment was four months' imprisonment with or without a fine not exceeding £50. Disqualification was mandatory, and it was made an offence to drive while disqualified. Hitherto drunken drivers had been charged under the Licensing Act, 1872, which provided for 'drunks' of all kinds, from those

71

in charge of steam engines to those in charge of firearms. The maximum penalties were only one month's imprisonment or a fine of forty shillings, but the Act was disliked by motorists since it empowered anyone to apprehend suspects.

The Royal Commission on Transport, 1929

By 1927 the Motor Car Act was ignored as generally as its predecessors are said to have been. The motoring organizations considered 20 mph to be an unrealistic limitation on the cars of the time, and they protested that such restrictions hampered the technical development of motor vehicles since high-performance cars could not be used legally on British roads; foreign competitors were thus given an advantage. But the opposition was equally active, and letters to the papers began to mount, complaining of the motorist's contempt for the law. Lords Cecil and Buckmaster introduced a Bill into the House of Lords 'to secure the comfort of the pedestrian: the motorist should get out of their way, and not the reverse'. The Bill proposed increases in penalties for dangerous driving and for speeding (*Hansard, Lords*, 12 December 1928).

However, the pressure for restricton was resisted by the government, and the Bill was shelved so that it could be taken into consideration by the Royal Commission on Transport which reported in 1929. The terms of reference were 'to consider the problems arising from the growth of road traffic', and what measures, if any, should be adopted to secure 'the employment of the available means of transport to the greatest public advantage' (*Royal Commission on Transport, First Report*, 1929).

Since the previous Royal Commission some things had changed, notably the attitudes of justices and juries who the motorists feared would be prejudiced against them. On the contrary, their opponents complained that motoring offenders were being treated much too leniently; and this view seems to have been shared by the County Chief Constables' Association whose spokesman told the Royal Commission that 'a very strong point advanced by members was of the insufficient penalties imposed by magistrates as a deterrent in cases of driving to the danger' (ibid. *Minutes of Evidence*, 1928, p. 547).

Otherwise the main arguments heard by the Commissioners for and against motorists were much the same as they had been in 1906 and before. The motoring organizations wanted the abolition of speed limits, but were prepared to accept a stiffening of the law regarding dangerous driving; their opponents wanted the latter, together with the retention of speed limits. Moreover, the situation was complicated by a government proposal to introduce a new offence: that of careless driving, carrying a lower penalty than driving recklessly or to the danger of the public. The government witness, Lord Russell, said that the proposal was consequent upon the intention to increase the maximum penalty for second or subsequent offences of reckless or dangerous driving, and to make endorsement and disqualification mandatory unless there were special reasons for not doing so. It was thought that this would operate unfairly against some offenders whose second offence might not, in itself, be such as to justify disqualification; hence it was proposed to give the prosecution a lesser offence upon which to proceed if they thought fit, and to give the courts power to convict on this lesser offence when dangerous driving was charged but the facts suggested a mild case only. Otherwise, Lord Russell said, there might be no conviction at all (ibid. *Minutes of Evidence*, p. 241).

The Commissioners' response to this proposal is noteworthy in view of the controversy raised by making a distinction between driving that is reckless or dangerous on the one hand, and careless on the other. They reported that they 'cannot understand the object of this clause, nor how any distinction can be drawn between [dangerous driving and careless driving] . . . we believe it would be impracticable. Moreover, careless driving could only be held to be an offence if it resulted in danger, and if it did this would clearly be dangerous driving. We are afraid that if this proposal became law it would have the effect of rendering nugatory the severe penalties which can be imposed for dangerous driving. We think it should be deleted from the Bill' (ibid. *First Report*, 1929, p. 12).

The Commissioners followed their predecessors in recommending that speed limits should be abolished if the penalties for dangerous driving were increased. They also considered that the offence of driving under the influence of drink should be transferred to the Road Traffic Acts, with increased penalties for second and subsequent offences.

Two other important recommendations were that third-party insurance should be compulsory for all vehicles, and that driving while disqualified should become a specific offence in its own right. Both recommendations were stimulated by the Cyclists' Touring Club, among others; on the subject of disqualification the Club's secretary told the Commissioners that disqualified drivers took little or no notice of the restriction and flouted it regularly; he thought that the only adequate punishment was imprisonment, and it should be mandatory on the courts to impose it: a view with which the Commissioners concurred (ibid. *Minutes of Evidence*, p. 574).

The proposal for compulsory third-party insurance met, however, with

73

strong resistance from the motoring organizations and, oddly enough, from the insurance companies. The secretary of the Automobile Association, Mr Stenson Cooke, thought that the proposal militated against the unlucky driver who had several accidents, and that it made the insurers the real arbiters as to who should or should not drive. The spokesman for the Royal Automobile Club objected because the good driver would be subsidizing the bad, and premiums would be forced up unfairly; for the Royal Scottish Automobile Association it was said that the element of compulsion made the proposal objectionable (ibid. *Minutes of Evidence*, pp. 209, 229).

As space does not permit a more detailed account of the Royal Commission's report, it must suffice to say that it was sensible and far-sighted. Most of its recommendations – with the notable exception of that dealing with the deletion of the proposed new offence of careless driving – were included in the Road Traffic Act, 1930. Moreover, much of the evidence cited foreshadowed future developments in the law: e.g. driving tests – which were strongly opposed by the motoring organizations – and the setting up of specially trained police traffic squads.

1930 and after

The Road Traffic Bill, which passed through parliament shortly after the Royal Commission reported, and became the Road Traffic Act, 1930, had a long and tortuous career. It had been drafted originally in 1922, but was shelved until 1927, when it was produced again and circulated to local authorities and other interested parties; during that year there was no time to deal with it and it was again shelved pending the Royal Commission's report. In the event it took a further seven months to pass through the legislative stages, and few bills of a non-political nature could have had such a prolonged examination and so much amendment, mainly because of the non-party but controversial issues of the abolition of the 20 mph speed limit for cars and motor cycles, the introduction of compulsory third-party insurance, and the increased penalties for dangerous and for drunken driving.

The pressure groups were very active, and the motoring organizations had spokesmen in both Houses. As Lord Sumner said in the Lords: 'Nobody who has witnessed the enormous driving force of the organized motoring organizations could believe that it was possible to choke off the attacks on the speed limits.' Earl Howe, a famous racing motorist of the day, spoke also of 'the great motoring organizations being against driving tests', though he himself was not opposed to the idea (*Hansard, Lords,* 12 December 1929). But the opposition to motoring was as active as ever, especially now that it was reinforced by a new pressure group – the Pedestrians' Association – founded in 1929 by an Oxford don, A. L. Goodhart, and with a chairman who had the intriguingly apt name of George E. Startup. One of the Association's spokesmen in the Commons was a Dr Salter who said that he spoke also for the Cyclists' Touring Club (which, incidentally, did not favour speed limits), the National Cyclists' Union, the Federation of Rambling Clubs, and the Holiday Fellowship Union; he wanted the speed limit retained, and he cited in support of his plea 'a scandalous state of things, a gathering of a number of cars called "The Monte Carlo Rally" to which some cars came across England at 90 mph, touching 95 mph through parts of London'. And, for good measure, Dr Salter expressed suspicion 'that the Minister himself is guilty of some recklessness' (*Hansard, Commons,* 18 February 1930).

By 1934 it seemed that the response by motorists to the de-restrictions of the 1930 Act was disappointing, and *The Times* of 11 April 1934 took note of the increasing number of complaints in its correspondence columns by publishing a leading article alleging that 'the effect of appeals made in 1930 for greater caution among drivers has worn off', and accusing the courts of undue leniency towards motoring offenders. In the same year the Pedestrians' Association sent a memorandum to the Minister of Transport asking for restoration of the speed limits on all vehicles, and for the abolition of the new offence of careless driving together with the 'soft option' clause enabling courts to convict for this offence in dangerous driving cases; the memorandum also urged that the distinction between 'criminal' and 'ordinary' negligence should be abandoned, stressing the view that all negligence resulting in death should be punished.

The outcome of all this pressure was the Road Traffic Act, 1934, which passed through parliament relatively quickly despite vociferous opposition from the motoring organizations. It contained sections reimposing speed limits in built-up areas, requiring all new drivers to pass tests, and establishing the pedestrian crossing. But the Act gave drivers some compensation for these further restrictions by enabling juries to convict for dangerous driving in manslaughter cases; this was seen as advantageous to motorists though the real intention was to make conviction of the guilty more certain where juries shrank from convicting for manslaughter.

During the war years, and until 1950, petrol rationing and other impediments to motoring kept the motorist's critics fairly quiet. But with the abolition of rationing and the increased home marketing of cars and motor cycles motoring began to boom again, and so did deaths, injuries, motoring offences, and the inevitable letters of complaint to the press. These carried

75

the traditional allegations of selfish and dangerous contempt for the law by drivers, and of magisterial leniency; there was also a remarkable number of complaints about juries failing to convict in cases of motor manslaughter and drunken driving. Pressure began to mount once again for the law to be given more teeth in dealing with drivers.

The answer was the Road Traffic Bill, 1954; this aimed to increase road safety, to introduce experiments to relieve traffic congestion, and to clear up anomalies in the law. Its important clauses concerned proposals for a new offence of 'causing death by dangerous driving'; the separation of the offence of driving under the influence of drink from that of being in charge under the influence; compulsory tests for ten-year-old cars; the liability of cyclists to charges of dangerous or careless driving; and the application of the traffic law to pedestrians.

The Bill had a chequered career; it did not become law until 1956, partly because it was 'killed' by the dissolution of parliament in 1955, but mainly because there was so much wrangling in committee over its clauses.

The two most controversial were those dealing with causing death by dangerous driving; and being in charge of, but not driving, a vehicle while under the influence of drink or drugs. The former was not, of course, a new offence at all as it had previously been called manslaughter. In the debate on the Bill the Lord Chief Justice (Lord Goddard), welcoming the clause, said that he had suggested the necessity for it to the Minister of Transport in 1933 after being continually astounded by the 'perverse' decisions of juries in manslaughter cases; Major Lloyd-George made a similar suggestion for the same reasons in the debate on the 1934 Bill (*Hansard, Lords,* 15 February 1955; *Hansard, Commons,* 11 April 1934).

Controversy about the apparent injustice of arresting a driver for being 'drunk in charge', though he had not been actually driving, had been intense in the debates preceding the Criminal Justice Act, 1925, which penalized a person accused of being drunk in charge in terms as severe as if he had been driving. A motorist who decided to 'sleep it off' in the forecourt of a public house before going on his way would be liable to the same penalty as if he had driven off on leaving the bar. Also it was pointed out that the police could walk into a bar and arrest any customer who seemed to be drunk unless he could prove to their satisfaction that he did not intend to drive. The motoring organizations disliked this measure intensely and the Home Secretary was sympathetic, but the government submitted to strong pressure from the police who felt that many guilty persons would escape justice if prosecution had to be confined to those who were driving (*Hansard, Lords,* 22 January 1930).

76

The Law and the Motorist

The 1956 Act met some of these objections by separating the offences of driving under the influence and being drunk in charge, giving a lower maximum penalty for the latter. But this change, and the new offence of 'causing death', were regarded by the anti-motoring groups as concessions to motorists who were thereby given more loopholes through which to evade justice. In fact, as in 1934, the intention of the legislature was misinterpreted by its critics since it was hoped that juries might be more willing to convict when the charge was causing death by dangerous driving than if it were the 'barbarous-sounding charge of manslaughter' (*The Times*, 30 May 1956.)

Perhaps the only real concession to the motorists in this Act was the very odd decision to cease requiring disqualification in all cases of failure to insure, unless there were 'special reasons' (as had been instituted by the 1930 Act); the issue was left to the court's discretion, and the proportion of such cases in which disqualification was imposed dropped immediately – whereas the insurance offences rose and continued to rise at an increased rate.

Otherwise the Act increased penalties for dangerous and careless driving, but evidently not sufficiently to deter the errant driver. By May 1960 the Lords were debating the same issue of speed limits versus a stiffer law against dangerous driving as they had done in 1895. But this time there was much more criticism of justices and juries for untoward leniency. The Pedestrians' Association increased pressure in favour of tightening up the law against drunken driving and against failure to stop after, or to report, an accident; and its chairman, Mr Graham Page, MP, introduced a private member's Bill which would have made it an offence for a person to be found in charge of a vehicle with a blood-alcohol content of ·15 per cent or more. Increases in the maximum penalties for failure to stop, etc., were also proposed, but the timing of the Bill was inopportune and it did not get beyond its second reading.

This unsuccessful attempt was a disappointment to the Pedestrians' Association and to others who wanted to see the law tightened up; and a further disappointment followed when the Road Traffic Act, 1960, became law. For this was really not much more than a re-enactment of the Acts of 1930, 1934, and 1956 in a single statute, though it did introduce parking meters and fixed penalties for not using them.

The Act did not increase penalties for drunken or dangerous driving although a propaganda campaign had been conducted to secure the former. The drunken driver seemed to become a particular target in the popular press during 1960 and 1961, and the impression given by press reports of

77

cases was most unsympathetic to motorists. Criticism of drivers also seemed to increase on radio and television, and the courts again came in for much castigation on grounds of inconsistency and excessive leniency.

During the period 1960 and 1961 traffic offences and road casualties continued to increase and to provide support for increased pressure by the Pedestrians' Association and its supporters for more severe legislation. It came with the Road Traffic Bill, 1961, which was eventually to become the current Act of 1962.

For British motoring law it is severe, and it is a more formidable measure than any before Parliament since 1903. Its principal weapon is disqualification, and it lists six serious offences for which the courts must disqualify for not less than one year unless there are special reasons for not doing so. The offences are:

Manslaughter
Causing death by dangerous driving
Reckless or dangerous driving if committed within three years of a similar offence
Driving under the influence of drink or drugs
Driving while disqualified
Racing

A further twenty offences are then listed for which disqualification is discretionary, including failing to stop after or to report an accident, which was not a 'disqualifying' offence under previous Acts. Moreover, disqualification is compulsory, for a period of not less than six months, unless there are special reasons, for a third or subsequent conviction for any of the twenty-six offences, and there are substantial increases in maximum penalties.

Even so, the Act is much less severe than the Bill, which left the courts little or no discretion in imposing disqualification for subsequent offences. The opposition of the motoring organizations to this extension of disqualification was fierce, and they and their supporters secured not only the qualification that 'special reasons' could excuse disqualification, but that these could refer to both the offender *and* the offence; hitherto 'special reasons' could relate to the offence only.

Opposition was intense also to the more stringent measures for dealing with drunken drivers, especially the provision that a 'person shall be taken to be unfit to drive if his ability to do so properly is for the time being impaired'. This is much less demanding than the older requirement that the offender should 'be under the influence of drink or drugs to such an extent as to be incapable of having proper control'. Equally strong objections were raised to the provision allowing the use of tests for the presence of alcohol in the body; these are voluntary, but the Act states that refusal to submit to a test can constitute evidence against a defendant.

The Act is now operating, and it has brought into the open once more the bitter struggle that has endured since 1896 between the motoring organizations and their opponents. The struggle has continued for three reasons: first, the continuous and rapid technical advance of the motor vehicle; second, the refusal of many drivers to obey a law which they think to be out of touch with contemporary conditions, and hence irksome and stupid; and finally, the difficulty which those who enforce the law have in interpreting it and in maintaining a sentencing policy which is consistent and just.

It is not the aim of this study to discuss the technical development of motor vehicles or of road construction, and the attitudes and behaviour of drivers will be considered later. But the problems of enforcing and interpreting the law follow logically from a historical account of it; so it seems to be essential to illustrate the law and analyse it in relation to the serious offences with which this study is concerned. It must be stressed, however, that this is being undertaken without legal training, and hence the risk of misunderstanding is considerable. On the other hand, it is a useful exercise, if only to show some of the difficulties in understanding the law that a layman-driver encounters; for a motorist cannot be expected to obey the letter and the spirit of a law which he cannot understand. And, as the writer is no more than an ordinary motorist, it may be that the things which bewilder him may bewilder others also.

THE SERIOUS OFFENCES

Homicide

When the driver of a motor vehicle causes someone else's death he may be said to have committed homicide by murder, or manslaughter, or causing death by dangerous driving. Each of these offences is treated separately in law, and the differences between them will now be discussed. The first step is to distinguish between the older offences of murder and manslaughter since, until 1956, a driver against whom homicide was alleged had to be charged with one of these.

Murder has been defined as 'when a person of sound memory and discretion unlawfully killeth any reasonable creature in being under the King's

79

peace with malice aforethought, either express or implied' (3. *Coke's Institutes*, 47). Manslaughter is 'the unlawful and felonious killing of another without any malice, either express or implied' (*Archbold*, 1962, para. 2468). In other words, it is manslaughter to kill another while behaving unlawfully but without any intention to kill or do grievous bodily harm; if there were such an intention, it would be murder.

Hence the distinction between these two offences rests on the interpretation of a rather difficult legal concept, i.e. 'intention', defined by Kenny (1962) as 'the state of mind of a man who not only foresees but also wills the possible consequences of his conduct'. Yet, as Kenny shows, one can foresee possible consequences, or be indifferent to them, *without* willing or desiring them, and still persist with a course of action; thus taking a risk, and behaving in a manner that is, in legal usage, 'reckless', and would be manslaughter if death were caused. As, for example, when a driver in a great hurry overtakes on a blind bend and causes a collision from which fatal consequences result.

A further requirement in murder and manslaughter is that the *mens rea* should be established; and this, according to Kenny (op. cit.), means that there must be in the guilty mind either 'intention' or 'recklessness': the two essential elements in this important legal concept.

From what has been said so far it will be observed that for behaviour to be reckless, in the legal sense, it must be advertent. And, indeed, Kenny makes a distinction between recklessness and negligence in that the latter implies inadvertence and cannot be relevant to manslaughter. He takes to task those who would speak of negligence as being 'criminal', 'gross', or 'culpable', since the term means that there was a complete absence of thought – and hence of intention or foresight – in the mind: a nullity, 'and of nullity there can be no degrees'.

According to Kenny's lucid analysis there could be no homicide if there were no advertence; no murder without intention; and no manslaughter without recklessness. But, unfortunately, the law is not so unequivocal, and Glanville Williams (1961, pp. 100–19) has shown that it is possible to commit manslaughter by behaving with 'inadvertent gross negligence'; gross, in that the behaviour departs considerably from that which might be expected of a reasonable man, and inadvertent in that the fatal consequences were not foreseen. He shows that criminal liability can be incurred for behaviour wherein there is no more than 'mere neglect to exercise due caution and the the mind is not actively but negatively or passively at fault' (op. cit. p. 100).

In most cases of motoring homicide it seems at first to be easy to say whether the death was caused by the accused's intention, recklessness, or negligence; but, in practice, it is not so, as we shall see later.

In manslaughter the problem seems to be, in the last analysis, one of degree: the degree to which the accused is blameworthy. Thus Lord Kilmuir, a recent Lord Chancellor, has postulated – despite Kenny – that there are at least four degrees of negligence to be considered in motoring offences: the first as required in manslaughter; the second as required in reckless or dangerous driving; the third as in careless driving; and the fourth as required to establish a pecuniary claim in civil actions (*Hansard, Lords*, 2 July 1956). However, a little thought may show this to be of no particular help to justice or jury, and one turns back with some relief to 1930 when the then Solicitor-General said that 'in practically every case ... a finding of reckless driving coupled with a resulting death contains all the ingredients of manslaughter, and that would be the proper verdict. It would be inviting a jury to derogate from the law if they were to be entitled to say that although a man had killed a victim outright he might be convicted only of dangerous driving' (*Hansard, Commons*, 25 March 1930).

Yet, according to Glanville Williams (op. cit. p. 110), 'a requirement of recklessness in motor manslaughter would exempt nearly all motorists who cause death, because the negligent motorist is usually the optimist who expects by his cleverness to avoid the danger he creates'. Hence it would not be easy to establish the advertence needed to prove recklessness.

Although insistence on recklessness as a central element in manslaughter seemed to make it more difficult to secure convictions, it was evidently no easier when the law relating to this offence was interpreted more widely. For, until 1930, there were precedents to support a view that any unlawful act resulting in death was manslaughter if it did not amount to murder; but this conception proved difficult to apply in practice because juries thought it unjust and would not convict. Hence, apparently, the inclusion of a provision in the Road Traffic Act, 1934, to enable juries to 'derogate from the law' and convict for dangerous driving in manslaughter cases if they thought fit.

This enabling provision derived from a leading case, *R. v. Stringer* ([1933] 24 Cr. App. R. 30), which is worth citing since it illustrates particularly well some of the problems that arise in cases of motor manslaughter.

The facts were that Stringer was driving his lorry along a main road in daylight when he came upon a bend where the road was under repair and was partially obstructed; another vehicle was approaching and, in avoiding it, Stringer's lorry struck a tarring machine and a road worker who was standing beside it, killing him. According to witnesses, Stringer's speed was 'fast', and he was charged on two counts: manslaughter, and driving in a manner dangerous to the public. He was acquitted of the former, but found guilty of the latter, and he appealed on the ground that a conviction for dangerous driving was incompatible with an acquittal for manslaughter since the two charges were, in this case, based upon the same facts. In other words, Stringer pleaded that if his driving had been dangerous he would have committed manslaughter, but since he had been acquitted of this charge his driving could not have been dangerous.

On appeal before Lord Hewart and four judges, counsel for the Crown cited *R. v. Bateman* ([1925] 19 Cr. App. 8), in which Lord Hewart had held that evidence of careless or incompetent driving was insufficient to justify a verdict of manslaughter unless it could be established that there had been 'such disregard for the lives and the safety of others as to constitute a crime against the State'. This pronouncement prompted another member of the court (Branson, J.) to inquire: 'How are you to differentiate between the degree of negligence sufficient to find a verdict of manslaughter, and the degree sufficient to find a verdict of dangerous driving?' However, Stringer's conviction was upheld, and the precedent was established that although a death had been caused, it could have been through dangerous driving that was not serious enough to constitute manslaughter. That was the ruling which parliament sanctioned in section 34 of the Road Traffic Act, 1934, enabling juries to 'write down' charges of manslaughter and convict for dangerous driving.

Ostensibly this section permitted juries to convict for dangerous driving in manslaughter cases although no notice of intended prosecution for the former offence had been served; it also allowed for the possibility that there could have been dangerous driving which had not, in itself, caused the death. But the real effect of the measure was to increase the number of 'degrees of negligence' which juries must consider, as in *Andrews* v. *DPP* ([1937] 26 Cr. App. 34, p. 39), wherein the arguments were concerned entirely with the degree of danger or recklessness in the defendant's driving, and not with whether it had caused the victim's death – which was not in doubt.

The facts were that the defendant, a bus driver, took a light van from his bus depot late at night to go to a bus that had broken down. While driving down a lighted road in a built-up area he overtook a private car at what was said to be a fast speed, and while on his wrong side of the road knocked down and killed a man who was crossing the road and was just about to reach the pavement on the defendant's offside. The deceased was carried on the bonnet of the defendant's van for some yards until he was thrown forward under its wheels and again run over, but Andrews did not stop. He was traced by description, but denied that he had been in the vicinity at the time. He was convicted of manslaughter, sentenced to 15 months' imprisonment, and disqualified for life.

Andrews appealed to the Court of Criminal Appeal against his conviction for manslaughter on the ground that the judge had not directed the jury so as to leave them a choice between finding manslaughter or, alternatively, dangerous driving. The trial judge had said, in summing up, that 'if you think that the defendant was driving recklessly and in a dangerous manner, within the meaning of those words, and it was because of that that the deceased was killed, then it is your bounden duty to convict of manslaughter'.

The court dismissed the appeal, and the defendant then took his case to the House of Lords, where it was again dismissed. Giving judgement, Lord Atkin said that dangerous driving, as expressed in the Road Traffic Act, 1930 (section 11), *covered* driving with such a high degree of negligence that if death resulted it would be manslaughter; but he held that it was quite possible for a driver to drive at a speed or in a manner which was dangerous, and cause death, and yet not be guilty of manslaughter. The question, he said, was whether or not the high degree of negligence required to constitute manslaughter was present; this was a matter of degree rather than of epithets, and it was one which the jury must decide on the facts before them.

A 'matter of degree' is not much different from one of opinion, and juries continued to be confused when the evidence in manslaughter cases was based more on opinion than upon fact. Moreover, according to Lord Goddard, they were also failing to convict in cases of 'what seemed to be most horribly dangerous driving', and he referred to 'shocking cases' in which juries had brought in unsound verdicts. Since it seemed that juries still thought manslaughter too grave a charge to be applied to motorists who killed, and so refused to convict, something less serious than manslaughter, but more serious than dangerous driving, would have to be devised if the guilty were not to go free. Hence the introduction of the offence of causing death by dangerous or reckless driving in the Road Traffic Act, 1956 (section 8).

Welcoming the new offence in a speech in the Lords, Lord Goddard said that juries would now be presented with a simple issue – 'Has there been death caused by dangerous driving? If you think that the man *was* driving dangerously, there is the offence. You will not be taken up with nice distinctions between dangerous driving, driving sufficiently dangerous to justify manslaughter, and so on' (*The Times*, 16 February 1955, p. 12). However, he did not welcome the section of the Act enabling juries to find the accused guilty of dangerous or reckless driving only in 'causing death' cases; he assured the House that 'they will always do so' (*Hansards, Lords*, 14 March 1955).

It seems strange, however, that simply because a victim happens to die, an offender is liable to be charged with causing death by dangerous driving and sent to prison for up to five years; yet, had the victim not been killed but 'only' maimed for life, the accused would have been charged with the lesser offence of dangerous driving and could not have been sent to prison for more than two years. It will be evident that driving that results in a death need not be more heinous than that which results in an injury, and this observation is amply supported by the evidence in the five cases of causing death by dangerous driving which are reported in the documentary study; none of these cases is worse than some of those in which there was dangerous driving but no death or even injury. So the practice of attaching different maximum penalties to causing death on the one hand, and dangerous driving on the other, seems to be absurd when the real distinction between the two offences depends almost entirely on chance.

In actuality the introduction of 'causing death' virtually ended prosecutions for manslaughter in motoring cases; but, in 1955, it became evident that it was the intention to retain the latter charge, with all its disadvantages, and use it 'in exceptional cases, such as those in which robbers, for example, had run down a policeman and were trying to escape' (the Lord Chancellor speaking in the Lords, *Hansard, Lords*, 14 March 1955). So it would seem that manslaughter was to be reserved for those who might be called 'real criminals', as a kind of ultimate sanction against those who use vehicles as instruments of crime. But, in fact, the offender who found himself in the awkward circumstances which the Lord Chancellor foresaw would place himself in jeopardy of being charged not with manslaughter, but with murder. Such was the case in *DPP* v. *Smith* ([1961] A.C. 290), which introduced yet another dimension into the problems of classifying homicide by driving.

The facts were that Smith, while driving his car, was signalled to stop by a police officer whom he happened to know; because he was carrying stolen goods, Smith did not pull into the kerb as requested but drove away. The officer clung to Smith's car which swerved so sharply that he lost his grip and fell into the path of an approaching car which ran over him and caused fatal injuries. Smith then drove on some two hundred yards, dumped the

84

stolen goods, and returned to the scene; there he admitted that he had been involved, and showed much remorse at the officer's fate which he denied having intended to cause in any way whatsoever.

Smith was charged with murder, it being submitted by the prosecution that a 'reasonable man' would have known that the consequences of attempting to shake off the police officer as Smith had done would be such as to cause death or grievous bodily harm; and, since the defendant had not pleaded insanity or diminished responsibility, it could be supposed that his expectations would have been the same in the circumstances as those of a 'reasonable man'. If this were so, the trial judge told the jury, Smith would be guilty of murder since he could be presumed to have intended the natural and probable consequences of his action. Attention was drawn to the defendant's report of his state of mind at the time, namely that he was panic-stricken at the thought of arrest while in possession of stolen goods and accelerated away without realizing that the officer was clinging to the car; but the test was whether a reasonable man would have taken this course. The jury decided that a reasonable man would not have acted thus, and found against Smith. He then appealed on the ground that the judge had misdirected the jury in applying the test of what a reasonable man would have intended, rather than inquiring into what he, the *defendant*, could have been expected to intend; the appeal was successful and the court substituted a verdict of manslaughter for that of capital murder, and a sentence of ten years' imprisonment for the death sentence. But, on appeal to the Lords by the prosecution, the Appeal Court's decision was reversed and the original verdict restored though, in anticipation, Smith had been reprieved. The reason given for the reversal was that the 'objective test' – the hypothetical intention and behaviour of a reasonable man – was applicable in this case and in others of its kind.

This decision excited much legal controversy since, as Glanville Williams demonstrated, it restored a state of affairs which existed before the Homicide Act, 1957, and which that Act was designed to end: i.e. the paradox that murder could be committed without intention, and literally by accident, if an accused person's intentions or behaviour differed grossly from what might be expected of a 'reasonable man' (*The Times*, 21 October 1960; see also subsequent correspondence in *The Times* during October and November 1960). Moreover, as Blom-Cooper (1960) had pointed out, the decision meant that a defendant who was stupid or very uneducated might be placed at a grave disadvantage if charged with murder in circumstances of this kind, since the conception of an ordinary man's judgement would be wholly inapplicable to him.

The implication of Smith's case for motorists are formidable, because murder could be alleged if fatal consequences resulted from circumstances in which a notional driver – the 'reasonable man' – might have expected the probable infliction of grievous bodily harm. For example, an elderly company director who became exasperated at being held up in a queue of traffic by a police pointsman and drove his Bentley at him would have been liable to a charge of capital murder had the officer not jumped out of the way; but, in fact, he was fined £25 for dangerous driving, and was disqualified until he had passed a driving test (an actual case from the 653 offences discussed in Chapters 7 and 8 below).

So, although the law seems to have become relaxed in its severity towards the driver who commits homicide with his vehicle, it retains a painful sting in its tail for some. Moreover, since the Act of 1956, it has become even more difficult than it was before to decide whether the behaviour of an offender whose driving has caused death constitutes manslaughter, causing death by dangerous driving, dangerous driving only, or murder.

One thing is clear, however: in murder and manslaughter the courts regard the defendant's state of mind to be relevant to the issue. But it is doubtful whether this is also true of causing death by reckless or dangerous driving.

From one point of view it would appear that the defendant's state of mind in these cases is not relevant. This could be inferred from the ruling in *Hill* v. *Baxter* ([1958] 1 All E.R. 193), when Lord Goddard distinguished between offences that were 'absolute prohibitions', in which the state of mind was irrelevant, and those wherein it was essential to establish that there was *mens rea*. He included reckless or dangerous driving among the absolute prohibitions, saying that it was no defence to such charges to say 'I did not intend to drive dangerously' or 'I did not notice the Halt sign'. Moreover, Kenny (1962, para. 25) inferred that there is no need for advertence or *mens rea* to be established in order to convict, if the statutes exclude the necessity to do so.

This view was reinforced by another decision in *R.* v. *Parker* ([1958] 122 J.P. 17), which was upheld on appeal by Lord Goddard and others. In this case the facts were that an elderly man had been driving his car down a busy main street when he crossed a dangerous road junction with the traffic lights at 'red' against him; he collided with a bus which had, quite properly, begun to move forward, and the end of his car swung round, killing a pedestrian. In directing the jury, Mr Justice Streatfeild said that a momentary disregard of safety precautions, or a momentary act of negligence could amount to dangerous driving. The defendant was convicted, but it is clear that his state of mind could not have been regarded as relevant to the causing of the victim's death. The case was, however, the subject of an article in which the learned writer noted that the judge's direction had omitted the term 'reckless', though not, it was thought, deliberately. But the writer drew attention to the fact that 'reckless' and 'dangerous' driving seem to be regarded in the statutes as being equally heinous, since they are linked together in the same section and the maximum penalty is identical for both (*Justice of the Peace & Local Government Review*, 19 March 1960).

Yet it is evident that recklessness must involve advertence, if the definitions used above have any meaning. So it would seem that recklessness that results in a death would be manslaughter. Hence Lord Kilmuir, in the debate in which he enumerated the four categories of negligence appropriate in motoring offences (see p. 81 above): 'Where you have reckless driving, that is, driving with reckless disregard, you have *mens rea*' (*Hansard, Lords*, 2 July 1956). This is reinforced by Wilkinson (1960, p. 73), an authority on traffic offences, who suggests that a defendant's state of mind is immaterial when the charge is causing death by dangerous (as opposed to reckless) driving; and he supports this view by a reference to *R. v. Scates* (*Crim. L.R.* [1957] 406).

It seems to follow that causing death by reckless driving requires deliberate intention and is, therefore, the same as manslaughter except – for the benefit of juries – in name and in penalty. Perhaps that is why most defendants are charged with 'causing death by driving at a speed or in a manner which is *dangerous*', etc.; the offence is then made an 'absolute prohibition' in which it is not necessary to establish any deliberate intent.

The confusion does not, however, end here since Glanville Williams has suggested that it is no longer justifiable to regard dangerous driving as an absolute prohibition, despite the ruling in *Hill v. Baxter* above. He cites a decision in *Spurge* ([1961] 45 Cr. App. R. 191), where it was held that the existence of an unforeseeable mechanical defect, such as to cause a vehicle to become out of control, constituted a defence to a charge of dangerous driving (Williams, G., 1961, p. 234). Yet an analysis of *Spurge's* case seems to suggest that the main issue was whether the offence (driving dangerously) was committed by the driver, Spurge (without regard to his state of mind), by the vehicle, or by both Spurge and his vehicle: the fundamental question was whether the defendant was in control of his vehicle. If he was not in control, because of a mechanical defect which he could not possibly have foreseen, then he could not have been *driving* it either dangerously or recklessly, and could not be guilty of that offence.

87

Legal and Social Background

In *Hill* v. *Baxter* the issue was slightly, but significantly, different from that in *Spurge*. In the former case the defence was that the defendant had been taken ill unforeseeably and had 'blacked out', so that he passed an illuminated Halt sign without seeing it and collided with another vehicle. Here the suggestion was that the defect arose in the driver, not in the vehicle, but it was not submitted that he was not in control, and so was not driving. However, the court was not able to agree with this view, nor with the submission that his illness was unforeseeable, and the defendant was convicted.

This problem of 'automatism' is particularly well illustrated in the following case, in which one Lewendon was acquitted of a charge of causing death by dangerous driving. The prosecution's case was that the defendant, while travelling at a speed in excess of 50 mph, pulled out onto his wrong side to overtake slow-moving traffic despite the fact that the road was obstructed by a string of racehorses being led slowly along the de-fendant's offside. Before reaching the horses his car hit the offside kerb, regained the road, and then ran straight through the line of horses and grooms, flinging the latter into the air. Afterwards the car hit a wall, shot up into the air, and finished up on its side facing the direction from which it had come. Moreover, it was said that the accused had been noticed immediately before this incident when he 'cut in' very sharply after passing a cyclist and passed over a busy crossroads in such a manner that the police pointsman had to step aside rapidly to avoid being hit. For the defence it was said that Lewendon had a petit mal at the time of the incident, and that he was not in control of the car but in a state of automatism. Evidence was given that he had been an epileptic since childhood though he had possibly not realized it; indeed his doctor said that he could not remember having told his patient, especially since he was not aware that he (Lewendon) was a weekend driver. It seemed incredible that the defendant had been under medical treatment since childhood without suspecting that he was an epileptic, yet the jury gave him the benefit of the doubt and found him not guilty. However, the judge recommended that the licensing authority should not renew the defendant's driving licence; it is interesting to note that the court had no authority to do more than 'recommend' that this be done (*The Times*, 14, 15, and 16 December 1961).

Lewendon's case demonstrates the great difficulty in dealing with motor-ing cases involving homicide, and also the implications which decisions made in them may have for a wide range of non-motoring cases. Whether these defences of automatism or of mechanical defect do, or do not, shake the doctrine of absolute prohibition is beyond this writer's competence, but

88

some weird implications would arise if they had no validity since it would seem that a vehicle could commit an offence more or less by itself. Its driver is liable only because he is in charge of it, and so we have a conception that is reminiscent of primitive law, as exemplified in the practice of trying and condemning objects or animals for crimes committed, and in the ancient principle of the 'deodand', according to which an object with which a killing was done could be made forfeit.

Further doubt is cast on the application of absolute prohibition to dangerous driving, and *ipso facto* causing death also, by the admissibility of evidence in such cases as to the effect of alcohol on the defendant's state of mind (*R. v. Fisher* and *R. v. Richardson, Crim. L. R.* [1960] 135). Yet in another case (*R. v. Norrington*, ibid. 432) the judge would not admit such evidence. If there were an absolute prohibition, the effect of alcohol on the accused's state of mind would be quite irrelevant; but this is not, apparently, the case.

These questions of intention, and of relative heinousness as between dangerous or reckless driving, are made all the more difficult and confusing by the fatal consequences in homicide cases; yet it would seem that the mere fact of the victim's death is irrelevant where the alleged offence is other than murder. In fact the problems still remain when the offence is reckless or dangerous driving, uncluttered by a victim's death; and they are complicated even further by the difficulty in drawing distinctions between reckless, dangerous, and careless driving.

Driving Dangerously or Recklessly

Section 2(1) of the Road Traffic Act, 1960, makes it an offence to drive a motor vehicle on a road 'recklessly, or at a speed or in a manner which is dangerous to the public, having regard to all the circumstances of the case, including the nature, condition and use of the road, and to the amount of traffic which is actually at the time, or which might reasonably be expected to be, on the road'. And under section 3(1) it is an offence 'to drive a motor vehicle on a road without due care and attention, or without reasonable consideration for other persons using the road'.

Under the 1960 Act the maximum penalties are the same for dangerous and for reckless driving, and somewhat less for careless driving; disqualification is usual for the first two but not so usual for the last, though the courts may disqualify for all these offences.

Much has been written about the difference between dangerous and careless driving, and most authorities have inferred that it is all a matter of degree. This sounds trite, but no other interpretation is possible from the history of the careless driving clause in the Road Traffic Act, 1930, which, it will be remembered, was retained despite the Royal Commission's advice that it was impracticable. Speaking of the clause in the House of Lords, the government spokesman, Lord Russell, said: 'I do not know what exactly is meant by driving without due care and attention, but no doubt benches of magistrates will have no difficulty in construing it. I think it will serve as an educational clause and a first offender's act for the driver who might otherwise become criminal' (*Hansard, Lords,* 16 December 1929).

Lord Atkin, speaking in the same debate, was not so sanguine; he expressed 'alarm' about the clause, and about the words 'without due care and attention' in particular. He pointed out that those words meant 'negligence', and 'it would be better to confine the clause to driving without consideration for others, as if you say that a motorist who drives a car negligently is only committing a minor offence, you are giving away a great deal of what you intended to do by creating the offence of dangerous driving'. Appreciating this point, Lord Russell replied that the clause was not intended to supply an alternative offence to dangerous driving, it was put in to cover minor offences; a somewhat equivocal statement, but it is clarified by some earlier remarks of Lord Russell's in which he said that the government wanted to make dangerous driving a 'disgraceful offence', which it could not be if it were to cover trivial offences.

Lord Atkin was not alone in having reservations about the careless driving clause; the anti-motoring faction had them also, and Lord Cecil called it a 'bolt hole in a motorist's protection bill which undermines the one thing we have got out of this Act: a somewhat increased severity for dangerous driving' (see *Hansard, Lords,* 16 and 17 December 1929, for the relevant speeches).

The position was exacerbated in 1934 when section 34 of the Act of that year enabled juries to convict for careless driving in 'danger' cases if they thought the facts did not justify the graver charge; this was the same kind of writing down that they were able to do in manslaughter cases where they could find dangerous driving rather than manslaughter. The effect was to widen considerably the choices open to those with powers to charge and convict for motoring offences, and these were considerable enough already. For example, it would seem that a driver who passed a Halt sign could be charged with driving recklessly, driving dangerously, driving without due care and attention, driving without reasonable consideration, or failing to obey a traffic sign. All these offences are matters of opinion, except the last which is one of fact; and it is from these two positions – fact and opinion –

that the opponents and supporters of motoring have argued and are still arguing.

Twenty-three years after the creation of the careless driving offence the *Justice of the Peace Journal* published an analytical article in which the learned writer tried to find criteria that might distinguish careless driving as something in its own right, but the best that could be done at the end was to say: 'We have tried to lay down hard and fast rules by which benches can be guided (in distinguishing careless from dangerous driving) but it is not possible to do so. The facts of the particular case must decide as to which definition should apply.' He continued: 'The Act clearly treats dangerous driving as more serious than careless, and it is, therefore, important that the courts should distinguish as clearly as possible between the two . . . in practice this is difficult' (*Justice of the Peace Journal*, 1953, 117, pp. 766–7).

The contrary view is expressed by Wilkinson (1960, p. 98): 'Parliament has shown that what lay magistrates, exercising their common sense as reasonable men and users of the highway, regard as "dangerous" driving shall merit the greater penalty, and what they do not regard as "dangerous" may nevertheless yet be careless driving. We all know what we ourselves regard as justifying a conviction under [the dangerous driving section] and what we regard as mere lack of due care and attention, and there is no need to elevate or debase into a question of law what is really a question of fact for a tribunal of fact.' Then, after this vague and rather irritatingly complacent dissertation, he quotes Mr Justice Winn's definition of dangerous driving as a *deliberate* choice of a course of driving from which danger arises; we are thus returned to the uncertain supposition that deliberate intention must be established in dangerous, but not in careless, driving. Some support for this latter view is offered by an article in the *Criminal Law Review* (1955, p. 238), in which the writer quotes an unreported decision by Mr Justice Sellers that there must be some deliberate act to constitute dangerous driving as an offence. But there is no case law cited on this decision and the writer concludes that 'the difference between these two offences has not, to this day, been authoritatively defined'.

Hence there seems to be no point in having a separate offence of careless driving unless the behaviour needed to establish it is different in kind and essence from that required to establish danger or recklessness. If it were only a matter of degree it would surely be possible to achieve justice by having one offence and adjusting the sentence within the very wide limits allowed; they are, after all, maxima.

If there is any real difference it would seem to depend on the presence or absence of the *mens rea*, with its twin elements of intention and reckless-ness. To establish the more serious offence it would therefore be necessary to show that there had been a deliberately taken risk which was, in itself, dangerous in the circumstances. This, of course, amounts to reckless driving; so it may be advisable to omit the term dangerous altogether, since it is not only superfluous, but also probably responsible for most of the confusion and doubt that now exist when one reflects that all reckless driving must be dangerous, and so must all careless driving. If there were only two offences, reckless driving on the one hand and careless driving on the other, we would have Kenny's distinction between recklessness and negligence: one that would not be hard for anyone to apply. Indeed it might be made even more direct and to the point if, instead of 'driving without due care and attention', the offence became one of 'incompetent driving'. An alternative would be to abolish the 'due care' offence and return to the principle of the 1903 Act which recognized only reckless or negligent driving. (The term negligent was inserted in this Act, section 1, but it was omitted from the sections of the 1930 Act dealing with dangerous and careless driving. The reason is not clear; it may have been to make the 1930 offences sound less heinous, or to turn them into absolute prohibi-tions by making it irrelevant whether there was negligence or not.) Differ-ences in heinousness could then be allowed for by using the full range of sentencing power. In any case, the increased penalties for careless driving in the 1962 Act seem to bring the two offences more closely together so that the separation will be only a fiction in the future.

Driving under the Influence of Drink or Drugs

Of all serious motoring offenders, the drunken driver is one of the most controversial and least popular, and the impression is that he has now replaced the 'road hog' as a target.

Until 1930 drunken driving was handled as a summary offence under either the Intoxicating Liquor (Licensing Act), 1872, or the Criminal Justice Act, 1925. The former placed drivers at the mercy of anyone who thought that another person was drunk 'while in charge of any carriage, horse, or steam engine'; the latter stiffened the penalties but it did require that arrest should be by a police officer.

The real problem in the early legislation was, as it is now, the acute difficulty in defining the terms apropos of 'drunkenness': by what standards was someone 'drunk' so as to be a danger when in charge of a vehicle, and what requirements must be met before a driver could be said to be in charge of a vehicle? How could the safety of other road users be protected, and at the same time drivers themselves be protected from foolish or over-zealous accusations of unfitness to drive through drink?

Giving evidence to the Royal Commission of 1929, the chief constable of Kent stressed the difficulty of getting convictions on a definition of drunkenness, since justices' ideas as to what constituted this condition were too extreme to include the driver who, although not falling all over the place, was unable to exercise the judgement needed to drive a vehicle safely. That was why the Royal Commission, and later on the government, adopted a form of wording derived from recommendations by the Cyclists' Touring Club and Lord Buckmaster, thus: 'Any person found, when driving or attempting to drive a mechanically propelled vehicle, to be so under the influence of drink or drugs as to be incapable of having proper control of such vehicle . . .' etc. (*Royal Commission on Transport, First Report*, 1929, p. 12). In the 1930 Act the final wording was: 'Any person who, when driving or attempting to drive, or when in charge of a motor vehicle on a road or other public place is under the influence of drink or drugs to such an extent as to be incapable of having proper control of the vehicle . . .' etc. In 1956, being in charge, but not driving, while under the influence of drink or drugs was made a separate offence, and it still is so, leaving the wording of subsequent statutes virtually the same until the Act of 1962 introduced the view that a driver would be committing an offence if he drove when his ability to do so properly was for the time being 'impaired' through consumption of drink or drugs.

Although this study does not include the 'in charge, but not driving' offence as such, it would be unsound to dismiss it without comment: if only to emphasize why it was omitted. The charge has been controversial ever since it came into the Act of 1930, because it penalizes drivers for their condition and not for their driving. Moreover, this is one of the exceptional cases wherein the burden of proof lies on the defence to show that the accused had no intention of driving while in the alleged condition. Indeed it has led to some extraordinary cases, as for example that of one Bentley, a lorry driver, who appealed against conviction on the ground that he had been too drunk to have been capable of even trying to drive; he had gone out with friends intending to get as drunk as he could, and he had succeeded. His appeal succeeded also, and although it is not known whether there was a counter-appeal, this case demonstrates, with many others, that this particular offence often makes the law look rather silly (*Daily Mail*, 27 September 1960).

In drunken driving the problem is much the same as in dangerous or careless driving; guilt depends on a matter of opinion (impairment) rather than on a matter of fact, since no minimum consumption of alcohol (or drugs) is specified. The central issue is the accused's condition, not the manner in which he drove; though that can be described in evidence to establish or to rebut the charge. It would appear also that it is not essential to prove any deliberate intention in these cases since the offence seems to be another in which there is 'absolute prohibition' whether the offender intends to become 'unfit' or not; this was the view of Mr Justice Humphreys in *Harding* v. *Price* ([1948] 1 All E.R. 283). Yet it may be reasonable to suppose that an offender would know that he was in a condition that would render him liable to a charge of 'driving under the influence', and that he would know this to be wrong. But, of course, he may not realize his state of mind until he has already committed the offence by driving even the smallest distance. And it is enough to substantiate the charge to see the offender move away from a stationary position; hence it is expected of 'the reasonable man' that he would always form the conclusion that he was unfit to drive *before* setting his vehicle in motion.

Because of the non-factual basis of the allegation, this is a particularly difficult charge to prove. Hence the many attempts to introduce a factual criterion by employing machines, such as the 'breathalyzer', and tests of urine. The latter are generally accepted, but the former are still said by some to be too liable to error to be acceptable in evidence; however, it is clear that the authorities intend to make some kind of objective test more or less compulsory since they made provision in the 1962 Act for refusal to take a test to be used in evidence. In any case, none of these tests does more than show that a driver has consumed a certain amount of alcohol; they do not indicate the extent of his 'impairment', and that is the essential criterion in the offence. A quantity that will cause impairment in one person will not do so in another, and we are then back to relying on opinion unless it is decided to give 'the reasonable man' a tolerance level and make anything in excess of that evidence of impairment. Tests of memory or agility given by the police or their surgeons are also open to objection because they may not be standardized, and there is often no proof that they were administered properly with the interests of the accused under safeguard.

But perhaps the greatest difficulty lies in establishing the condition of the accused on arrest, since there may be an interval between then and an examination by a police doctor, during which the driver may have sobered. That is why some police authorities, including the one in whose area this research was done, rely entirely on police evidence as to incapacity to drive, leaving the doctor to say only that the accused was, or was not, suffering from any illness that might have affected his driving. The procedure has advantages in that it requires the doctor to give evidence only on matters in which he is expert, namely the presence of illness, and he is not concerned with questions about driving. Problems have arisen nevertheless, since, in London, justices have been asking police doctors to say in addition whether or not they thought the accused was fit to drive; and, if the delay was substantial and the driver had sobered, the doctor had to say so and the result was usually an acquittal.

The difficulties of proving the charge do not, however, end there, for it has often been suggested that offenders escape conviction by being taken to hospital after accidents, thus being spared police inspection. A survey (*Daily Mail*, 21 December 1961) was carried out at Withington Hospital, Manchester, in which it was alleged that more than half the drivers taken in between midnight and 6 a.m. after road accidents had in their blood at least the maximum level of alcohol considered by the British Medical Association to be safe for driving. Indeed there is support for this allegation in this research: in one case of causing death by dangerous driving the offender, complaining of concussion, was taken to hospital with his victims before the police arrived. There was half a bottle of gin in his car, and the offender had been seen shortly before the incident to be driving with one hand and holding his head with the other. This is circumstantial evidence, but the impression was that drink played a greater part in the incident than it did in the court hearing.

It is not surprising that such difficulties should provide some of the best examples of 'perversity' among juries. One example was in *Dryden* v. *Johnson* ([1961] *Crim. L.R.* 551), in which the divisional court allowed the prosecutor's appeal against the justices' dismissal of a charge of driving while under the influence of drink. The defendant was seen by a police officer driving into a car park at ten minutes after midnight, and was said to have been unsteady on his feet and smelling of drink. Examined by a police surgeon thirty-five minutes later, he was said to have been unable to speak coherently, he wrote illegibly, and he could neither walk straight nor put on his shoes and socks while seated. A urine test showed that he had consumed at least five pints of beer, but the justices acquitted on the ground that the suspicious condition of the accused at the police station was not sufficient evidence that he was drunk thirty-five minutes earlier. In commenting on judgement, Mr Justice Salmon said that the argument on the accused's behalf would not have deceived an ordinarily intelligent child of twelve, let alone a bench of magistrates. The argument on the accused's behalf was not reported.

A further problem arises in that a driver's ability to drive can be impaired by other influences besides alcohol: he may have an excitable temperament or be in a neurotic state, or he may have taken drugs.

So far, driving under the influence of drugs has not been mentioned specifically since the elements needed to constitute the offence are the same as when the agent is drink. This is obvious when the drug has been taken for 'kicks', but the similarity may not be so clear when the offender has taken a medicament to alleviate a condition like hay fever, not realizing that his physical condition might predispose him to drowsiness from the drug. It may seem hard that such a driver is liable to prosecution, but the fact that he is liable illustrates the particular characteristic of this and some other driving offences: they are absolute prohibitions against certain behaviour that is held to be dangerous in itself, regardless of the actor's motives or intention. In cases where the action of the accused seemed to be entirely innocent and justifiable it would be open to the police either not to prosecute at all or to do so under some other offence, but otherwise it is unlikely that the driver's sickness or need for a medicament would prevent conviction.

Driving under the influence is one of the offences for which disqualification is an almost certain penalty, and indeed it is mandatory on the court to order at least twelve months' disqualification unless there are some special circumstances connected with the offence or with the offender. Hence there is here a move towards setting a minimum sentence (of some consequence, since a year's disqualification can be a serious matter for offenders who drive as part of their job) for a first offence. This puts it in a particularly serious category together with that of driving while disqualified, a rather different offence which will now be discussed.

Driving while Disqualified

This offence was first established in the Road Traffic Act, 1930, and it was preserved intact in the Act of 1960, which made it an offence to apply for, or to obtain, a licence to drive, or to drive a motor vehicle on a road if, at the time of so doing, the applicant was disqualified from driving. The penalty prescribed by the 1930 Act was imprisonment, unless the court found special reasons for imposing a fine only, and the 1962 Act made further disqualification mandatory.

It is another offence in which there is an absolute prohibition, and it would seem that no deliberate intention need be established since there is nothing in the section, such as the term 'knowingly', requiring foreknowledge that an offence is being committed. This illustrates another legal

96

peculiarity of motoring offences in that intention is not considered to be relevant to the offence, though it must be present; otherwise it would be virtually impossible to commit the offence at all. For this is, typically, a deliberate offence, as Lord Cecil pointed out in the debate leading to the 1930 Act, when he called it 'a very serious offence . . . that must be a deliberate attempt to evade the law' (*Hansard, Lords,* 22 January 1930).

It is also unique among motoring offences in that it is the only one in which the court has little or no option as to sentence for a first offence: the offender must go to prison unless there are special circumstances attached to the offence or to the offender. This may seem severe, but it derives from the rather special nature of the offence; that is to say, the offender not only breaks a clear prohibition by law, he also defies the court, despite a warning – which is always given – that such defiance must be punished by imprisonment. The offender then goes further, and beyond the point where there is a breach of the law, in that he endangers the public by exposing its members to the risk of injury by a person who may not be able to offer any compensation. For all British insurance policies exclude drivers from cover if they do not hold a current driving licence, which a disqualified driver does not. So there must be in these cases an associated and additional offence of driving while uninsured, though it does not appear to be the practice to charge it.

The nature and the implications of this offence are shown particularly well in *Lines* v. *Hersom* ([1951] 2 All E.R. 650), in which the defendant had been fined £5 and disqualified for twelve months for driving while uninsured some four months before being seen by the police to be driving his van. He was stopped, and at first gave a false name and address; later he admitted his identity, saying that he had been working so late that he had missed his last train and had to drive to get home. In mitigation he pleaded that he was a disabled ex-serviceman whose health and business depended on his being able to drive; but, despite an exemplary service record, he was imprisoned for one month and disqualified again. On appeal to quarter sessions it was held that his circumstances did constitute 'special circumstances' within the meaning of the statute, and fines totalling £30 were substituted for the imprisonment. However, the prosecution appealed, and the case was finally decided in their favour; giving judgement, Lord Goddard said that this was not a case where the defendant's circumstances could properly be taken into account, and that was not Parliament's intention: 'For this very serious offence a motorist should go to prison. It is about as serious an offence as he can commit: to set his disqualification at defiance and drive at a time when, if he cannot pay, nobody would get any compensation for injury received in an accident with which he may meet because no insurance company would be liable.'[1]

Even when the special circumstances are considered relevant, they have to be very strong to justify a sentence other than imprisonment. An example of a successful plea on these grounds is *R. v. Phillips* ([1955] 119 J.P. 499), when the defendant drove his car to get a doctor in the emergency of his wife's sudden illness; here the accused was not sent to prison.

In passing, it should be noted that disqualification is not a sentence as such: if it were it would be illegal to impose it with another penalty, e.g. a fine, for a single offence. It appears to be an order of the same kind as is made to endorse a driving licence or to require payments under a maintenance order (*R. v. Appeals Committee of Surrey Quarter Sessions* [1963] 1 Q.B. 990).

Now let us consider another offence where the issues are rather less complex.

Failing to Insure against Third-party Risks

This is another offence that originated in the proceedings of the Royal Commission on Transport, 1929, and appeared first in the Act of 1930. Since then it has become one of the most frequent of all motoring offences although it carries such potentially serious consequences for the victim when an incident occurs.

The offence is one of absolute prohibition, in which intention or foreknowledge is irrelevant; it is punished by either fine or imprisonment and, under the 1930 Act, it was mandatory to disqualify for twelve months unless there were special reasons connected with the offence. In the 1956 Act the offence was not altered in substance, but courts were no longer required to disqualify as they had been formerly. Before that the attitude to the offence was more severe, and in 1950 the courts were enjoined not to give conditional or absolute discharges in these cases where the offence appeared to be deliberate (*Taylor* v. *Saycell* [1950] 2 All E.R. 887).

In these offences it is, therefore, important to distinguish between the deliberate offence and the accidental offence, though both are inexcusable in law. Indeed a good many insurance offences are committed because of ignorance or because of inadvertence, but the main purpose of the law here is to protect the public and so to accept no excuse for using a vehicle on the road if there is no insurer to indemnify anyone injured by it.

---

[1] In 1955 the law was that the special circumstances had to be attached to the offence and not the offender; this was changed in 1962 to include both offence and offender.

Not much need be said about this offence; it is very specific and straightforward. It does not, therefore, make many demands on justices for its interpretation, and to that extent is very different from the last offence which it is necessary to discuss – failing to stop after, or to report, an accident.

Failing to Stop after, or to Report, an Accident

At the beginning of this lay analysis of the motoring law there was a discussion of one of the oldest motoring offences in the statutes, dangerous driving, and it may be that some confusion in its interpretation was exposed. We now come to another offence whose lineage is equally distinguished and whose interpretation has a parallel with dangerous driving in that it is not as simple as it looks.

Section 77 of the Road Traffic Act, 1960, repeats almost word-for-word a section of the 1930 Act, and of the Act of 1903 before, in that it reads:

'(1) If in any case, owing to the presence of a motor vehicle on the road, an accident occurs whereby personal injury is caused to a person other than the driver of that motor vehicle, or damage is done to a vehicle other than that motor vehicle or to a trailer drawn thereby, or to an animal other than an animal in or on that vehicle or a trailer drawn thereby, the driver of the motor vehicle shall stop and, if required so to do by any person having reasonable grounds for so requiring, give his name and address, and also the name and address of the owner and the identification marks of the vehicle.

'(2) If in the case of any such accident as aforesaid, the driver of the motor vehicle for any reason does not give his name and address . . . he shall report the accident at a police station, or to a police constable as soon as reasonably practicable, and in any case within twenty-four hours of the occurrence thereof'

. . . or an offence is committed, and the offender becomes liable to a fine for the first offence, and to a fine or imprisonment for a second and subsequent offence.

Although the wording of this offence differs little from the Motor Car Act, 1903, section 6, there is one significant omission: the 1903 Act specified that the driver must have acted *knowingly*. It thus emphasized the element of intention which was apparently essential to the offence; hence the burden was on the prosecution to show that the act was done knowingly. In 1930 when the expression 'knowingly' was omitted, the apparent purpose was to bring this offence into line with other motoring offences and make it an absolute prohibition in which guilty knowledge was irrelevant. But, as Lord Goddard said in *Harding* v. *Price* ([1948] 1 All E.R. 283), it can be a defence to show that a driver was unaware of an accident, and nobody could be expected to stop and to report something of which he knew nothing. In Lord Goddard's opinion the word 'knowingly' was omitted in 1930 to shift the burden of proof from the prosecution to the defence, upon whom it would now be incumbent to show that the accused knew nothing of the incident; hence some degree of deliberate intention is still implicit in this offence.

This ruling seems at first to be unexceptionable and common sense, but an academically analytical approach to the motoring law leaves some doubt as to whether this is so. For, if it is true that a driver cannot commit the offence if he was unaware of the incident upon which it is founded, is it not a defence to a charge of failing to stop at a traffic signal or Halt sign to say that one did not see it and hence did not know of it? Yet, in *Hill* v. *Baxter* ([1958] 1 All E.R. 193), Lord Goddard made it quite clear that such a defence was no answer to a charge where there was an absolute prohibition, and deliberate intention was not essential.

It would seem that it was the inclusion of 'knowingly' in section 6 of the 1903 Act that made this an especially heinous offence, and indeed it was so regarded, if the parliamentary debates and press correspondence of the time are any indication of public attitudes. In those days this offence was inserted to deal with the hit-and-run driver who, when number plates were not carried, sought to escape from the scene undetected and was often successful in so doing. But in the 1903 Act the really serious charges were brought under the section dealing with reckless or negligent driving, and the maximum penalties under section 6 were a fine of £10 for a first offence and either a fine of £20 or one month's imprisonment for a second or subsequent offence (with power to suspend the licence for a second or subsequent offence). The Act of 1930 increased the penalties but deleted the power to disqualify, so the trend seems to have been away from heinousness towards the quasi-criminal, as Mr Justice Humphreys called it in *Harding* v. *Price* (*supra*); but he did add that some justices thought it to be a 'public evil'.

It is probable that some change in attitude to this offence has been induced by the increasing number of vehicles on the roads and the tendency for them to hit each other rather than persons; indeed, the evidence presented later in this study suggests that the most common instances of the

offence are when a driver collides with another vehicle and drives on without stopping or reporting the matter. Another thing that may have softened
the impact of this offence is the advent of compulsory insurance, since some
offenders interviewed in this research thought, quite wrongly, that the
injured party had only to claim on his insurance company in order to have
the damage to his vehicle repaired, and so he did not suffer enough hardship to justify the offender's stopping and embroiling himself in counter-
claims and possible unpleasantness. The offender who thinks like this
omits to consider the victim's no-claim bonus, which he may lose unless he
can avoid blame; the victim may also have to bear a proportion of any claim
himself.

As it now stands, this is not an easy offence to prove, even though the
onus is on the accused to show that he was unaware of the incident; denial
is usual in these cases and there is often enough doubt for the defendant to
get the better of it. This was evident in *Butler* v. *Whittaker (Crim. L.R.*
[1955] 317). The accused's vehicle had collided with a cow and he had
driven on in the belief, so he claimed, that he had not caused any injury to
the animal although he admitted that he had heard a 'slight knock'. Later
the animal's leg swelled and the veterinary surgeon found a severe injury.
In the magistrates' court the defendant was convicted; he appealed to
quarter sessions, where his appeal was upheld on the ground that the
prosecution 'had to show that the defendant knew that there had been an
accident' (a direct contradiction of Lord Goddard's view in *Harding* v.
Price, supra) and 'that he knew, or in the circumstances a reasonable man
would have known, that an injury had been caused to the cow'. Perhaps it
is significant that the court refused the appellant's application for costs
because 'whatever might be his legal duty, a prudent driver [the reasonable
man?] would have stopped to assure himself that no injury had been
caused'. So here again we find deliberate intention accompanied by the
fictional 'reasonable man' of whom it is difficult enough to conceive in the
normal course of events; to put him into a motor vehicle does not make
matters easier.

Such are some of the problems of interpretation of the law relating to the
six motoring offences with which this study is mostly concerned.

The historical preamble shows very clearly a number of factors that
have contributed to produce this profusion of difficulties. In the last sixty
years the law has been under almost continual pressure from technological

influences, and from a public of increasing size who are irritated by constraint. Also it is possible that the law is not respected as it should be because it is not understood and it is not consistent. Moreover, it has been the result of continued compromise between two bitterly opposed factions: those who are against the motorist and will do all they can to constrain him, and those who oppose constraints unless they are relatively minor in their effects. Examples of both sides are, respectively, the Pedestrians' Association and the Automobile Association.

The survey shows also that the motoring law in 1903 and 1930 was framed by legislators who knew little of the motor vehicle. Some were drivers, but few had the expertise of Earl Howe, who, when he demanded driving tests and a speed limit in built-up areas, was dismissed as a Cassandra by the government spokesman, Lord Russell (*Hansard, Lords,* 4 February 1930). But Lord Russell seemed to be less ignorant about the technicalities of motoring than his predecessor, Lord Balfour, who piloted the 1903 Bill through the Lords, and while doing so said that it was impossible to attempt any interference by regulation with the character and construction of a motor car (*The Times,* 22 July 1903). Of the anti-motoring group in the House of Lords, Lord Cecil was prominent; yet he admitted in 1927 that he had never owned or driven a motor car, although he devised a very restrictive Bill and pushed it to a second reading in that same year.

The overall result has been a law that is almost incredibly vague and difficult both to interpret and to administer. It is therefore hardly surprising that judges, magistrates, and juries have found it virtually impossible to avoid decisions that have seemed to be perverse to victims, defendants, and public alike. The difficulties may have encouraged a tendency to increase the number of motoring offences that are held to be absolute prohibitions, since this device seems to make it easier to reach a definite conclusion; it cuts down time-consuming argument, and reduces the likelihood of offenders' escaping conviction by means of verbal skill; but, on the other hand, the absolute prohibition is bound to induce antagonism towards the law on the part of those who feel that they have good reasons for their actions. When a defendant thinks he is innocent, and his story is dismissed as irrelevant because the act is forbidden, a sense of injustice is bound to remain.

The confusion inherent in the law is probably felt most of all by the unfortunate juries in motoring cases, and their inability to grasp the subtleties of the law concerning homicide and dangerous driving is both evident and understandable. As Wootton (1957, p. 147), an experienced magistrate, has said, 'it can be extraordinarily difficult to disentangle the true facts' in motoring cases, in which so much evidence is given from a fleeting impression during a time of some excitement. The numerous cases that were heard in court in the course of this research lent much substance to Wootton's remarks: the evidence was often most bewildering, and when this was so, the defendant usually got the benefit of the doubt.

Hence it is easy to sympathize with the view expressed by 'A Barrister' in the *Observer* (25 February 1962), that juries do not constitute an effective means of deciding guilt when the issues are in the least complex. As he puts it: 'Juries are nowadays far too ready to acquit a guilty man: this is particularly so in cases where, such as in driving offences, they are prone to utter "there but for the grace of God go I", and acquit.' So it may be that the motoring offender would get a stricter but perhaps fairer deal before experienced magistrates, or before a judge with a specialized knowledge of motoring, than before an awed, confused, and insecure jury.

But whatever be the fate of juries in motoring cases – and it might be thought that it would have been sealed long ago by the scathing comments of such eminent judges as Lords Goddard and Atkin – it would seem that the law relating to the serious offences with which this research is concerned should be thoroughly renovated. However, it is not enough to say this without making some positive suggestions for renovation, though the task is undertaken here with some trepidation because this is a sphere of knowledge that can easily be misunderstood by people who have not had a formal legal training.

First, it seems desirable to limit absolute prohibitions to offences for which defendants can offer little or no excuse, such as parking and speed-limit offences. If it were practicable it would be as well if absolute prohibitions were the exception rather than the rule among motoring offences: such a situation would present problems owing to the volume of work, which might swamp the courts, but any other system risks antagonizing the very individuals whose cooperation is essential – the drivers or riders of motor vehicles.

Second, it is clear that much confusion arises from the existence of so many categories of unlawful driving, e.g. reckless, dangerous, and careless; and the confusion is increased when someone is killed. So it is suggested that there should be no distinct offence of dangerous driving, but two separate offences: reckless driving (which must be advertent), and careless or incompetent driving (which is inadvertent). If the driving is reckless and someone dies because of it, the charge should be manslaughter, since any alternative would serve only to confuse the issue. If someone dies in an incident caused by careless or incompetent driving, then careless driving ought to be the charge, since the inadvertence presupposes that the driver did not foresee the probability that anyone might be injured; as Kenny (1962, p. 25) has put it, inadvertence means a total lack of foresight, so there can be no degrees of inadvertence or degrees of heinousness. Moreover, Lord Devlin has made a similar distinction between 'wicked' and 'bad' driving, and he considers that it is pointless to distinguish between dangerous and careless driving since all careless driving must be dangerous also (address to the Magistrates' Association, *The Times*, 21 October 1960).

An alternative solution is to revert to the position in 1903 and have only one offence of dangerous driving with a high maximum penalty; then all degrees of dangerous driving could be dealt with according to their deserts. If death resulted, the offence could still be charged under the dangerous driving section, which would have a range of penalties to allow for its punishment. But this alternative would clearly be undesirable in practice since such a wide variety of behaviour would be included under a single offence that sentencing would seem to be highly inconsistent and variable. Moreover, previous offences read out in court when an offender appeared for a subsequent offence would have to be assessed solely by the penalties inflicted: a procedure that would be manifestly unjust.

Whichever solution is preferred, it is submitted that the law should not in any circumstances be distorted to make it acceptable to juries. Indeed this would be a strange course to take since it is to put means before ends, and the maintenance of a just and protective law is surely the end desired.

If judgements involving dangerous driving are often too complex for juries, then questions concerning impairment to drive through the influence of drink or drugs must be even more overwhelming. For, if this is a matter of opinion, the opportunities for inconsistency are unlimited whether the assessment is made by justices or by juries. It seems inescapable that an objective test based on a maximum permissible amount of alcohol in the blood is the only sound answer; the urine test and the breathalyzer are already available for such a purpose. If the permitted level were set so that it was appropriate for an individual with a 'weak head' for alcohol, the heavier drinker who 'can take it' might suffer; but what would he suffer in fact? Only the curtailment – in the public interest – of a little personal pleasure, by restricting alcohol consumption to, say, two pints of beer before driving. Surely this would be worth while in order to save lives.

Apropos of driving while disqualified, there is not much that could or need be done to the law as it is. But this is not true of the other relatively straightforward offence, driving without insurance. Here the law should be modified so as to exempt from liability the motor cyclist who pushes his machine on the road. For it is now an offence for someone to push an uninsured or unlicensed motor cycle from his house to a garage for repair, although the owner may not have any intention whatsoever of riding it; to proceed for failure to insure under such conditions – which does happen – does nothing to enhance the prestige of the law. On the contrary, it makes it look silly.

Finally, there is failing to stop after, or to report, an accident. In these cases it has been shown that the main duty of the law is to ensure the protection of others and their property; hence it is attractive to suggest that this should become an offence of absolute prohibition. If recklessness were evident it would always be possible to charge reckless driving instead of, or in addition to, failing to stop, etc. The key element in the offence is, it would seem, the decision whether or not to stop after the impact, and it does not appear unreasonable to allow the law to assume that a driver must know – if he has the 'feel' of his vehicle that is necessary for proper control – that he has hit, or has been hit by, something; then it would be his duty to stop and investigate. The matter of reporting is a consequence of stopping, and must depend on it.

It would be misleading to give the impression that all these difficulties in interpretation begin in the courts. In fact they become acute long before the hearing, when the crucial question is being decided as to whether to prosecute, and if so, for what.

It is, after all, the police who decide in most cases except homicide whether there will be a charge – and hence an offence – and of what kind it will be. Moreover it has been shown that the law allows them much latitude in making these decisions. So it seems to be almost beyond dispute that the attitude of the police to the motoring offender is a major factor in determining the social attitude to motoring offences. In other words, it is the way in which the police categorize motoring behaviour that is so important: if they charge behaviour that is relatively trivial under a serious offence they inevitably undermine the seriousness with which the public regard that offence and so reduce its deterrent power. Conversely, if they charge serious misbehaviour under an offence that is regarded as only quasi-criminal, they may undermine any social sanctions that exist against such misbehaviour. Of course this applies to offences of all kinds, but it affects motoring offences in particular, because they touch so many citizens so closely.

In the next chapter, therefore, there will be an examination of police methods in dealing with motoring offenders and offences, and an attempt to indicate some of the attitudes of police officers towards them.

4

The Police and the Motorist

ATTITUDES DEVELOP

Few inventions can have influenced relations between the police and the public more than that of the internal combustion engine. The image of the policeman has changed from that of a friend and protector of all but a small criminal minority, to that of a regulator and supervisor who is in close contact with all who use the roads, whether as drivers, passengers, or pedestrians; and in this role he has to enforce a law that is not regarded with much respect or sympathy by a substantial number of those whom it affects.

As the preceding chapter indicated, the relationship between police and motorist did not make a very good start, and this was no fault of the police. Their first task in 1905 was to enforce the 20 mph speed limit: a measure which the police did not like, and which was wished on them by a legislature singularly ignorant about motoring. Moreover it was a law that could be enforced in only one way: by the so-called 'speed trap' in which police officers were concealed at each end of a measured distance to time unsuspecting drivers.

It was to deal with these police traps that a band of enthusiastic motorists organized cyclist patrols to warn drivers of their presence, and these 'scouts', as they were called, were first employed on the London–Brighton road in 1905, with considerable success from the motorist's standpoint. The scouts and their sponsors were the forerunners of the Automobile Association, which soon became the powerful watchdog of the motorist's interests. Hence it could be said that our most powerful motoring organization owes its origin to a conflict with the police, though it is questionable whether the AA is particularly proud of the fact.

However, as more and more of the public became users of motor vehicles, they came to see the police in this light: as there to harass and prosecute, rather than to help and protect. And the impression was emphasized by the rapid growth of minor offences dealing with parking and obstruction until it seemed that the law was fast outpacing public conceptions of morality. Noting this, the chief constable of Huntingdonshire and Ely has pointed out that the effect was for both the law and the police to lose the respect and support of the public; he suggests that it is not surprising that offenders should feel public opinion to be on their side rather than on that of law and order, so loosening the constraints on unlawful behaviour of all kinds (Williams, C., 1961, p. 362). Some support for this view was given by an offender interviewed during this research, who said that his conviction for dangerous driving had turned out to be 'like joining a sort of club whose members discuss their offences with each other as people talk about their business deals'.

Although it is not uncommon to find agreement with a comment in the *Police Review* (24 June 1960) that the police (according to the public) spend so much time 'harrying motorists that they neglect their primary duty of preventing crime', relations between the police and the road user should not be regarded too pessimistically. In their *Memorandum to the Royal Commission on the Police* (AA & RAC Standing Joint Committee, 1960) the motoring organizations said that 'when account is taken of the exceedingly large number of occasions on which the police approach motorists in circumstances which can hardly be expected to secure an enthusiastic welcome, the number of serious complaints made to the motoring organizations against the conduct of individual police officers may be considered to be extremely small'. According to this *Memorandum*, most criticism is of the failure of police authorities to define a clear policy for enforcing the law, and of a lack of uniformity among police forces in this respect. But the traditional criticism is not absent: the *Memorandum* contains the inevitable suggestion that certain officers are more interested in getting convictions than in giving guidance, and there is marked concern about the practice of 'plain-clothes officers patrolling in cars which are not identifiable as police cars. . . . There is a marked distaste for this kind of activity, particularly when it results in prosecutions for minor offences.'

It may be inferred from this comment that the use of police cars in disguise is unfair in rather the same way as the earlier practice of concealing police traps. And indeed the use of these plain-clothes patrols is controversial among the police; but it does seem that a greater deterrent is needed than the appearance of a clearly marked police car to inhibit the behaviour of some drivers, if the experience of the present Minister of Transport, Mr Marples, is any indication of what really goes on. Speaking in the Commons he described motorists' reactions to his driving in the fast lane of Western Avenue out of London at the stipulated maximum of 40 mph. He said that he was passed repeatedly on the nearside; 'they flashed their lights at me, and they hooted their horns at me', thus earning a headline above the report of the speech 'They All Hoot Marples' (*Daily*

Mail, 1 March 1962). But Mr Marples's claims fall far short of those made by a barrister who noted how often he was overtaken during a sixty-day period in speed-restricted areas: in the 40 mph limit he was overtaken by more than 4,000 vehicles of all types, including two tricycles; and in the 30 mph limit by 3,700 vehicles, including three invalid chairs and one hearse. According to this motorist, his law-abiding driving brought forth a mixture of uncomplimentary names, advice to 'put your L plates up', 'V' signs, and so on (*Daily Mail*, 14 June 1961).

Such experiences would suggest that plain-clothes patrols would have a salutary effect on road discipline. But substantial correspondence on the subject in *The Times* shows that there are counter-arguments. For example, drivers might not think it safe to stop when signalled to do so by a plain-clothes patrol since bandits could easily adopt this as a ruse. It has also been said that the use of disguise would have an adverse effect on relations between the police and the motoring public because 'detectives are not generally operating against a whole sector of the community but against some particular wrongdoer, and the fate of such offenders does not have the same air of being something of a lottery where punishment is concerned as it does in the case of motorists' (see leading article, *The Times*, 5 May 1960, and correspondence on the subject in preceding issues).

It is rather hard to follow the logic of an argument suggesting that the police are being unethical in operating out of uniform unless seeking a particular quarry. For it would follow that it would be improper to use plain-clothes officers for duties involving protection or surveillance; yet this is frequently done without any outcry that policemen are being used as *agents provocateurs*. Indeed one suspects that no objections would be raised if the objects of attention were other than motorists.

This attitude towards the use of plain-clothes traffic patrols seems to be based on the same attitudes that were so evident in objections to the early speed traps, and perhaps also to the use of mechanical devices to check speed, noise, and blood-alcohol: that these, and any other methods, are justified when they are used to catch 'criminals', but motoring offenders – it is implied – are not 'criminals': they are in a category of their own.

The currency of this view in official and lay circles is particularly well illustrated by the 'courtesy cop' scheme, instituted in 1938 at the instigation of the Minister of Transport with the aim of educating rather than prosecuting the 'errant' motorist. Under the scheme prosecution was the last means to be employed; it was the ultimate force, to be used only when advice and admonition had failed. But this concept seems to demand a tolerance for those who break the motoring law that is in direct conflict with the will of the legislature, as expressed in the practice of making most of these offences absolute prohibitions. And it could be said, as it seems to be said of non-motoring offences, that the law is quite clear about what may or may not be done, and it is the business of the licence holder to know it. This is defensible in regard to 'moving' offences, but it would not be so if it were applied to the much more complicated and controversial offences of obstruction. A law, or manner of enforcement, which does not take human frailties into account is unlikely to be respected, so it would seem sound to rely mostly on preventive methods before having recourse to prosecution. However it does seem odd that such arguments are rarely put forward for non-motoring offenders.

A further confirmation that the police regard motoring offenders as in a category of their own emerged from interviews with some seventy police officers of nearly all ranks during this research. In discussion, considerable interest in the study was shown because officers thought that it was time to find out as much as possible about serious motoring offenders; whatever seemed to promise more knowledge, and hence more success, in tackling this ever-growing problem they were ready to support. But it was soon clear that, with one exception (a superintendent who had been a traffic officer for a long time), they could not see how motoring offenders could be of any interest to criminologists.

This attitude is implicit in police policy in motoring cases with regard to the production of evidence as to previous convictions: non-motoring offences are not revealed since they are regarded as irrelevant. This practice was accepted without question by the officers interviewed; but three senior officers thought that it would not be improper to produce non-motoring convictions if it were a bad case in which the offender deserved more of a lesson than he might get if only his motoring convictions were given. Some officers thought that they would be rebuked from the bench if they produced evidence of non-motoring convictions ('crime', as they called it), and the practice of not doing so appears to be universally accepted. But whence the convention came could not be discovered in the literature. It is, however, a subject of controversy from time to time among magistrates, as shown in a recent instance in which a defendant pleaded guilty to certain motoring offences and the bench was told that there were no previous convictions; moderate fines were, therefore, imposed. But the bench was informed, *after* the hearing, that the defendant had a thoroughly bad record of non-motoring offences. Another instance concerned a defendant found guilty of a serious motoring offence, upon whom the justices decided at first to impose a heavy fine but, after reconsideration, they substituted a more moderate fine with a period of disqualification. On hearing the decision the defendant informed us 'somewhat gleefully that only a few days previously he had been disqualified for a similar period by another court, so the sentence of disqualification was stultified and the fine was much smaller than would otherwise have been imposed'. In this case the police did not give out the defendant's full record, and withheld the details of a motoring conviction because it had occurred after the offence with which this particular bench was concerned. In a comment on these cases the editors of *The Magistrate* remarked that 'we believe it is usual for the police, in motoring cases, to give previous convictions for motoring offences only' (*The Magistrate*, May 1961, p. 68, citing these examples with commentary).

Two typical attitudes are illustrated here: first, that motoring offences and crime are different, and second that the police try to be almost abnormally fair in serious motoring cases.

The following comment, made by a senior police officer to the governor of a prison when writing about an offender, is cited to lend weight to the first attitude: 'He is a bad character, with four motoring offences and four of crime recorded against him.' Broadly speaking, the police definition of the terms crime and criminal seems to be bounded by the area of responsibility of the Criminal Investigation Department (CID); but the question 'What is crime?' caused a good deal of perplexity, especially among junior ranks, and particularly when coupled with the question 'What is a criminal?'. As the CID did not appear to be interested in motoring offences unless a stolen vehicle was involved, or there had been a hit-and-run killing, it was not usual to think of motoring offences as crimes, and that was that.

The second attitude – that the police are extremely scrupulous in their fairness in serious motoring cases – is one that will not, perhaps, be attributed to the police by many motorists, whether they have been offenders or not. Especially would it be contested by those who believe strongly that the police officer gets promotion if he is active in making charges and getting convictions – a view that is widespread, as suggested above.

THE POLICE POINT OF VIEW

It would be naïve to suppose that the police are not sometimes at fault, but there is some difficulty in disposing of the reply given by a chief constable to the suggestion that convictions and promotion go together. He pointed to the opportunities that exist on the roads now for any police officer to initiate proceedings if he wanted to, particularly where speeding and parking are concerned. If he did so it is unlikely that the zealot would find himself popular with any of his superiors who have to process the quantity of paper that is involved in each report: the amount of work is considerable and it is doubtful if officers would undertake it unnecessarily. Nor would such excessive zeal be looked on with favour by the courts which are already overloaded with motoring offences.

It is in fact the policy in the District under study that charges should not be preferred for carping or trivial reasons, and officers concerned with traffic are instructed that the friendly warning with some constructive advice is to be given where possible. And on mobile patrols that the writer accompanied, this policy was put into practice; there was certainly no over-readiness to say 'you will be reported' despite the unfriendly response of some of the people who were stopped. On the other hand, there was a tendency to stop young men of 'teddy-boy' aspect when riding motor cycles or driving old cars, to check that they had insurance or a driving licence; this was based on what the police called 'a good copper's sixth sense that something might be wrong', and they were often correct. But, to the offenders, this is 'picking on the working class', and any other explanation is a euphemism.

From the police point of view it is not quite as easy to catch and prosecute the serious motoring offender as is generally supposed. This is so even of the seemingly cut-and-dried offences, like driving uninsured or while disqualified; for in order to find such offenders it is necessary to stop drivers on suspicion, unless they are involved in accidents, and the police do not like doing this because of the detrimental effect on their relations with the public when a mistake is made. Contrary to the writer's previous opinions it was found that the institution of the 'routine check' was disliked by many senior officers because it was thought to be an unwarranted interference with the liberty of the subject; it was felt that it was justified only as a somewhat random means of catching criminals who were using vehicles for criminal purposes, and of deterring them from doing so.

Apart from routine checks, the police have to rely on reports from the public or on what they happen to see, unless there is an accident. And even when there is an accident it is not easy to get the necessary evidence to proceed, unless there are good witnesses who are prepared to come forward. Moreover, the investigation of cases is often quite difficult, especially on a crowded main road on a hot day, with vehicles queueing up waiting to get by; and it is no easier to take measurements and statements when it is pouring with rain, or dark and cold. Even if witnesses are prepared to come forward – and it seems that fewer are because of the time they would have to spend in attending court and because of the discomfiture of cross-examination – their memory of what happened is apt to be distorted by the excitement of the moment and the very suddenness of the incident.

If the 653 cases that have been studied in this research are an indication, then it would seem that about 60 per cent of prosecutions alleging serious offences derive from 'accidents'; of the remainder (excluding the un-insured and the disqualified), some 20 per cent were reported by members of the public, and the rest were seen by police officers. Clearly the difficulties are much greater where no accident has occurred, and this is so especially of dangerous driving and, to a lesser extent, of drunken driving also. Even when the public report a case it is hard to intercept the offender and get enough evidence to convict: an example is a case in which the residents of a suburban road in a built-up area had complained to the police about a motor cyclist who drove daily down their road about 8 a.m. at very high speeds with considerable noise. To catch him it was necessary to post one of the all too few motor cyclist officers, who had to lie in wait; after two days of waiting the offender appeared, and when chased was found to be travelling at 75 mph. He was very aggressive and uncooperative with the police, and maintained throughout that he was 'only doing thirty'. When considering whether to prosecute, the superintendent noted that 'our difficulty, as always, will be to show the danger when in fact nobody appears to have been inconvenienced'. However, there was a conviction for dangerous driving (fined £35), and for speeding (fined £5); but it is possible that this offender might have avoided conviction altogether had the decision in *Tribe* v. *Jones* been known, in which it was held that speeds of 65 mph were not necessarily dangerous in themselves in the absence of other dangerous circumstances (*The Magistrate*, January 1962, p. 7).

Another example is that of an offender who was seen by a patrol to drive across a zebra pedestrian crossing while a woman was walking over it, and she had to halt to avoid being hit. When stopped the defendant refused to give either his name or address, and said that it was a pity that the 'police had not something better to do' and that they should 'mind their own bloody business'. He offered to meet the observer of the police car off-duty at any time, and was alleged to have said 'I'll show you'. Egged on by a woman passenger, he kept repeating to the police that they were 'country yokels with nothing better to do'. He had no road fund licence, for which he was fined £2, and for the pedestrian crossing offence he was fined £3 – with 28 days to pay! Though no such comment escaped the police, it is doubtful whether all the unpleasantness involved in this case was recompensed by so trivial a fine, and the police may well ask sometimes: 'Is it worth it?'

Further illustration of the difficulty involved in getting sufficient evidence to prosecute for dangerous driving is provided by the following case. On a Saturday afternoon in August the attention of two bystanders was attracted by a 600 cc motor cycle travelling at 'great speed' towards a notorious bend (a well-known black spot for accidents); unable to round the bend on his correct side of the road the rider veered across the double white lines and collided with an approaching scooter, injuring the scooterist's pillion passenger. On reaching the spot the police took statements to the effect that the motor cyclist was travelling at a speed of 'at least 65 mph'; also his speedometer was jammed at 45: a speed that would be too great to round such a bend safely. On the spot the defendant admitted responsibility before the scooterist and the two witnesses, but before the magistrates he pleaded not guilty and elected for trial by jury at quarter sessions, where he was acquitted. Then the police proceeded again on a charge of careless driving and secured a conviction before the magistrates, who fined the offender £15.

But, if it is difficult to bring dangerous drivers to court, it is even harder to do so in the case of drunken ones, whose capacity to escape conviction is remarkable, especially before juries. A good example is of a woman driver whose case was examined during this research. She was stopped for a routine check at a road block on a trunk road shortly after midnight, and it was alleged that she was incoherent, that her breath smelled of alcohol, and that she staggered visibly on getting out of her car; also it was said that she was most 'awkward' and uncooperative. In evidence she admitted that she had been at a bar from 6.30 p.m. until midnight, and had had at least nine gins. But she told the jury that she had driven for twenty-one years and knew when she was fit to drive; she thought herself quite fit then, but had the misfortune to stumble in her high heels when she got out of her car and the police drew the most convenient conclusion. Also it was submitted on her behalf that there had been no accident, nor was there evidence of dangerous driving. She was acquitted, but her case is typical of at least a dozen cases in which the accused 'got off' although there was clear evidence of a considerable consumption of drink.

An indication has been given in the preceding chapter of the difficulty in proving to the satisfaction of the court that the accused was too drunk when arrested to have proper control of his vehicle (see pp. 93–5 above). It seems that the dice remain loaded against the police, as illustrated by a recent case before the London sessions. In this instance the defendant was certified by the police doctor to be free from any illness that could have caused his behaviour. The evidence was given in writing, but the defence called the witness in person and asked him directly whether, in his opinion, the defendant was fit to drive. The reply was that the police had not asked for an opinion of this kind, but only one as to health; however, at the time of examination, the accused did not seem unfit to drive. The chairman then asked the jury if they wished to hear any more, and said 'he (the doctor) was not called by the police, and now he says that the man was fit to drive. Now we have the full facts, which we did not have before.' The jury acquitted, and the chairman concurred with the verdict.

The case provoked a leading article in *The Times* (12 March 1962) to call the practice of limiting medical evidence to health 'a bad rule', and it stressed that 'it is patently essential in these cases that there should be medical evidence. It is the most important evidence of all, and to exclude it merely on the grounds that the doctor is on the spot only as soon as he can be is absurd.'

On the other hand, there was strong support for the police, notably from magistrates, and it does seem a pity that a perfectly reasonable procedure was so misunderstood as to imply that the police deliberately misled the court by not calling medical evidence on the question of sobriety. On the contrary, it would be misleading the court to produce evidence as to fitness by someone who had not seen the accused within a reasonable time of the initial arrest; it could also be thought irrelevant to do so. This is not to say that it is not best evidence to have a medical opinion when a doctor can be on the spot; it is – but doctors are rarely on the spot and are often incredibly difficult to obtain at short notice. A lady magistrate made this point in writing of a case before her in a rural area when the police tried twelve doctors before they could find one prepared to examine, and she said that it was often at least three hours before a doctor could attend (*The Magistrate*, correspondence, April 1961, p. 57). Hence the urgent need for the development of adequate testing machines.

Discussions with general practitioners who have worked for the police suggest that fewer and fewer doctors are prepared to undertake the duties of a police surgeon. It can be unpleasant to examine a drunken person, and it often means being called out in the small hours to do so; the time that is lost through having to attend court, and the dislike of cross-examination, are factors that have already been mentioned with reference to non-medical witnesses. In addition, the doctor may receive threatening letters before a case, and anonymous telephone calls to the effect that he will be 'done over' if he dares to give evidence against X. He may also get a 'warning' from the defence solicitors that they intend to produce an eminent medical witness to rebut the evidence for the prosecution, implying that it would be wiser for the doctor to play down his evidence rather than look silly in court by seeming to oppose the view of an authority. This kind of threat is also used by the prosecution against doctors appearing for the defence, so that medical witnesses for the defence are not in a much happier position. It is not, therefore, surprising that doctors dislike involvement in cases of drunken driving on either side. Consequently the police may have to manage increasingly on their own.

Quite apart from the difficulties of handling cases in court, the business of arrest in drunken driving incidents can be most disagreeable. The accused is sometimes aggressive and violent, and even more often is likely to vomit or urinate in the police car or on the charge-room floor. The reports of the cases in this study reveal the utterly wretched condition of some of the defendants, who soiled themselves and gave way to other regressive tantrums of tears and self-recrimination while on the way to the station (see p. 229 below). On arrival, the standard of behaviour deteriorates even further, and it is often necessary to put offenders in the cells to sober up. In circumstances of this kind the police are frequently accused of trickery in persuading accused persons to admit guilt by promising that they will present the case in as favourable a light as possible.

In fairness to the police it must be said that, in the course of this research, only eight instances were encountered of offenders' alleging that the police had suggested that a guilty plea would 'make things better for everyone'. Two cases were, however, rather disturbing if the offenders can be believed. In one instance the informant said that he was disorientated by a bright light being shone in his eyes; owing to a previous injury, this stimulus was exceedingly distressing, and he said that the tearful and disturbed behaviour induced by it was used in evidence against him (see p. 281 below). In the other case the respondent said he was kept at the police station in a cell for several hours after arrest, and was not allowed to contact his parents or his solicitor; when brought before the stipendiary magistrate next morning this worried and inexperienced young man readily believed a housebreaker he met in the cells of the court, who said that he would be sent to prison for three months. As he had no chance to prepare a defence he pleaded guilty, on, he said, police advice, but it is fair to say that he did not think his treatment was unjustified in the circumstances.

In *R.* v. *Morgan* ([1961] *Crim. L.R.* 538) the Lord Chief Justice expressed strong disapproval of 'the usual practice' of the police (in this case, in Carmarthen) of detaining drunken drivers all night in the cells without charging them, another abuse of power by the police, it might properly be thought. But, here again, it must be said that many drunken drivers are in no state to be charged until many hours after arrest, and it would clearly be wrong to charge anyone until he was able to understand what was being done. Paradoxically, one respondent interviewed in this study criticized the police for letting him have his ignition key and enabling him to leave after a few hours, 'long before I was really sober'.

The police answer to these allegations is, of course, that there are bad elements in every force; but, on the whole, they plead that it would be stupid to act in such a way since it would present the defence with telling evidence that would surely be to the prosecution's disadvantage, and would, in any case, be bad for police-public relations, about which the police are now quite sensitive. This is one of the reasons for the care with which the police consider and prepare cases for prosecution; indeed it is doubtful if the public realize just how much detailed and laborious work has to go into the preparation of even the most minor charges. If they did, it may be that they would not so readily subscribe to the view that the police are over-eager to get convictions.

First there has to be a report made on the spot, often in very unpleasant weather and uncomfortable circumstances, and it is frequently necessary to record details meticulously and take statements from witnesses. All this has to be typed out later by the officer handling the case, together with personal recommendations upon which senior officers can rule; and the latter are quick to reject any papers that are untidy, or badly composed, with a 'do again' in red ink. Subsequently, in most districts additional forms have to be completed in typescript, and all the statements must be checked and re-checked. Often it will be necessary to draw plans of the scene and take photographs, and these are likely to be challenged if in the least inaccurate or unsatisfactory. Then there is the tedious business of calling on witnesses and taking statements at home, and if any of the individuals concerned live outside the Police District, it means writing to the local police and asking for their assistance. Licensing and insurance details have to be checked, previous convictions obtained, and finally summonses have to be served. And even then there may be several adjournments, to make it more than a month, or sometimes several months, before a case is heard. All these tasks are the responsibility of the officer initiating the report, since 'following through one's case to the end' is a police tradition. Thus it is not hard to believe police officers when they say that they do not provoke or encourage prosecutions.

Yet, onerous as this preparatory work may be, it is only supportive administration; an equal, if not greater, burden rests on the senior officers who make the decision to prosecute.

The Decision to Prosecute

In most motoring cases the decision whether to prosecute, issue a written warning, or drop the matter altogether is made by the superintendent (or equivalent) in charge of the police division, probably on the recommendation of the chief inspector, who may specialize up to a point in traffic cases, and on that of the inspector in charge of the subdivision in which the offence occurred. There are, however, certain exceptions, such as cases of alleged manslaughter, or of causing death by dangerous driving, in which the papers are sent through the chief constable to the Director of Public Prosecutions for advice. It is also normal for unusual cases to be referred to police headquarters for the chief constable's instructions, and it may be that counsel's advice is sought, especially where the evidence seems to be insubstantial but it is thought to be in the public interest to proceed.

Mainly, however, the decision to proceed or, in police parlance, to 'issue process', is made by the superintendent; and because most motoring offences are 'absolute prohibitions' it may not seem to be a difficult one. In the less serious cases it is largely a problem of deciding whether the public interest and respect for the law will be served best by a written warning or by prosecution, because the police are anxious not to appear over-zealous in prosecuting, and so influence police-public relations adversely. In the group of serious offences with which this study is concerned there is little or no choice between prosecution or dropping the matter, though it may well be decided to warn where there is insufficient evidence to prosecute an offender whose behaviour is known to deserve it.

In motoring cases some of the most difficult decisions at divisional level concern the vexed question as to whether to proceed for dangerous driving, careless driving, or both. And discussion with senior officers showed up some differences of opinion on this matter: some held the view that dangerous driving was a 'sin of commission', and careless driving a 'sin of omission'; and others based their decision on whether someone could have been, or had been, injured. But the main factor seemed to be the expected attitude of the justices: where they were inclined to severity there was little hesitation in preferring 'danger', but it was usual to insure by charging 'due care' as an alternative to 'danger'.

This practice of charging offenders with both dangerous driving and an alternative of careless driving is widespread, and is known among the police as the 'two bites at the cherry'. But it might be asked why it is used at all since justices can convict for 'due care' in cases of alleged dangerous driving, without any alternative charge being made, if they do not think that the facts support the graver charge. Moreover, the practice of the 'two bites' was the subject of some implicit criticism in court by Mr Justice Lynskey, who said that the police ought always to bring the more serious charge if the facts supported it: a statement that drew the comment from a learned writer that 'the police are entitled to leave the decision (as to whether to convict for the lesser offence) to the court in the ultimate, but when they do prefer two charges it is reasonable to infer that they are in doubt about which charge to prefer' (*Criminal Law Review*, 1954, p. 939).

However, discussions with the police suggested to this writer a rather different reason for using the 'two bites' procedure: that it can help to prevent the guilty from 'getting away with it'. The typical situation is where a defendant accused of 'danger' elects trial by jury, who can only convict or acquit on the 'danger' charge; they cannot convict for 'due care' since this is a summary offence outside the purview of higher courts. If the alternative of 'due care' is charged, it can be adjourned at the hearing in the magistrates' court when the defendant elects trial; then, if the jury acquit him, he can be brought back to the lower court and tried on the lesser charge. Otherwise he would go free. The procedure can be used also when an accused is convicted by the jury, but appeals successfully against this. Hence the 'two bites at the cherry' are a safeguard against the probability that an accused, faced by a reputedly severe bench, will elect trial and escape conviction. The practice is also used sometimes when it seems likely that the defence will agree to a guilty plea on the lesser charge, and thus save the calling of witnesses and much other time-consuming business.

It may be thought by drivers that this is a typically unfair police trick of catching offenders 'coming and going', and another example of the often quoted business of 'throwing the book' at the offender. But the facts do not support such a view; the main concern seemed to be the public interest in that a guilty man should not escape justice by the skill of his advocate.

On the contrary, the fairness of the police superintendents was often striking, especially over the question of the influence of drink in cases of dangerous or careless driving. They would not allow any reference to drink in the prosecution case when there was not to be a charge of driving under the influence, unless the accused tried to assert that his behaviour was due to ill health or tiredness. Hence in most cases there was no mention of drink once it had been decided not to proceed for drunken driving; and this tended to obscure the real extent to which alcohol was a factor in the dangerous and careless driving charges.

It is, however, often done to couple a charge of driving under the influence with an additional (not alternative) charge of dangerous driving. This is no second 'bite at the cherry'; there are here two distinct offences, and the outcome is frequently a conviction on both. Moreover it would, of course, be quite rational to acquit on the drink charge and convict on that of dangerous driving, and vice versa. It will be remembered that both driving under the influence and dangerous driving can be indictable offences; they become so if the accused elects trial, or if the police prefer the charge on an indictment in the first instance and leave him no option but to go before a jury. There is no need to dwell on the reason why the police are disinclined to take the latter course; for one thing they do not tend to expect better justice from a jury than from the magistrates in these cases, and for another – as one superintendent put it – such a course would carry an implicit criticism of the magistrates and some lack of confidence in them.

Decisions to proceed in failing to stop or to report cases are apt to be difficult because of the need to establish that the offender knew that there had been an accident; while the onus of this lies on the defence (*Harding* v. *Price* [1948] 1. All E.R. 283), there would be little point in proceeding where it was reasonably clear that there was a defence of this kind. There is also the problem of tracing the offender, which can take considerable time; but it offers a chance to do some interesting detection, and many of these cases demonstrate that there has been sound and thorough police work to find an elusive person.

Nevertheless, it would seem true to say that this offence does not present anything like the difficulties associated with charges for dangerous or drunken driving, and it is these that cause the most trouble. Hence it is usual for the police to use counsel to prosecute in these offences even when the case will almost certainly be dealt with summarily; in most other summary cases the police superintendent or inspector will prosecute in person, and this is another role of the police officer that is not often appreciated by the layman. It requires considerable legal knowledge, and the capacity to marshal and present facts, together with a grasp of detail that would defeat other than sound intelligence. It should perhaps be realized that brains in the police are not concentrated entirely in the CID – an impression that laymen are apt to have. Motoring cases impose considerable strain on the more junior police officers also, for they often have to give evidence and withstand severe cross-examination quite early in their careers.

Legal and Social Background

RELATIONS BETWEEN THE POLICE AND THE COURTS

Generally speaking, there was hardly any criticism by police officers of magistrates in their handling of cases; their criticism was mainly of the higher courts, and in particular of juries and their over-readiness to acquit. There was, however, among the police a marked respect for the independence of justices: they showed no sign of being confident that the police case would be believed, or that they would even have the benefit of the doubt. This was particularly marked in a division in which the chairman of the magistrates was a Queen's Counsel: here the officers made it plain that it kept them up to the mark to appear before legally qualified magistrates. In contrast, the opinion of offenders with whom the matter was discussed was otherwise: they were almost unanimously convinced that the police and the bench were in league; and as one of them pointed out, the impression is hardened by the habit of calling the courts 'police courts', and by having police officers as court ushers.

A certain amount of dissatisfaction was expressed by police officers over the difficulty of convincing benches, and even more so juries, of the credibility of police evidence in cases of speeding or drunken driving. There was strong support for the use of instruments such as the radar speed meter and the breathalyzer, provided that they are simple to operate and easy to test for accuracy. From the police standpoint, however, even the use of accurate instruments can be frustrating, as it has been found that some justices, the motoring organizations, and the motoring press are apt to allege that the devices were being operated improperly. As the *Autocar* put it in a leading article (27 November 1959), when a motor cyclist was convicted at Southend on the evidence of a noise-level meter: 'Electrical measuring machines carry for many people an aura of mystery and infallibility which is quite unjustified. When one group of human beings – the police for example – operates radar devices in an endeavour to trap motorists driving too fast or, as now at Southend, making too much noise, there should be definite assurances on behalf of the other human beings in cars that the intervening magic boxes are being operated fairly and the results are being interpreted properly.'

In conclusion it must be said that the fairness and good sense with which the police were observed to handle the offences studied were most impressive. Indeed it seemed all too easy to infer that no case was brought without good reason and that the police could usually be believed in contrast to the defendant. It is true, of course, that most of the cases reviewed resulted in conviction; but the impression persisted even when cases that

120

were dismissed were heard. It was soon evident that there was a marked danger of making a one-sided judgement; hence it became increasingly necessary to interview offenders to see what they thought about their treatment by the police. Police officers had no doubt whatsoever that interviews of this kind would produce one salient point of view: that the offender had done no wrong, and that he was the victim of other people's bad driving, poor roads, and police vindictiveness. How right they were will be evident later.

5

The Size of the Problem[1]

Before considering in detail the serious motoring offences that form the basis of this research, it is advisable to try to see their relation to the general picture of crime in England and Wales during the period under study.

THE SOURCES AND THEIR INTERPRETATION

To construct an overall picture it is necessary to draw primarily on statistics, the most reliable being the official *Criminal Statistics*, their *Supplementary Tables*, and the Home Office Returns of *Offences relating to Motor Vehicles*. There are some other useful statistical sources that deal with motoring offences, notably the reports of chief constables, but the figures they contain are invariably embodied in the official statistics compiled by the Home Office. These offer what is probably the best evidence, but – like all social statistics – they do not tell the whole story, showing as they do only those offences that are officially 'known', and leaving undocumented a proportion of unknown size. As Lodge (1953) has said, the criminal statistics do not show the real state of crime but only figures related to it, and their interpretation is not unlike 'attempting to draw a man's shadow on the wall or, if non-indictable offences are in question, from his shadow on wire-netting'.

Moreover, it is difficult to augment the statistical information given in one official source with the data from another, since methods of compilation differ in each case. For example, the *Criminal Statistics* for England and Wales present *persons* dealt with for motoring offences by the courts, whereas the Home Office Returns of *Offences relating to Motor Vehicles* give data in terms of *offences*, showing only a grand total of persons dealt with for *all* kinds of motoring offence, so that it is impossible to deduce from the figures the number of particular offences attributable to any one person. Nor can this be calculated from the *Criminal Statistics*, since, for motoring and most other offences, they specify only the *principal* offence with which

[1] Because of their quantity, the statistical data are presented at the end of this chapter, to avoid undue disruption of the text. For ease of reference, the page on which a particular table or figure can be found is given the first time it is mentioned in the text.

an offender was charged – accompanying offences are not mentioned unless they were of a different degree of 'indictability' (e.g. a non-indictable offence accompanying an indictable offence *would* be shown separately). Because the *Criminal Statistics* are based on principal offences, they tend to underestimate the incidence of motoring offences; and this can be seen very clearly from a comparison of the total number of persons found guilty whose principal offence was a motoring offence as given in the *Criminal Statistics*, with the total number found guilty of motoring offences, whether principal ones or not, as shown in the Home Office Returns. The comparison is made in *Table 5* (p. 145) for the years 1954 to 1959, and it shows that the differences between the two sets of totals are not inconsiderable. In 1958 the Home Office Return total exceeded that of the *Criminal Statistics* by over 7,000.

It is, therefore, the Home Office Return total of persons found guilty of motoring offences that is subtracted from the total number of persons found guilty of offences of all kinds, as given in the *Criminal Statistics*, in order to indicate the motoring offender's contribution to the total picture of known crime (*Table 6*, p. 146). Yet even here there is a difficulty, in that data for *persons* convicted are available only for the magistrates' courts; for the higher courts, findings of guilt have been used, which do not necessarily reveal the numbers of offenders involved. Since, however, the proportion of cases heard by the higher courts is small, it is unlikely that the inclusion of these figures for 'convictions' has resulted in distorting the general picture.

Another rather confusing feature of motoring offences is that they are not easily classified as 'indictable' or 'non-indictable', since most of the serious ones (except manslaughter and causing death by dangerous driving) can be tried either on indictment before a jury or by magistrates, according, usually, to the defendant's choice. They are what Lodge (1953, p. 285) has called 'hybrid' offences.

From a research standpoint it is unfortunate that the *Criminal Statistics* group the majority of motoring offences under the vague heading 'Other motoring offences'; though, no doubt, this course is forced on the compilers by the very high incidence of these offences. The Annual Reports of the Prison Commissioners go even further by grouping all motoring offences under 'Offences against the Highway Acts', which renders a potentially valuable source virtually useless for this kind of inquiry.

So far it might be inferred that the official statistics, and the *Criminal Statistics* in particular, tend markedly to underestimate the actual number of motoring offenders. There are, however, two counter points that must be

123

made. First, in the *Criminal Statistics* there is no apparent distinction between *one* individual who commits *eight* offences – for example, speeding – in the course of one year, and *eight different* individuals who each commit only *one* offence of the same kind in the same year; that is, for these two examples together the total number of offenders shown in the tables would be sixteen, not nine. The same individual can thus swell the total very considerably, and this can be seen to some extent from the Home Office Returns which, as mentioned already, give the grand total of persons found guilty *and* the grand total of offences for which they have been responsible; but it is impossible to see what the position is for the different kinds of motoring offence. Second, none of the sources shows the ratio of motoring offences to the population at risk, to the number of driving licences in issue, or to the number of vehicles on the roads. These are clearly weighting factors of the first importance, and it will be seen that they tend to have a fairly considerable effect on the statistical picture.

These observations serve to underline the caution given in the opening paragraph of this chapter: that statistics of crime can tell but a part of the story. They can only indicate what the real state of affairs is likely to be, and no more than this can be claimed for the analysis that follows.

MOTORING OFFENCES IN GENERAL

Bearing in mind the limitations of these statistics, let us ask just how much motoring offenders contribute towards the rising total of crime in England and Wales today. Wootton (1959, p. 25) has said that their contribution is considerable enough to label the motoring offender the typical criminal of our time; and if we consider a criminal to be anyone who offends against the law of the state, the figures would support her view.

Table 6 and *Figure 1* (p. 146) present these statistics in their raw state: it can be seen that motoring offenders constituted 46 per cent of all offenders in 1954; since then the proportion has increased steadily until it reached 55·5 per cent in 1959.

The case against the motoring offender looks even worse when offences are calculated per 100,000 of the population aged 14 and over – a perfectly fair procedure since it is unusual for persons under 14 to commit motoring offences. (However, the number of offenders aged under 14 rose from 40 in 1954 to 131 in 1959, an increase that merits investigation, but official statistics do not facilitate any analysis.) *Table 7* and *Figure 2* (p. 147) compare the numbers of motoring offenders calculated in this way with the numbers of offenders who have committed other kinds of offence during the period 1954–59. Motoring offenders are seen to be substantially in the lead with an increase of 69·2 per cent over the period in contrast to the relatively small increase of about 15 per cent for the non-motoring offenders.

The two graphs (*Figures 1* and *2*) show that the dominance of the motoring offender is of fairly recent origin; motoring offenders took the lead about 1955.

In considering reasons for this development the obvious factor to be taken into account is the increase in the number of drivers and vehicles licensed during the period 1954–59. These are tabulated in *Table 8* (p. 148), in which the data are shown in index form for ease of comparison, and it will be seen that after 1956 offenders seem to move increasingly ahead of both licences and vehicles.

However, the real picture is not clearly illustrated until offenders are shown per 100,000 vehicles and per 100,000 drivers licensed, as in *Table 9* and *Figure 3* (pp. 148–9). The data give little comfort to those who would hope that the curve showing the incidence of motoring offences could be smoothed out by this quite legitimate operation, though both curves declined slightly in 1959. The graph suggests that there is a functional relationship between the number of motoring offenders and the numbers of drivers and of vehicles licensed, since the curve for offenders per 100,000 driving licences follows a similar course to that per 100,000 vehicles licensed until the latter rises more sharply in 1957–58.

Clearly an increase in congestion on the roads is likely to produce a big rise in such motoring offences as those connected with parking and lighting. But have these risen to such an extent that they could be said to be responsible for the much higher total of motoring offences? If this were so we would expect to find them increasing at a much faster rate than any other group of motoring offences. However, a comparison of parking and lighting offences with the most frequent driving offence – driving without due care – all calculated per 100,000 driving licences over the period 1954–59, shows that convictions for parking and lighting offences increased by only 16 per cent, whereas those for careless driving rose by 32 per cent – a marked difference. Moreover, the Home Office Returns show that the contribution of obstruction, parking, and lighting offences to the total of all motoring offences did not change very much during the period, ranging from 22·5 to 19·8 per cent, and reaching its lowest point in 1959 – a peak year for motoring offences.

There does not, therefore, seem to be adequate evidence for saying that parking and lighting offences account for the marked rise in motoring offences. Nor is it possible to blame those who 'exceed the speed limit in a built-up area', another very common offence; here there is a *decrease* over the period of just below 5 per cent when the incidence is calculated per 100,000 driving licences in issue.

So much for the offences that could be expected to move directly with a rise (or fall) in the number of vehicles on the roads. But this is not to say that the great increase in traffic has not been influential; for it is bound to bring with it an additional element of stress in driving and so make drivers more prone to commit offences. It is, however, noticeable that *Figure 3* shows that the increase in the numbers of vehicles and drivers licensed in 1954 and 1955 did not bring about a rise but a *fall* in the number of motoring offenders. This phenomenon is even more apparent when indictable offences are treated separately as in *Table 10* and *Figure 4* (pp. 149=50). Although the scale of the graph may overestimate changes in the offence rates, the point remains that an increase in vehicles and drivers licensed was accompanied by a decrease in the offence rate at one stage in the period.

Another explanation of the marked increase of motoring offences would be an intensification of police activity in dealing with these offences. The only statistical indication of this would be an increase in the proportion of motoring offences 'known to the police' that resulted in prosecution. Unfortunately, however, there are no published records of motoring offences known to the police because the official statistics group them with many other kinds of offences known, under a 'Miscellaneous' heading, except for the minority offence of causing death by dangerous driving. So it is necessary to rely once again on the Home Office Returns which give data for 'Total offences and alleged offences'; but these are not the same thing as offences known to the police since the latter include all offences reported, whether the offender is traced or not. The Home Office Return offences and alleged offences, on the other hand, seem to include only those where the offender is traced, because each is the subject of either prosecution or a written warning; such traced offences are obviously only a proportion of the total number known to the police. The percentage of prosecutions out of the offences alleged and reported in the Home Office Returns is not, therefore, a very meaningful proportion to use for this purpose, but for what it is worth it is shown in *Table 11* (p. 150). The striking feature of this table is the remarkable stability of the proportion of prosecutions at around 70 per cent over the period under review. The same is to be said of the proportion of prosecutions that result in findings of guilt: here again there is a very small range, from 95·2 to 96·4 per cent. So there does not seem to have been any noticeable increase in severity on the part of the police in terms of prosecuting rather than issuing written warnings; nor have the courts tended to find a higher proportion of offenders guilty. At present, no more can be said with any confidence, and though the possibility of increased police activity cannot be dismissed completely, there are reasons for thinking it unlikely.

One explanation of the increase in motoring offences that is often heard is that the sentences imposed by the courts do not deter the offenders. Hence Lord Lucas of Chilworth's accusation that magistrates were guilty of 'culpable negligence' themselves in their treatment of the motoring offender (*The Times*, 17 October 1959). Indeed *Table 12* (p. 151), which shows how the courts disposed of motoring offenders of all kinds, does not suggest undue severity, and sentencing remains remarkably stable despite the manifest increase in the incidence of offences, though it does show some signs of stiffening in 1959. There is, however, one exception to this consistency: the very marked decrease in the proportion of offenders disqualified, which fell from 6·1 per cent in 1956 to 3·8 per cent in 1957, remaining at much the same low percentage in 1958 and rising only to 5·2 per cent in 1959. The reason for this drop in the small proportion of offenders disqualified would seem to be the change in the law effected by the Act of 1956, which made it no longer compulsory for disqualification to be imposed for driving uninsured unless there were 'special reasons'. As *Table 13a* (p. 153) shows, the proportion of offenders disqualified for this offence fell from 83 per cent in 1956 to 39 per cent in 1957.

Another reason for the failure to 'crack down' on the increasingly numerous offenders could be the kind of attitude expressed by the Hon. Ewen Montagu, speaking from the bench in 1959, when he said that the drinking driver, in many cases, 'has not been drinking a lot, and is an eminently responsible man to whom a small fine means a lot'. He continued: 'Neither is enough stress paid to the fact that a disqualification means considerable hardship as far as wage earning goes. In the majority of cases the important thing is that there should be a conviction, not necessarily an enormous fine' (*The Times*, 12 December 1959). So there are justices who firmly believe that heavy sentences are not a solution to the problem, and Mr Justice Stable was speaking in this vein when he is quoted as saying in court, 'If I thought that by sending people to prison I should save thousands of people killed on the roads every year, then I would do it. Personally I don't believe that sending bad drivers to prison is going to achieve that result' (*The Times*, 27 October 1959).

Those who would be severe may find support for their attitude in the figures for the disposal of persons convicted for driving while disqualified:

after a very substantial rise in the number of offences and alleged offences, reaching a peak of 2,895 in 1956, there was a fall to 1,615 in 1957. This accompanied a marked increase in the proportion of offenders sent to prison (34·5 per cent in 1956 and 61 per cent in 1957), and a substantial increase in the proportion further disqualified (see *Tables 13a* and *19a*). On the other hand, it must be noted that the number of motoring offenders who were disqualified fell considerably after the 1956 Act made it no longer mandatory to disqualify insurance offenders; hence the number of disqualified drivers 'at risk' was much smaller. So the increased severity of sentencing is not the complete answer in this instance, which will be considered again later in this chapter.

Table 12 shows that the courts still use the fine as their principal weapon, and it is because of this that many of their critics, for example Lord Lucas (in a letter to *The Times*, 27 October 1959), point to movements in the 'average fine' as an indication of changes in the severity of the bench towards motoring offenders. And, indeed, the average fine is still low, though it increased steadily from 48*s.* in 1954 to 74*s.* in 1959. But it should be emphasized that only the figures for the magistrates' courts are available in the statistics, and the bigger fines of the higher courts are excluded. Moreover, we are here witnessing the distorting effect of using an arithmetic mean to find the average – in fact, there is no option – in which the many small fines for trivial offences may well conceal quite a few substantial ones for the more serious offender. For instance, the average fine for dangerous and reckless driving moved from just over £10 in 1954 to just over £15 in 1959, and the fine for driving or being in charge while 'under the influence' increased from a little over £17 to nearly £23.

There seems to be little doubt that the courts are not using anything like the maximum powers at their disposal to deal with motoring offenders. The most usual prison sentence for magistrates' courts is from two to three months, and for the higher courts it is under one year, though there was one offender in 1954 who received two or three years' corrective training for driving recklessly or dangerously. But the very low proportion of offenders sent to prison suggests that many on the bench are inclined to agree with Mr Justice Stable.

Some discussion of the comparative treatment of offenders by the higher and the lower courts might seem appropriate here, but it has been left until later because statistical records permit only the comparison of the two offences of dangerous and reckless driving and driving or being in charge while 'under the influence', and both of these offences will be looked at in detail below.

The evidence presented and discussed so far has done little to explain the considerable rise in motoring offences during the period under review, and their overtaking of other offences after 1955. Let us now consider the further possibility that this may be a manifestation of the general increase in crime during the period. If so, we might expect to find repeated within this rather special and distinctive field of offenders a marked feature of the overall criminal picture – that is, the dominant part played by the age group 17 to 21.

This expectation is confirmed by the data presented in *Table 14* and *Figure 5* (p. 154), which show the age distribution of motoring offenders before all courts. From the graph it is easy to see the lead that the age group 17 to 21 has achieved since 1956 when it overtook the group aged 21 and over. It would seem that the 14 and under 17 age group has the lowest proportion of motoring offenders, probably because the number of drivers in this group is much smaller. When indictable offences are considered (*Table 14* and *Figure 5a*, p. 155) the trend is even more evident. There is a striking increase in the number of offenders under 21 between 1958 and 1959, owing to a rise in convictions for causing death. Proportionally they exceed the 30 and over age group and move very close to the here dominant 21 and under 30 group.[1] So it is the young offender before the magistrates' courts who appears to be responsible for a high proportion of the increase in motoring offences; and, as has been said already, it is possible that the figures for these offenders are an underestimate since they have been derived from the *Criminal Statistics*. It is also quite clear from the tables giving details of offences by this age group that motor cyclists are the principal culprits, producing a steady 60–65 per cent of the total convictions in every year during the period.

The hypothesis that the motor cyclist is one of the principal offenders is further supported when an attempt is made to rank offenders according to the type of vehicle they were driving. This is possible, up to a point, since the *Criminal Statistics* group motoring offences by kind of vehicle, though not after 1957. From these figures we find that between 1954 and 1957 there were the following percentage increases in convictions: 14 per cent for drivers of goods vehicles, 27 per cent for drivers of private cars, and 49 per cent for motor cyclists. But, of course, convictions relating to private cars are by far the most numerous, totalling 177,400 in 1957 as compared with 104,207 for goods vehicles and just over 75,000 for motor

---

[1] For comparison, see *Table 15* and *Figure 6* (pp. 155–6), showing the incidence of non-motoring offenders of all kinds; and *Table 16* and *Figure 7* (pp. 156–7) giving the same details for indictable non-motoring offenders.

cycles. Convictions for offenders who were drivers of public-service vehicles and taxis decreased during the period (by 17 and 10 per cent respectively) but so did the numbers of licensed vehicles in these two categories. So, here again, the numbers of the various classes of vehicle on the roads must be taken into account. A calculation of convictions per 1,000 of the particular type of vehicle shows that the number of offenders in each category fell, except in the case of taxi drivers whose conviction rate increased slightly, and of motor cyclists whose conviction rate increased considerably from 45 per 1,000 vehicles licensed in 1954 to 53 in 1957. It may be, therefore, that motor cyclists are largely responsible for the upward movement of the curve in *Figure 3*, showing offenders per 100,000 vehicles licensed.

There are, then, grounds for thinking that motoring offences are tending to follow the general pattern of crime in that deeper analysis shows that the under 21 age group has the highest proportion of offenders. Moreover, it is shown later that among the offences with the higher rates of increase are those which might sensibly be regarded as characteristic of younger offenders – failing to insure and offences with motor cycles.

In further pursuit of the question whether the general picture of crime is reflected in motoring offences it will be useful to look at these offenders differentiated by sex. Is there here the usual male dominance that is found in crime generally?

As males are known to be in the great majority among holders of driving licences, one would expect to find them outnumbering females to a greater degree among motoring offenders than among other offenders. But it is a little surprising to find the ratio as high as between 18:1 and 22:1, compared with the 8:1 ratio of males to females in crime of all kinds (*Tables 17* and *18*, pp. 157–8).

THE MORE SERIOUS ASPECT – SPECIFIC OFFENCES

Having considered motoring offences of all kinds, it is now intended to separate out the six specific classes of offence with which this study is concerned, in order to indicate the contribution made to the general picture by the more serious offenders. These classes of offence are:

1. *Causing Death by Dangerous Driving*
   Road Traffic Act, 1960, section 1. An indictable offence.

2. *Driving Recklessly or Dangerously*
   Road Traffic Act, 1960, section 2(1). A 'hybrid' offence that may be dealt with on indictment or summarily.

The Size of the Problem

3. *Driving a Vehicle while under the Influence of Drink or Drugs*[1]
   Road Traffic Act, 1960, section 6(1). Also a 'hybrid' offence.

4. *Driving while Disqualified*
   Road Traffic Act, 1960, section 110. A non-indictable offence.

5. *Failing to Insure against Third-party Risks*
   Road Traffic Act, 1960, section 201(1). A non-indictable offence.

6. *Failing to Stop after, or to Report, an Accident*
   Road Traffic Act, 1960, section 77. A non-indictable offence.

Tables 19 and *19a* (pp. 159–60) show the raw data for these six offences as a group; and with one exception – driving while disqualified – all the offences show a sustained rise in incidence, especially causing death by dangerous driving, and failing to insure. But these data are particularly susceptible to the influence of the three weighting factors: population size, number of vehicle licences, and number of driving licences. When the last factor is taken into account, the picture revealed by *Table 20* (p. 161) and the accompanying graph (*Figure 8*,[2] p. 162) is radically different. Only one offence, failing to insure, retains a manifest increase, and the remainder are 'steadied' considerably by the operation.

Unfortunately, it is not possible to show here the breakdown of offenders by age and sex for each of these offences since, as already mentioned, this information is given in the official statistics for indictable offences only; for the non-indictable or 'hybrid' offences the grouping of offences prevents isolation for separate study. Hence *Figures 4* and *5a*, dealing with indictable offences, exclude a high proportion of the six offences now under discussion. It is unfortunate also that the presentation of the official statistics does not permit a comparison between the higher and the magistrates' courts in respect of their treatment of each offence; this is possible only for dangerous driving, and for driving under the influence, and it will be discussed when dealing with these offences.

Let us begin by looking at the offence with the highest percentage increase during the period: Causing death by dangerous driving (formerly charged as Manslaughter).

---

[1] It should be noted that the tables in this chapter include offences of being in charge of (but not driving) a vehicle while under the influence of drink or drugs, because, until 1956, the statistics for this offence were combined with those for driving under the influence.

[2] The data for causing death are not shown on the graph because the number of offences is too small to be compared with the other offences in graph form.

Legal and Social Background

Causing Death by Dangerous Driving (RTA, 1960, section 1), and Manslaughter

The striking thing about the data for these offences is the very substantial increase in the numbers of both prosecutions and convictions after 1956, when the necessity to charge motoring offenders involved in fatal incidents with manslaughter was removed owing to the introduction of the new offence, causing death by dangerous driving. The real key to the increased incidence would appear to be the fact that after 1956 a much greater proportion of those prosecuted were found guilty; in 1956, only 10 per cent of those prosecuted were convicted, but in 1957 the percentage rose to 58. In the twelve months between 1956 and 1957 the number of prosecutions increased nearly ninefold, and there seems to be no doubt that this was a result of the greater confidence felt by the Director of Public Prosecutions and the police in the possibility of securing convictions by juries, who had hitherto been notoriously reluctant to find a motorist guilty of manslaughter, with all its sinister implications.

Having drawn attention to the increase in the number of prosecutions, it may seem inconsistent that *Table 19* shows that, in every year of the period 1954–59, all offences and alleged offences of this kind were prosecuted. But it will be remembered, as explained on p. 126 above, that the figures in the Home Office Returns refer only to offences that have been cleared up.

A comparison of the percentages of findings of guilt for this offence and for the other five offences suggests, however, that juries are still hesitant to find a motorist guilty of an offence carrying a maximum punishment of five years' imprisonment. Compared with other offences the rate of conviction is low, and after a marked fall in 1958 it has remained steady in 1959 and 1960 at just over 60 per cent.

It is possible to separate persons found guilty of this offence by age and by sex. The latter classification does not yield any useful result since there were only twelve women convicted in the whole period, but the former shows that the greatest number convicted for this offence were in the age group 40 and over, with those 21 and under 30 following closely. When calculated per 100,000 of the population in each age group, however, the mode is in the group 21 and under 30, with the 14 and under 21 group next, and the lowest number in the over 30s. So here the teenage group loses its lead.

The change in attitude towards this offence following the change in its legal nomenclature is apparent also in the treatment of those convicted.

Until 1957 prison was not only the principal punishment, it was the *only* punishment; in that year, imprisonment gave way to the fine and, in contrast to the preceding years, when no fines were recorded, 44 per cent of offenders were so treated and 44 per cent were sent to prison; in 1959 the respective proportions were 50 and 37 per cent. Even so, imprisonment is still used more for this offence than for any other except driving while disqualified, for which it is mandatory.

As it is grouped with other offences against the person, causing death by dangerous driving is perhaps the only offence that can be compared *a priori* with other non-motoring offences – at least so far as treatment is concerned. For this purpose, *Table 21* (p. 163) gives the sentences of fines or imprisonment imposed for certain offences in this group:

Manslaughter (other than motoring cases)
Felonious and malicious wounding
Assault, aggravated assault, assault against a constable
Common assault

The figures for the higher courts show that the lowest proportion of the offenders found guilty of any one or more of the above offences who were sent to prison was 58 per cent in 1954, compared with 37 per cent of offenders convicted for causing death by dangerous driving. And, with the single exception of cases of driving while disqualified, both the higher and the magistrates' courts are much more severe with these other offenders against the person than they are with any of those found guilty of the serious motoring offences under study. It may, however, be felt that the comparison made here is unsound, in that offences in which death occurred are not, from some viewpoints, comparable with offences in which there were no fatalities. But, even when the offences against the person are restricted for purposes of comparison to murder and non-motoring manslaughter, it is still found that the courts seem to deal with them with greater severity than the motoring cases: in the three years, 1957, 1958, and 1959, fines were imposed on less than 5 per cent of the offenders in this restricted group, and between 51 and 86 per cent of them were sent to prison.

This, it may be thought, is common sense since the non-motoring offender against the person is likely to be a greater danger to the community than his motoring equivalent, and so he is more suitable for incarceration. Also it may be said that protection from dangerous motoring offenders can be secured by disqualifying them, without imposing a further load on an overworked prison system by sending more of them to prison.

But society has no guarantee that such offenders will not drive although disqualified, and it may be that the more 'criminal' of them would be more inclined to do so. Hence, if protection is a requirement, the practice of fining and disqualifying does not seem adequate. There is also the question of deterrence, and if this is thought to be important it is curious that the more extreme punishment of imprisonment does not figure more prominently among motoring cases where there has been an 'offence against the person', e.g. causing death by dangerous driving.

Driving Recklessly or Dangerously (RTA, 1960, section 2 (1))

Between 1954 and 1959 convictions for this offence increased by 69 per cent from 4,380 to 7,410 (*Table 19*). This is quite a remarkable increase considering the difficulty that is encountered in convincing juries or benches that driving is 'dangerous or reckless' rather than 'careless', and also the probability that a number of cases that would now be prosecuted under the new offence of causing death by dangerous driving were, until 1956, dealt with under reckless or dangerous driving because of the general reluctance to convict for manslaughter. This probability is supported when the number of offences per 100,000 driving licences in issue is calculated (*Table 20*): the data reveal a slight fall in convictions for these offences in 1956 and 1957, but in 1958 they began to rise again. Thus when the weighting factor of licences in issue is taken into account, the impression made by the raw data is considerably changed – the increase in these offences between 1954 and 1959 is shown to be 16 per cent when presented in this way.

But there is no room for complacency on account of this rather better picture, since the offences are increasing again, and there is reason to suppose that a real overlap exists between them and the common and rapidly increasing offence of careless driving. A proportion, probably a fairly substantial one, of charges preferred under section 2(1) is reduced at trial to careless driving, a label that conceals a very wide range of driving behaviour, as will be demonstrated at a later stage in this study by case histories of instances where the modified charge was brought. Indeed it would seem that the dividing line between the two offences is one of opinion or of pure chance only; hence the seriousness of the increase in convictions for careless driving from 423 per 100,000 driving licences in 1954, to 558 in 1959 (*Table 20a*, p. 162).

Driving dangerously is one of the offences for which the sentencing of higher and magistrates' courts can be compared (*Table 22*, pp. 164–5). The first point to note is that the percentage of findings of guilt is slightly

134

higher in the magistrates' courts than in the higher courts, especially since 1956. It is possibly due to the known tendency of juries to give motoring offenders the benefit of the doubt – a tendency that is found also in cases of driving under the influence – but there is also the obvious point that offences tried in the higher courts may be more difficult to decide. The decrease since 1956 in the percentage of offenders sent to prison by the higher courts is striking, falling from 18·4 in 1956 to 5·4 in 1957; and here again there is substantial support for the belief that many cases that would now be charged as 'causing death' were formerly heard under the dangerous driving section. Even so, the higher courts appear to be more severe in treatment than the magistrates' courts, in which the proportion of the guilty sent to prison in 1958 is lower than at any time in the period, despite the increase in the number of offenders. The fine seems to have become slightly more popular in both types of court. However, this would appear to be one of the offences in which it does not pay to elect trial by jury, even though there is a slim chance that one is more likely to escape conviction.

As regards disqualification, *Table 23* (p. 166) shows that there has been an increase in the proportion of offenders thus dealt with, from 31 per cent in 1954 to just over 47 per cent in 1959, although there has been a slight fall in the proportion of motoring offenders disqualified by all courts during the period (*Table 12*). Unfortunately, it is not possible to compare the proportions of offenders disqualified by the higher and magistrates' courts respectively, because details of disqualifications are not available for the former. This is one of the deficiencies of the Home Office Returns from the point of view of attempting an analysis of the sentencing of the higher courts; another is the fairly large number of cases for which no details of sentence are given, apparently because no separate punishment was imposed. That is the reason for the exclusion of a number of cases from *Table 23*, in which it will be seen that a proportion of the offences is unaccounted for.

However, it does not say much for the seriousness with which this offence is regarded when it is found that only 167 sentences of imprisonment were passed out of 7,410 findings of guilt in 1959 by all courts – only 2·2 per cent (*Table 13*). This is very nearly the lowest proportion during the six-year period, although 1959 was a peak year for this offence. One cannot help comparing this with the proportion of offenders against property who are committed to prison by the higher courts, which never falls below 50 per cent throughout the period (*Criminal Statistics*, 1954–59, Table III). Truly it would seem that the motoring offender is 'different'.

135

Driving or in Charge of a Motor Vehicle when under the Influence of Drink or Drugs (RTA, 1960, section 6(1)).

Like the two offences just discussed, driving or being in charge under the influence of drink or drugs was also affected by the changes in the law brought about by the Road Traffic Act, 1956, which, in this case, separated the elements of 'driving' and being 'in charge' into two specific offences. Taken together, the raw figures show an increase of 67 per cent in the findings of guilt over the period (*Table 19*), with the steepest increase in 1959: possibly an aftermath of the change in the law. Again, though, the operation of weighting by the number of driving licences in issue shows a less alarming picture, reducing the increase to just over 18 per cent (*Table 20*).

When the offences are separated and calculated per 100,000 driving licences in issue, it appears that there has been an increase since 1956 in findings of guilt for 'in charge' cases, from 7·8 offences in 1957 to 9·7 in 1959; and for 'driving under the influence' cases, from 39 offences in 1957 to 41 in 1959.

Although it is encouraging that the raw or weighted figures for these offences do not show the steep rise between 1956 and 1959 that is evident in the other offences (except driving while disqualified), it must be remembered that they are probably the most difficult of all motoring offences in which to secure a conviction. Perhaps that is why the proportion of findings of guilt among offenders charged with either offence did not increase immediately after the change in the law in 1956 (*Table 19*). On the contrary, where just over 86 per cent were convicted in 1955, 84·6 per cent were found guilty in 1958. This rather static picture is confirmed also by *Table 22*, comparing the handling of these offences by the higher courts and the magistrates' courts. In both higher and magistrates' courts the proportions found guilty are almost the same for the years 1955 and 1958: in the higher courts 51 per cent were convicted in 1955 and 50·8 per cent in 1958 after a fall in the proportion between these years; in the magistrates' courts the respective percentages are 90·4 and 90·2. A slight rise is, however, evident in 1959 for both higher and magistrates' courts.

The difference in the proportion of offenders convicted by the higher and the magistrates' courts respectively is worth comment. It is so striking that it seems to support the belief that an offender who elects trial by jury will have a better chance of getting off. No doubt some cases sent for trial are more difficult to decide and so more difficult to convict, but in addition it would seem that the role of the jury as the deciding agent must have a considerable effect on the number of convictions. In contrast to the higher courts, the proportion convicted by the magistrates is very high, but this difference is mitigated somewhat when it is remembered that it is in these courts that many offenders plead guilty, which they do not tend to do in the higher courts; also there is the possibility that these cases are easier to decide, which has been mentioned above. Before a proper estimation of the effect of a jury can be made we need to know the proportion of offenders who plead guilty in the magistrates' courts, and the proportion who elect to go for trial; and it is one of the aims of this study to look into this question.

Examination of the disposal of convicted offenders by all courts (*Table 13*) shows no increase in severity; rather do we find the fine steadily encroaching on other forms of punishment: the proportion sent to prison fell steadily from 5·8 per cent in 1954 to 4·1 per cent in 1959, but the proportion fined rose from 92·8 per cent in 1954 to 94·3 per cent in 1959. This, despite the marked increase in the 'raw' figures for these offences, which are the figures before the benches and the public! Comparison between higher and magistrates' courts shows the same trend, with a proportionately greater *decrease* in sentences of imprisonment by the higher courts than by the magistrates' courts, especially since 1955; in that year 11 per cent of the findings of guilt in the higher courts were the subject of prison sentences; in 1959 the proportion was 6·6 per cent. In the magistrates' courts these proportions were, at the highest, 5·9 per cent in 1955, and at the lowest, 3·9 per cent in 1959 (*Table 22*).

The trend towards leniency in dealing with these offences is given slightly more support by *Table 23*, showing the proportion of cases in which offenders are disqualified by magistrates (the data for the higher courts are unfortunately not available). It will be seen that there has been a reduction from 97 per cent of offenders disqualified in 1954 to 85·2 per cent in 1959. The reasons for this are hard to assess in view of the rise in the 'raw' incidence of these offences, and the rational appeal of disqualification as a means of dealing with this kind of offender that hits him hard and yet avoids inflicting a prison sentence. It may be that many of these offenders are persons whose livelihood depends on driving and that justices refrain from passing this sentence because of the numerous cases of hardship that would result from the loss of a necessary adjunct to their business.

Considering that the 'drink' offences appear to attract the most public attention and criticism, it is surprising to find the courts seeming to eschew the more severe forms of sentence. Though the point must be made that in real terms the greater leniency has not led to any immense rise in these

137

offences, yet they have not shown much sign of falling in incidence, and their steadily increasing total must cause grave concern – especially when one takes into account that the difficulty in proving this charge enables many a guilty driver to go free. As will be discussed later, a number of cases were encountered in this research in which drink could be seen from the evidence to be relevant to the offence, although it was not the subject of the charge preferred.

Finally, it should be mentioned that the stiffer penalties imposed for driving while under the influence may have made juries less inclined to convict for this offence. So, perhaps, as in the motoring charges under the manslaughter offences, severity may not necessarily be the solution, if the aim is to deter by the high probability of conviction.

Driving while Disqualified (RTA, 1960, section 110)

Earlier in this chapter it was noted that this is the one offence of the six under review that has not shown a general tendency to increase over the six-year period until 1959, i.e. right at the end. *Table 20* shows that convictions for this offence, per 100,000 driving licences in issue, rose steadily from 23 in 1954 to just over 30 in 1956; they then fell sharply to 16·4 in 1957 before rising again to 25·7 in 1959.

The incidence of the offence is clearly linked closely with the total number of offenders disqualified from driving, and the relationship is demonstrated by constructing an index (1954 = 100) showing the movement of disqualifications for all offences on the one hand, and of convictions for driving while disqualified on the other (*Table 24*, p. 166). It can be seen that until 1956 convictions for driving while disqualified increased faster than disqualifications: a 54 per cent increase in convictions compared with a 28 per cent increase in disqualifications. In 1957 both indices fell: disqualifications by 42 per cent but convictions by 67 per cent. After that the two indices rose by almost the same amount. The much greater fall in convictions for driving while disqualified between 1956 and 1957 was almost certainly a result of the change in the law under the 1956 Act, which allowed justices discretion in disqualifying for insurance offences where previously they had little or no option. *Table 13a* shows that there was a marked fall in disqualifications for insurance offences in 1957, hence it would seem that there is an obvious connection between these two offences. Whether this link is confirmed by the research findings can be seen later, when the records of those who drive while disqualified are studied.

A further point needing investigation is whether offenders become more

138

The Size of the Problem

vulnerable to this offence if they are disqualified for long periods. In other words, is the typical offender one who has been disqualified for a long time – over one year – or is he one who has lost his licence for only a few months? It is almost certain that he is the former, and if this is so the wisdom of long suspensions becomes questionable, because they may, in fact, 'encourage' people to commit this offence.

Failing to Insure against Third-party Risks (RTA, 1960, section 201(1))

As *Table 13a* shows, convictions for this offence have risen steeply over the period, especially since 1956 when the law requiring disqualification in most cases was modified to make disqualification discretionary. The raw totals of convictions rose from just over 18,000 in 1954 to 47,930 in 1959: an increase of about 165 per cent. And even when weighted with the driving licence factor the incidence of convictions rose from 257·3 in 1954 to 484·1 in 1959: a more realistic rise, perhaps, but still one of 88 per cent (*Table 20*).

The movement of convictions can be seen plainly from the following index, using the raw totals of convictions given in the Home Office Returns (base year 1954 = 100).

Year	No. of convictions (000s)	Index 1954 = 100	Annual increase
1954	18·0	100	
1955	20·2	112	+12
1956	22·8	127	+15
1957	26·2	146	+19
1958	35·2	196	+50
1959	47·9	266	+70

Figure 8 brings out more clearly the steep rise in convictions for this offence, especially from 1957, and it will be noticed that it bears comparison with *Figure 5*, which shows the incidence of motoring offences in general by age groups. In the latter figure the upsurge of offences by the group aged 17 and under 21 seems to reflect the increased incidence of these insurance offences, which Chapters 7 and 8 show to be especially common among young motor cyclists. And, indeed, this could well be an offence that typifies the young motoring offender since its usual elements include: some irresponsibility and lack of business sense; the tendency to be using a borrowed vehicle; and shortage of money to pay a premium – or unwillingness to spend it on anything so mundane as insurance.

Another causal element in the increase of insurance offences is the related increase in taking and driving vehicles away without consent, an offence that automatically carries with it a conviction for driving uninsured.

This has been said to be a teenage phenomenon, and it is evident that it is, from the following raw totals of convictions for taking and driving away by magistrates' courts, as given in the *Criminal Statistics*:

Year	21 and over	17 and under 21	14 and under 17
1954	1,998	1,561	572
1955	2,045	1,861	660
1956	2,329	2,377	899
1957	2,385	3,170	1,203
1958	3,076	4,268	1,911
1959	3,185	4,632	2,674

These figures show percentage increases over the six-year period of 59 per cent for the group aged 21 and over, 196 per cent for those aged 17 and under 21, and about 367 per cent for those in the age group 14 and under 17. However, *in toto* those who take and drive away provide only 25 per cent of all the findings of guilt for failing to insure.

Hence the majority of insurance offences are not, apparently, associated with 'taking and driving away', and are, therefore, committed by either borrowers or owners. Where it is the former the reason for the offence is obvious, and it is often a misunderstanding between lender and borrower; but where it is an owner and the cause is not genuine misunderstanding or forgetfulness, it could be inability to afford the premiums—which, incidentally, were raised in the period 1957–58 and so may have made the less well-off youngster more prone to take chances and commit this offence.

A further factor contributing to the increase in insurance offences may be the growing extent of car ownership among the lower income groups that has been apparent since 1945. This may mean a greater number of 'old crocks' on the road: vehicles which are attractively cheap to buy, but very expensive – if not impossible – to insure. But here one can only speculate, because data to support these inferences are not available.

Finally there is the obvious possibility that an apparent toleration of this offence by the courts has stimulated its occurrence. Certainly the marked drop in offenders disqualified, from 88 per cent in 1954 to 37 per cent in 1959, and the stability in the proportions sent to prison (about 4·6 per cent) during the period, despite the rise in offences and convictions, give an impression of leniency that may not have been lost on potential offenders (cf. the view of a police officer to this effect, mentioned on p. 50 above).

But, whatever the explanation of the greatly increased incidence of this offence, there can be little doubt that those who fail to insure are major contributors to the present swollen condition of the statistics dealing with motoring offences.

The Size of the Problem

Failing to Stop after, or to Report, an Accident (RTA, 1960, section 77)

With its sinister implication of hit-and-run driving, it is disturbing at first to find that the raw total of convictions for this offence has risen by nearly 120 per cent, from 5,066 to 11,019, between 1954 and 1959: and the weighted total per 100,000 driving licences in issue has risen by 54 per cent (*Tables 13a* and *20*).

This is, however, a peculiarly difficult offence about which to draw inferences from statistics. For here again we have an offence that is often ancillary to others that can be more serious: causing death, dangerous driving, driving under the influence, and so on. And, as Selling (1941) has pointed out, the *mens rea* that is essential to this offence is often derived from the commission of another more serious: e.g. a case in which a motorist knocked down and killed a pedestrian on a deserted road after having taken drink and, thinking there were no witnesses and being aware of his state, fled from the scene. A further difficulty is the tendency of the police to charge 'failing to stop' as one offence, and 'failing to report' as another; hence two offences, under the same section of the Act, arise from the same single incident; a feature that must swell the figures for these offences quite considerably.

As might be expected, the proportion of these offences that is prosecuted is about the lowest of all the six we have looked at, since there is often considerable doubt as to whether the suspect knew there had been an incident; but, considering this difficulty, the proportion of those charged that results in conviction is quite high: between 82 and 85 per cent (*Table 19a*). Over the period there has, with one exception, been little change in the disposal of these offenders, though there was a slight increase from 94 to 96·7 per cent in the proportion fined (*Table 13a*). The exception is again in the proportion disqualified which, as in cases of failing to insure, has fallen considerably between 1954 and 1959, from ·30 to ·03 per cent, having risen to ·58 per cent in 1955; but, as *Table 13a* shows, the numbers disqualified are amazingly small. Perhaps this is once more the effect of linking this offence with others more serious, for which heavier penalties are awarded – a necessary procedure since, under the Acts of 1930 and 1960, disqualification could not be ordered for this offence by itself.

RECIDIVISM AMONG MOTORING OFFENDERS

Reference has been made already to the probable influence on the picture of motoring offences of those who offend repeatedly, and no survey of

Legal and Social Background

this kind would be complete without more discussion of this problem. An objective examination of the subject is, however, extremely difficult, if not impossible, because the data available are confined to indictable offences. The majority of motoring offenders are thus excluded. Moreover, no information is available from the official statistics after 1958, when methods of recording were changed.

Nevertheless, it is quite useful to consider the position among this small minority of offenders who committed indictable motoring offences, since enough has been said already to indicate that, by and large, these are the extreme element with whom the magistrates' courts do not feel competent to deal; though it must be remembered that there are a number of offenders who elect to be tried in the higher courts.

Table 25 (p. 167) shows the number of *different* persons convicted of indictable motoring offences who have records of previous indictable offences, and it distinguishes between previous motoring offences and indictable offences of other kinds. It reveals that about 15 per cent of all those convicted for indictable motoring offences between 1954 and 1958 had one indictable offence or more, *other* than motoring offences, on their records; and 10 per cent had two or more.

The proportion of offenders with one indictable motoring offence or more proved against them is much smaller, at about 3 per cent over the period, and only 1 per cent had two or more offences on their records. This difference may be because there is some tendency to select for indictment those with bad records for non-motoring offences, most others being dealt with summarily unless they choose otherwise. Chapters 8 and 10 show that very few motoring offenders appear before the higher courts unless they elect trial by jury. Hence a more likely explanation is that these 'experienced' offenders prefer trial by jury.

That there are some extremely persistent offenders is shown by the presence in both 1957 and 1958 of 27 persons with a history of five or more non-motoring indictable convictions; and in 1955 there were two persons with more than twenty. There is also one remarkable individual who, in 1955, had over twenty previous indictable *motoring* convictions.

Indeed it is of some interest that the actual number of persons with previous convictions for non-motoring offences increased from 40 in 1954 to 86 in 1958, having touched 99 in 1957. Though this evidence is slender, it would suggest that there is an increasing number of cases before the courts in which the motoring offender is not exactly devoid of criminal tendencies.

As mentioned above, no information is available from official sources

142

about the previous convictions of motoring offenders dealt with by magistrates' courts – an omission that the next part of this study will seek to rectify. It may be that there has been no real interest in the motoring offender's previous conduct off the road, since it is now usual for the police to produce in court only records of previous motoring offences unless the case is sent for trial or sentence to a higher court. Such a policy seems to reflect the idea that these offences are essentially different from the usual 'criminal' charge, and that it would be both unfair and irrelevant to produce evidence of previous non-motoring offences; though, of course, it must be added that the formidable administrative task of searching for records for so many offenders may have had much to do with the adoption of this policy. In the event, however, as this practice is the rule for the vast majority of motoring offenders, whose non-motoring offences are thus left unmentioned, it is hardly surprising that a stereotype is created of an 'otherwise blameless and respectable citizen who is only a criminal in a strictly technical sense'.

CONCLUSION

Having completed this general survey, we will now ask two questions. First, to what extent can the statistical picture be considered reliable; and second, which aspects of it should be singled out for special mention?

In answering the first question it is hardly necessary to underline the two major difficulties that seem to beset the presentation of the data, and certainly do beset their interpretation. One difficulty, common to all statistics of crime, arises from the number of different offences that can result from a single incident; as, for example, when a car that has been taken without the owner's consent is driven at a speed dangerous to the public, without being insured, by an unlicensed driver, who hits and causes bodily harm to another person, and does not stop or report the incident – a constellation of six motoring offences that could easily arise from one instance of 'taking a vehicle without the owner's consent'. Hence if the same individual takes several vehicles in the same year, he can do much to swell the statistics for all motoring offences. And a similar difficulty affects the one situation that the statistics should be able to depict with some accuracy: the treatment of offenders by the courts. Here it is hard to assess the degree of severity or leniency, since apparent leniency towards certain offences may stem from their accompanying other offences which carry the major punishments.

But, against this, one must offset the numerous motoring offences that never reach the courts; a 'dark number' that observation suggests is very considerable. They are, of course, an unknown quantity and it would be quite unsound to use them to support conclusions in a study that aims to be objective. All that can be said at this stage is that their existence must undermine any argument that the statistics here presented show an inflated and unduly pessimistic picture.

In answer to the second question posed above, four points are selected for special mention:

(a) The remarkable increase in motoring offences overall during the period, and especially in 1957, 1958, and 1959. This persists despite the 'weighting' of the totals by such factors as population and the number of current driving or vehicle licences. And it has been shown that, for a time (from 1954 to 1957 for indictable offences), the rise in the number of *vehicles* licensed did not affect the situation adversely (*Table 10*).

(b) Next for emphasis is the very high incidence of young offenders per head of the population since 1956. Their substantial lead among motoring offenders – a fairly recent phenomenon – puts a rather different complexion on the whole problem. For it suggests that motoring offences may proceed from the same set of attitudes that influence the other offences to which this age group is the dominant contributor.

(c) There is no evidence to show that the courts have responded to the manifest increase in motoring offences by the use of more severe treatment. On the contrary, it has been found that the one measure that has been strongly advocated – disqualification – was applied less as the period studied progressed. It also seems that there is substance for the belief that the probability of conviction is lower when an offender is sent for trial by jury than it is when he is dealt with by magistrates; though the sympathy of juries may be largely responsible, there are other incalculable factors: the complexity of the cases sent for trial, and the varying attitudes of judges to motoring offenders.

(d) Finally there is the prominence of the motor cycle as a means by which motoring offences are committed. This fact tends to be obscured by the much greater number of private cars involved. But the issue is plain when the numbers of each kind of vehicle are taken into account. And here again the spotlight falls on the younger offender.

Table 5

CRIMINAL STATISTICS FOR ENGLAND AND WALES COMPARED
WITH HOME OFFICE RETURNS OF OFFENCES RELATING TO
MOTOR VEHICLES: PERSONS FOUND GUILTY OF MOTORING
OFFENCES

(England and Wales 1954–59, all courts)

Year	Persons of all ages found guilty, whose principal offence was a motoring offence (Crim. Statist.)	Persons found guilty of motoring offences (Home Office Returns)	Difference between Column (b) and Column (c)
(a)	(b)[1]	(c)[2]	(d)
1954	335,124	337,077	1,953
1955	352,781	355,010	2,229
1956	397,562	400,438	2,876
1957	431,136	434,672	3,536
1958	532,040	539,743	7,703
1959	572,673	577,857	5,184

[1] Column (b) excludes offenders found guilty of a motoring offence where this was not the principal offence.

[2] Column (c) shows *all* offenders found guilty of motoring offences, including those where the motoring offence was dealt with in conjunction with another kind of offence.

Table 6

MOTORING OFFENDERS AND OTHER OFFENDERS
(*England and Wales 1954–59, all ages*)

Year	Total all offenders	Persons guilty of motoring offences[1]	Persons guilty of non-motoring offences	Motoring offenders as percentage of all offenders
	(*Crim. Statist.*)	(*Home Office Returns*)	(*Column (b) – Column (c)*)	(*Column (c) as % of Column (b)*)
(*a*)	(*b*)	(*c*)	(*d*)	(*e*)
1954	725,578	337,077	388,501	46·4
1955	735,288	355,010	380,278	48·2
1956	784,197	400,438	383,659	51·0
1957	864,475	434,672	429,803	50·3
1958	993,445	539,743	453,702	54·3
1959	1,040,796	577,857	462,939	55·5

[1] These figures are subject to a slight error since the totals included for the higher courts are convictions, not persons. It is unlikely, however, that the error would be such as to distort the picture at all.

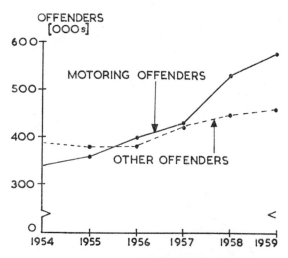

Figure 1. Offenders found guilty of motoring offences and those found guilty of other kinds of offence

(*England and Wales 1954–59, all courts*)

The Size of the Problem
Table 7

(*England and Wales 1954–59*)

Year	Population aged *14* and over[1]	Offenders found guilty of motoring offences (Home Office Returns)[2]		Offenders found guilty of other offences (Crim. Statist.)	
		Total	Per *100,000* of population aged *14* and over	Total	Per *100,000* of population aged *14* and over
1954	34,878,000	337,077	966	359,726	1,031
1955	34,943,000	355,010	1,016	351,296	1,005
1956	35,075,000	400,438	1,141	351,250	1,001
1957	35,274,000	434,672	1,232	393,142	1,114
1958	35,440,000	539,743	1,523	414,015	1,168
1959	35,655,000	577,857	1,621	422,694	1,185

[1] Population figures are derived from those used in the *Criminal Statistics* for England and Wales.

[2] These figures are subject to a slight error since the totals included for the higher courts are convictions, not persons. It is unlikely, however, that the error would be such as to distort the picture at all.

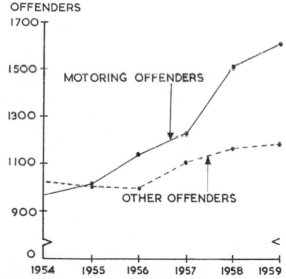

Figure 2. Offenders per 100,000 of the population aged 14 and over
(*England and Wales 1954–59, all courts*)

147

Table 8

COMPARATIVE INDICES OF MOTORING OFFENDERS, DRIVING
LICENCES IN ISSUE, AND MOTOR VEHICLES LICENSED
(*England and Wales 1954–59, 1954 = 100*)

Year	Motoring offenders		Driving licences		Motor vehicles licensed	
	Total	Index	Total	Index	Total	Index
			millions		millions	
1954	337,077	100	7·0	100	5·0	100
1955	355,010	106	7·6	108	5·6	112
1956	400,438	119	8·1	116	6·0	120
1957	434,672	130	8·4	120	6·5	130
1958	539,743	160	9·1	130	7·0	140
1959	577,857	171	9·9	142	7·6	152

Source: Home Office Returns and Ministry of Transport Returns of Motor
Vehicles Licensed and Driving Licences in Issue, 1954–59.

Note: Figures for licences and vehicles licensed were estimated to the nearest
hundred thousand by the Ministry of Transport Statistics Division.

Table 9

OFFENDERS FOUND GUILTY OF MOTORING OFFENCES PER
100,000 DRIVING LICENCES IN ISSUE AND 100,000
VEHICLES LICENSED
(*England and Wales 1954–59*)

Year	Offenders per 100,000 driving licences	Offenders per 100,000 vehicles licensed
1954	4,815	6,686
1955	4,671	6,316
1956	4,943	6,583
1957	5,174	6,648
1958	5,931	7,752
1959	5,836	7,600

Source: As *Table 8.*

The Size of the Problem

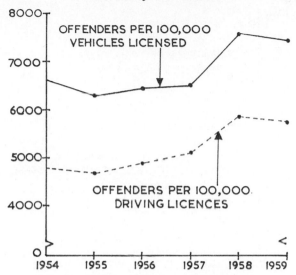

Figure 3. Offenders found guilty of motoring offences per 100,000 driving licences in issue and vehicles licensed
(*England and Wales 1954–59, all courts*)

Table 10

OFFENDERS FOUND GUILTY OF INDICTABLE MOTORING
OFFENCES PER 100,000 DRIVING LICENCES IN ISSUE AND
100,000 VEHICLES LICENSED

(*England and Wales 1954–59, all courts*)

Year	No. of offenders found guilty of indictable motoring offences	No. of driving licences in issue	No. of vehicle licences in issue	Offenders per 100,000 driving licences	Offenders per 100,000 vehicles licensed
		millions	*millions*		
1954	7,401	7·0	5·0	105·7	146·8
1955	8,084	7·6	5·6	105·5	143·8
1956	8,696	8·1	6·0	107·3	142·9
1957	9,173	8·4	6·5	109·2	140·3
1958	10,654	9·1	7·0	117·1	153·0
1959	12,667	9·9	7·6	127·9	166·6

Source: As Table 8.
Note: This table shows findings of guilt for causing death by dangerous driving, manslaughter, dangerous or reckless driving, and driving or being in charge while under the influence of drink or drugs.

149

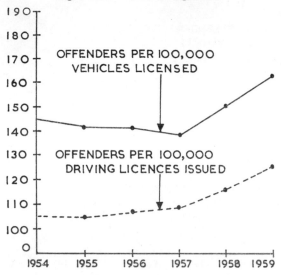

Figure 4. Offenders found guilty of indictable motoring offences per
100,000 driving licences in issue and vehicles licensed
(*England and Wales 1954–59, all courts*)

Table 11

NUMBER OF MOTORING OFFENCES REPORTED AND PROSECUTED
SHOWING PERCENTAGE OF FINDINGS OF GUILT
(*England and Wales 1954–59, all courts*)

Year	Total offences and alleged offences[1]	Offences prosecuted		Findings of guilt	
		Total	% of total offences and alleged offences	Total	% of offences prosecuted
1954	608,640	417,578	68·8	398,828	95·5
1955	643,855	446,451	69·4	426,315	95·5
1956	712,962	502,274	70·4	482,018	95·9
1957	776,609	542,711	69·8	522,658	96·2
1958	1,004,085	698,924	69·6	673,853	96·4
1959	1,070,633	772,003	72·2	744,783	95·2

Source : Home Office Returns, 1954–59.

[1] These are offences 'cleared up', where the alternatives were either to prosecute or
to issue a written warning. They are not, therefore, quite the same thing as 'offences
known to the police', which include offences *not* cleared up.

Table 12

DISPOSAL OF MOTORING OFFENDERS WHERE DETAILS OF SENTENCE ARE RECORDED

(England and Wales 1954–59, all motoring offenders – magistrates' courts)

Year	Total findings of guilt	Absolute or conditional discharge		Fined		Imprisonment without the option of a fine		Disqualified	
		Total	% of those guilty	Total	% of those guilty	Total	% of those guilty	Total	% of those guilty
1954	336,628	8,235	2·4	327,242	97·2	988	·29	18,878	5·6
1955	354,506	7,644	2·1	345,507	97·5	1,186	·33	21,683	6·2
1956	399,867	7,435	1·8	390,799	97·7	1,305	·32	24,301	6·1
1957	433,972	7,259	1·6	424,965	97·9	1,297	·29	16,323	3·8
1958	538,874	8,187	1·5	525,544	97·5	1,619	·30	18,843	3·5
1959	576,853	8,703	1·5	565,155	98·0	2,089	·36	29,016	5·2

Source: Home Office Returns, 1954–59

Table 13

SENTENCES PASSED FOR SERIOUS MOTORING OFFENCES WHERE DETAILS OF SENTENCE ARE RECORDED

(England and Wales 1954–59, all courts)

Year	Total findings of guilt	DETAILS OF SENTENCE					
		Absolute or conditional discharge		Fined		Prison or Borstal	
		Total	% of those guilty	Total	% of those guilty	Total	% of those guilty
MANSLAUGHTER AND CAUSING DEATH							
1954	9					9	100
1955	3					3	100
1956	4					4	100
1957	147			65	44·2	65	44·2
1958	175	2	1·1	90	51·4	68	38·8
1959	228			115	50·4	84	36·8
DRIVING RECKLESSLY OR DANGEROUSLY							
1954	4,380	43	·98	4,161	95·0	113	2·5
1955	4,770	28	·58	4,513	94·6	156	3·3
1956	4,948	23	·46	4,712	95·2	148	2·9
1957	5,084	28	·55	4,864	95·6	117	2·3
1958	6,195	32	·51	5,969	96·3	113	1·8
1959	7,410	18	·24	7,124	96·1	167	2·2
DRIVING OR IN CHARGE UNDER THE INFLUENCE OF DRINK OR DRUGS							
1954	3,012	10	·33	2,796	92·8	177	5·8
1955	3,311	5	·15	3,059	92·3	209	6·3
1956	3,795	8	·21	3,543	93·2	210	5·6
1957	3,942	13	·32	3,703	93·9	182	4·6
1958	4,284	12	·28	4,042	94·3	180	4·2
1959	5,029	8	·16	4,747	94·3	209	4·1

Notes: (i) Details of disqualifications cannot be shown in this table because they are not recorded for the higher courts. Nor are disposals shown for driving while disqualified, failing to insure, or failing to stop, in cases heard in the higher courts.

(ii) Where the percentages do not total 100, as in causing death, no separate punishment was recorded for a number of offences.

(iii) In the Home Office Returns a few cases of causing bodily harm are shown. These are *not* included in *Table 13*.

Table 13a

SENTENCES PASSED FOR SERIOUS MOTORING OFFENCES WHERE DETAILS OF SENTENCE ARE RECORDED

(England and Wales 1954–59, magistrates' courts)

Year	Total findings of guilt	Absolute or conditional discharge		Fined		Prison		Disqualified	
		Total	% of those guilty	Total	% of those guilty	Total	% of those guilty	Total	% of those guilty
DRIVING WHILE DISQUALIFIED									
1954	1,612	136	8·5	836	51·8	558	34·6	190	11·7
1955	1,987	142	7·0	983	49·5	733	36·8	272	13·6
1956	2,455	226	9·2	1,203	49·0	845	34·5	326	13·2
1957	1,385	25	1·8	362	26·1	846	61·0	441	32·0
1958	1,708	36	2·1	458	26·7	988	57·8	494	28·9
1959	2,543	54	2·1	750	29·5	1,424	55·9	862	33·9
FAILING TO INSURE AGAINST THIRD-PARTY RISKS									
1954	18,011	824	4·6	16,135	89·6	849	4·7	15,961	88·6
1955	20,202	705	3·5	18,168	89·9	1,008	5·0	17,973	89·0
1956	22,857	713	3·1	20,585	91·0	1,148	4·4	19,061	83·1
1957	26,228	1,978	4·1	23,400	89·3	1,167	4·4	10,255	39·1
1958	35,232	1,365	3·8	31,652	89·8	1,439	4·0	12,089	34·3
1959	47,930	1,894	3·9	42,694	89·0	2,249	4·7	17,628	36·7
FAILING TO STOP AFTER, OR TO REPORT, AN ACCIDENT									
1954	5,066	304	5·9	4,759	93·9	1	·02	15	·30
1955	6,360	329	5·2	6,027	94·7	2	·03	37	·58
1956	6,849	325	4·7	6,517	95·1	4	·06	34	·49
1957	7,090	294	4·1	6,795	95·8	0		7	·01
1958	8,703	322	3·7	8,377	96·2	2	·02	4	·05
1959	11,019	349	3·2	10,663	96·7	7	·06	3	·03

Source: Home Office Returns, 1954–59.

Note: This table excludes causing bodily harm and offences shown as 'not accounted for' or 'otherwise disposed of'.

Table *14*

OFFENDERS AGED 14 AND OVER WHOSE PRINCIPAL OFFENCE
WAS A MOTORING OFFENCE, PER 100,000 OF THE
POPULATION IN THE AGE GROUP
(*England and Wales 1954–59*)

Age group	1954	1955	1956	1957	1958	1959
ALL COURTS						
14 and under 17	102·7	135·6	175·1	224·8	262·4	441·4
17 and under 21	698·3	912·1	1,082·6	1,535·5	2,195·9	2,766·9
21 and over	1,026·4	1,063·8	1,189·0	1,256·7	1,528·2	1,592·3
HIGHER COURTS						
14 and under 17	–	–	–	–	–	·05
17 and under 21	·13	·23	·21	·63	·73	2·8
21 and under 30	·92	1·10	1·53	2·02	2·33	3·2
30 and over	1·05	1·15	1·20	1·45	1·95	2·0
MAGISTRATES' COURTS						
14 and under 17	102·7	135·6	175·1	224·8	262·4	441·4
17 and under 21	698·2	911·9	1,082·4	1,534·9	2,195·2	2,764·3
21 and over	1,024·4	1,061·6	1,186·3	1,253·2	1,523·9	1,593·6

Source: Criminal Statistics, *England and Wales,* 1954–59
Note: The figures do not take into account those charged with manslaughter;
and those charged with causing death by dangerous driving appear only in the year
1956 and thereafter.

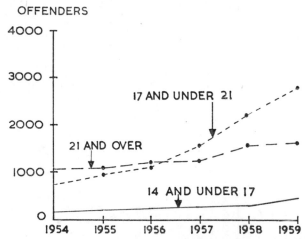

Figure 5. Offenders aged 14 and over whose principal offence was a
motoring offence, per 100,000 of the population in the age group
(*England and Wales 1954–59, all courts*)

154

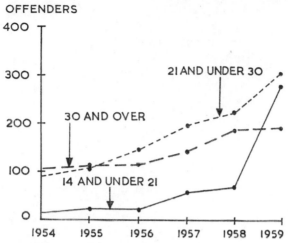

Figure 5a. Offenders aged 14 and over whose principal offence was an indictable motoring offence, per 100,000 of the population in the age group

(England and Wales 1954–59, higher courts)

Table 15

OFFENDERS AGED 14 AND OVER WHOSE PRINCIPAL OFFENCE
WAS A NON-MOTORING OFFENCE, PER 100,000 OF THE
POPULATION IN THE AGE GROUP
(England and Wales 1954–59, all courts)

Age group	1954	1955	1956	1957	1958	1959
14 and under 17	1,962·5	1,775·1	1,956·3	2,343·0	2,472·3	2,596·9
17 and under 21	1,927·9	1,925·6	2,128·3	2,617·2	3,144·8	3,112·3
21 and over	989·9	908·5	881·9	965·5	977·7	971·8

Source: Criminal Statistics, England and Wales, 1954–59

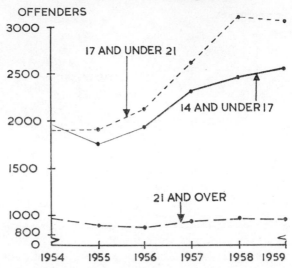

Figure 6. Offenders aged 14 and over whose principal offence was a non-motoring offence, per 100,000 of the population in the age group (*England and Wales 1954–59, all courts*)

Table 16

OFFENDERS AGED 14 AND OVER WHOSE PRINCIPAL OFFENCE
WAS AN INDICTABLE NON-MOTORING OFFENCE, PER 100,000
OF THE POPULATION IN THE AGE GROUP

(*England and Wales 1954–59, higher courts*)

Age group	*1954*	*1955*	*1956*	*1957*	*1958*	*1959*
14 and under 21	103	104	123	153	207	207
21 and under 30	112	110	122	141	172	184
30 and over	25	23	24	26	28	30

Source: Criminal Statistics, England and Wales, 1954–59

156

OFFENDERS

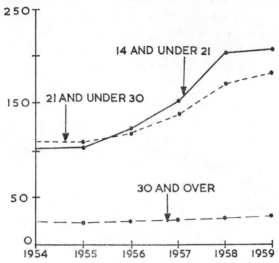

Figure 7. Offenders aged 14 and over whose principal offence was an indictable non-motoring offence, per 100,000 of the population in the age group

(*England and Wales 1954–59, higher courts*)

Table 17

OFFENDERS WHOSE PRINCIPAL OFFENCE WAS A MOTORING OFFENCE – COMPARISON OF MALE AND FEMALE RATES PER 100,000 OF THE POPULATION AGED 14 AND OVER

(*England and Wales 1954–59, all courts*)

Year	Males	Females	Ratio of male to female
1954	1,934	88	22·0:1
1955	2,012	109	18·4:1
1956	2,265	115	19·7:1
1957	2,440	124	19·6:1
1958	2,997	152	19·6:1
1959	3,218	153	21·0:1

Source : Criminal Statistics, England and Wales, 1954–59

Table 18

OFFENDERS WHOSE PRINCIPAL OFFENCE
WAS NOT A MOTORING OFFENCE – COM-
PARISON OF MALE AND FEMALE RATES PER
100,000 OF THE POPULATION AGED 14 AND
OVER

(England and Wales 1954–59, all courts)

Year	Males	Females	Ratio of male to female
1954	1,733	301	5·7:1
1955	1,703	278	6·1:1
1956	1,841	262	7·0:1
1957	2,050	293	7·0:1
1958	2,148	325	6·6:1
1959	2,223	279	7·9:1

Source: Criminal Statistics, England and Wales, 1954–59

Table 19

INCIDENCE OF SERIOUS MOTORING OFFENCES

(England and Wales 1954–59, all courts)

Year	Total offences and alleged offences[1]	Offences prosecuted		Findings of guilt	
		Total	% of total offences and alleged offences	Total	% of offences prosecuted
MANSLAUGHTER AND CAUSING DEATH					
1954	35	35	100	9	25·7
1955	29	29	100	3	10·3
1956	41	41	100	4	10·0
1957	251	251	100	147	58·5
1958	357	357	100	175	49·0
1959	376	376	100	228	61·0
DRIVING RECKLESSLY OR DANGEROUSLY					
1954	5,865	5,794	98·7	4,380	75·5
1955	6,071	6,023	99·2	4,770	79·1
1956	5,972	5,920	99·1	4,948	83·5
1957	6,092	6,051	99·3	5,084	84·1
1958	7,447	7,407	99·4	6,195	83·6
1959	8,823	8,715	98·7	7,410	85·0
DRIVING OR IN CHARGE UNDER THE INFLUENCE OF DRINK OR DRUGS					
1954	3,609	3,608	99·9	3,012	83·4
1955	3,869	3,867	99·9	3,311	86·1
1956	4,458	4,456	99·9	3,795	85·1
1957	4,656	4,654	99·9	3,942	84·7
1958	5,073	5,066	99·8	4,284	84·6
1959	5,720	5,715	99·9	5,029	88·0

Source: Home Office Returns, 1954–59.

[1] These are offences 'cleared up', where the alternatives were to prosecute or to issue a written warning. They are not, therefore, quite the same thing as 'offences known to the police', which include offences *not* cleared up.

Legal and Social Background

Table 19a

INCIDENCE OF SERIOUS MOTORING OFFENCES

(*England and Wales 1954–59, magistrates' courts*)

Year	Total offences and alleged offences[1]	Offences prosecuted		Findings of guilt	
		Total	% of total offences and alleged offences	Total	% of offences prosecuted
DRIVING WHILE DISQUALIFIED[2]					
1954	1,900	1,803	94·8	1,612	89·4
1955	2,321	2,216	95·2	1,987	89·9
1956	2,895	2,776	95·8	2,455	88·4
1957	1,615	1,611	99·9	1,385	85·9
1958	1,918	1,909	99·8	1,708	89·4
1959	2,885	2,866	99·1	2,543	88·7
FAILING TO INSURE AGAINST THIRD-PARTY RISKS[2]					
1954	20,209	19,385	95·9	18,011	92·9
1955	22,769	21,687	95·1	20,202	92·3
1956	25,556	24,495	95·8	22,857	93·3
1957	29,317	28,091	95·8	26,228	93·3
1958	38,864	37,279	95·9	35,232	94·5
1959	52,503	50,707	96·5	47,930	94·5
FAILING TO STOP AFTER, OR TO REPORT, AN ACCIDENT[2]					
1954	10,322	6,196	59·0	5,066	81·7
1955	12,355	7,626	59·2	6,360	83·4
1956	13,185	8,204	62·0	6,849	83·5
1957	12,750	8,424	64·5	7,090	84·1
1958	14,885	10,185	68·0	8,703	85·4
1959	18,178	13,023	71·6	11,019	84·6

Source : Home Office Returns, 1954–59.

[1] These are offences 'cleared up', where the alternatives were to prosecute or to issue a written warning. They are not, therefore, quite the same thing as 'offences known to the police', which include offences *not* cleared up.

[2] These offences are shown for magistrates' courts only; figures are not available for higher courts, but few are committed for sentence.

160

Table 20

FINDINGS OF GUILT FOR SERIOUS MOTORING OFFENCES PER
100,000 DRIVING LICENCES IN ISSUE

(*England and Wales 1954–59, all courts*)

Offence	1954	1955	1956	1957	1958	1959
Causing death or manslaughter	·12	·04	·05	1·3	1·9	2·3
Driving recklessly or dangerously	62·0	62·7	61·0	60·6	68·0	72·1
Driving or in charge under the influence of drink or drugs	43·0	43·5	46·8	47·0	47·0	50·8
Driving while disqualified	23·0	26·1	30·3	16·4	18·7	25·7
Failing to insure against third-party risks	257·3	265·8	282·1	312·2	387·1	484·1
Failing to stop after or to report an accident	72·3	83·6	84·5	84·4	95·6	111·2

Source : Home Office Returns and Ministry of Transport Returns of Vehicles Licensed and Driving Licences in Issue, 1954–59.

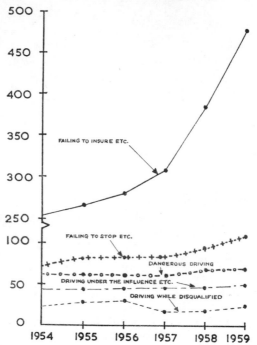

Figure 8. Findings of guilt for serious motoring offences per 100,000
driving licences in issue
(*England and Wales 1954–59, all courts*)

Table 20a

FINDINGS OF GUILT FOR CARELESS DRIVING PER 100,000
DRIVING LICENCES IN ISSUE

(*England and Wales 1954–59, magistrates' courts*)

Offence	1954	1955	1956	1957	1958	1959
Careless driving	423·0	461·2	462·4	461·0	516·5	558·3

Table 21

FINES AND PRISON SENTENCES IMPOSED ON THOSE AGED 14
AND OVER FOUND GUILTY OF CERTAIN OFFENCES AGAINST
THE PERSON

(England and Wales 1954–59)

Year	Total guilty	Fined		Imprisoned	
		Total	% of those convicted	Total	% of those convicted
ALL COURTS					
1954	14,595	8,305	57·0	1,800	12·4
1955	15,065	8,756	57·8	1,944	12·9
1956	15,959	9,426	59·0	2,111	13·2
1957	17,514	10,571	60·1	2,332	13·3
1958	18,091	11,181	61·6	2,615	14·5
1959	20,161	12,149	60·3	2,772	13·7
HIGHER COURTS					
1954	831	83	9·3	494	58·1
1955	871	91	9·8	545	60·2
1956	993	110	10·4	619	59·8
1957	1,162	132	10·6	719	61·4
1958	1,338	151	10·8	863	65·1
1959	1,558	176	11·3	984	63·2
MAGISTRATES' COURTS					
1954	13,664	8,222	60·1	1,306	9·5
1955	14,194	8,665	61·0	1,399	9·8
1956	14,906	9,316	62·5	1,492	10·0
1957	16,352	10,439	63·9	1,613	9·8
1958	16,753	11,030	65·8	1,752	10·4
1959	18,603	11,973	64·4	1,788	9·6

Source: Criminal Statistics, England and Wales, 1954–59.

Notes: (i) The offences included in the above are principal offences charged under manslaughter (except where death was caused by driving), felonious wounding, malicious wounding, assault, aggravated assault, assault against a constable, and common assault.

(ii) Where the offender was aged 14 and under 17, 'imprisonment' means all committals to approved schools and detention centres. For those over 17 Borstal sentences are also included.

163

Table 22

A COMPARISON OF HIGHER AND MAGISTRATES' COURTS IN RESPECT OF TREATMENT ACCORDED TO TWO SPECIFIC MOTORING OFFENCES

(England and Wales 1954–59)

Year	Total offences handled	Total findings of guilt	% of offences handled	SENTENCES			
				Prison Total	Prison % of findings of guilt	Fines Total	Fines % of findings of guilt
DRIVING RECKLESSLY OR DANGEROUSLY – HIGHER COURTS							
1954	237	186	78·5	32	17·2	87	46·8
1955	182[1]	186[1]	—	39	21·0	85	45·7
1956	248	196	79·0	36	18·4	107	54·6
1957	242	185	76·4	10	5·4	119	64·3
1958	276	195	70·7	14	7·2	121	62·0
1959	309	233	75·4	24	10·4	120	51·5
DRIVING RECKLESSLY OR DANGEROUSLY – MAGISTRATES' COURTS							
1954	5,557	4,202	75·6	81	1·9	4,074	96·9
1955	5,841	4,584	78·4	116	2·5	4,428	96·3
1956	5,672	4,752	83·7	112	2·3	4,605	97·5
1957	5,821	4,899	84·1	107	2·1	4,745	96·8
1958	7,131	6,000	84·1	99	1·7	5,848	97·5
1959	8,406	7,177	85·4	143	2·0	7,004	97·4

DRIVING OR IN CHARGE UNDER THE INFLUENCE OF DRINK OR DRUGS – HIGHER COURTS

1954	486	206	19	43·4	166	80·0
1955	476	243	27	51·0	189	77·7
1956	570	254	26	44·6	201	79·1
1957	609	247	19	40·6	194	78·6
1958	731	371	23	50·8	306	82·5
1959	718	394	26	54·9	319	81·0

DRIVING OR IN CHARGE UNDER THE INFLUENCE OF DRINK OR DRUGS – MAGISTRATES' COURTS

1954	3,122	2,806	158	89·8	2,630	93·7
1955	3,391	3,068	182	90·4	2,870	93·5
1956	3,886	3,541	184	91·1	3,342	94·3
1957	4,045	3,695	163	91·3	3,509	94·9
1958	4,335	3,913	157	90·2	3,736	95·4
1959	4,997	4,635	183	92·7	4,428	95·5

Source: Home Office Returns, 1954–59.

1 This is a statistical mystery; the reason for it is not clear, unless four cases heard in higher courts were held over from cases sent up for trial in the previous year, or a number of cases sent for trial on other charges were convicted of dangerous driving as an alternative.

Notes: (i) Total offences handled in the magistrates' courts are exclusive of those sent for trial to the higher courts.
(ii) Disposals not included in the table are those recorded as 'no separate punishment' or 'otherwise disposed of'.

Table 23

USE OF DISQUALIFICATION IN THE MAGISTRATES' COURTS FOR TWO OFFENCES

(England and Wales 1954–59)

Year	Total findings of guilt	Total disqualified	% of findings of guilt
DRIVING RECKLESSLY OR DANGEROUSLY			
1954	4,202	1,322	31·4
1955	4,584	1,593	34·7
1956	4,752	1,949	41·0
1957	4,899	1,994	40·7
1958	6,000	2,187	36·4
1959	7,177	3,414	47·5
DRIVING OR IN CHARGE UNDER THE INFLUENCE OF DRINKS OR DRUGS			
1954	2,806	2,723	97·0
1955	3,068	2,981	97·1
1956	3,541	3,426	96·7
1957	3,695	3,231	87·4
1958	3,913	3,349	85·5
1959	4,635	3,951	85·2

Source: Home Office Returns, 1954–59.
[1] Details of disqualifications are not shown for the higher courts.

Table 24

THE RELATIONSHIP BETWEEN DISQUALIFICATIONS AND CONVICTIONS FOR DRIVING WHILE DISQUALIFIED

(England and Wales 1954–59, magistrates' courts)

Year	Number disqualified for all motoring offences	Index 1954 = 100	Number of convictions for driving while disqualified	Index 1954 = 100
1954	18,878	100	1,612	100
1955	21,683	115	1,987	124
1956	24,301	128	2,455	154
1957	16,323	86	1,385	87
1958	18,843	100	1,708	106
1959	29,016	154	2,543	158

Source: Home Office Returns, 1954–59

The Size of the Problem

Table 25

SERIOUS MOTORING OFFENDERS AND PREVIOUSLY PROVED INDICTABLE OFFENCES

(England and Wales 1954–58,[1] *all courts)*

The number of *different* persons aged 14 and over found guilty whose principal offence was an indictable *motoring* offence: showing the number of indictable *motoring* offences and the number of indictable offences of *all* categories previously proved against the offenders.

Year	Number guilty	Previous indictable motoring offences						Previous indictable offences – all categories						
		0	1	2	3	4	5/10	0	1	2	3	4	5/10	11/20
1954	322[2]	309	10	2	–	–	1	282	8	11	5	4	7	5
1955	357[2]	341	8	3	3	1	1[3]	305	12	8	4	5	15	8[4]
1956	400	391	7	1	–	–	1	332	26	11	8	3	14	6
1957	503	490	8	4	1	–	–	404	39	19	9	5	19	8
1958	627	604	17	3	2	1	–	541	34	11	7	7	22	5

Source: Home Office Supplementary Statistics relating to Crime and Criminal Proceedings in the years 1954–58.

[1] Information is not available for 1959 owing to changes in the structure of the statistical tables.

[2] Totals for 1954 and 1955 exclude motoring offenders found guilty of manslaughter.

[3] This offender had over 20 previous offences proved.

[4] Two offenders had over 20 previous offences proved.

PART TWO

The Documentary Study

653 SERIOUS MOTORING OFFENDERS
AND THEIR OFFENCES

6

The Police District

The Police District chosen for this study has been disguised to some extent in the description that follows, since it is desirable that offenders and informants should not be identified. This consideration has limited the information that could be presented.

The District lies in one of the Home Counties. It includes a number of boroughs and some rural districts, but most of its local authorities are urban districts. In 1961 the population of the District was just over half a million.

Some idea of the sociological composition of the District can be obtained from the percentages of occupied and retired males in the Registrar-General's occupational groups as shown in the 1951 census. One of the major hypotheses in this study concerns occupational distribution, and relevant data may be obtained by comparing the District in this respect with England and Wales as a whole (*Table 26*).

Table 26

PERCENTAGE OF OCCUPIED AND RETIRED MALES
AGED 14 AND OVER, 1951

Registrar-General's occupational class	Police District	England and Wales
	%	%
I. Professional, etc.	7	3
II. Intermediate	17	15
III. Skilled	53	53
IV. Partly skilled	14	16
V. Unskilled	9	13

Source: Census England and Wales, 1951 (data for 1961 not available at time of writing).

Although the Registrar-General's occupational distribution has been much criticized, as mentioned above (p. 44), there is relatively little dispute about the representative nature of Groups I and V, and it is in respect of these two classes that the Police District shows the greatest divergence from the country as a whole. In other words, it is highly probable that the upper occupational classes are *over*-represented, and the lower classes *under*-represented in the District. Hence the hypothesis that the serious motoring offender comes typically from the ranks of the well-to-do is being examined under conditions that are not ideal.

For police purposes the District is divided into eight divisions, each centred upon a town and coming under the jurisdiction of one or sometimes two magistrates' courts. Two courts of assize and two of quarter sessions provide the higher courts for the district. The great majority of the magistrates' courts are manned by lay justices, and there are no stipendiaries.

The eight divisions and the courts are linked as follows:

Division	Court
A	Opsley
B	Batwick; Treeford
C	Batwick; Elston
D	Barchet; Seabridge
E	Lesdon
F	Sefford; Mesley
G	Sefford; Mesley
H	Frockton; Barling

Let us now look at each of the divisions in detail.

Division A is probably the most built-up of all the divisions; it includes three urban districts in which the Registrar-General's Classes III, IV, and V are unusually well represented for this Police District. There are several council housing estates and caravan sites, as well as expensive residential areas. The traffic is at a high density all the year round; it is of all kinds, including a substantial holiday flow along two major trunk roads which pass through the division. It has a single magistrates' court at Opsley, which is one of the busiest in the District for motoring cases. A depot of the police mobile squad is located in the division, so it is probably subject to more police attention than most of the other divisions.

Division B tends to be more residential and suburban than Division A though the population does not contain an unduly high proportion of white-collar residents. Two major trunk roads pass through this division also and both are much used by holiday traffic; one is narrow and winding for a major road and it has more than its share of stretches where overtaking is very dangerous: long slow-moving queues of traffic are common, especially in the summer. The division also includes a large race-course which adds to its traffic problems. It has two courts: Batwick, the business of which is confined to the division; and Treeford, the cases for which come mostly from another police district. It was the fifth busiest division for offences in this study.

Division C includes a large borough, and its population is well balanced according to the Registrar-General's classification, since about 76 per cent of occupied and retired males are in Classes III, IV, and V. It lies astride two major trunk roads, one of which is shared with Division B, and the other is a holiday route that is one of the busiest roads in Britain in all seasons. Though it ranks seventh for activity so far as the serious offences dealt with here are concerned, it is a busy division for motoring cases and it makes full use of two magistrates' courts: Batwick, which is shared with Division B; and Elston, which deals mostly with divisional cases.

Division D lies on the boundary of the District and its parent county, and is considered by the police to be the quietest division; indeed it did produce the lowest number of offences for this research. However it also has two trunk roads passing through it that have particularly heavy traffic during the holiday season, and there is a very busy bottleneck junction where they meet. The division tends to be more rural and residential than the others, but it includes a substantial council housing estate and 'overspill' housing area in which Classes IV and V are prominent, as well as a large military training establishment and depot on its borders. It has two courts: Barchet, which is exclusive to it; and Seabridge, which is shared with another police district.

Division E is another well-balanced area sociologically since it is mostly urban and built-up, with a very large council estate for London's overspill population. There is also a large military training establishment in the division, and a number of summer camp sites used by the army and youth organizations. It contains a high proportion of busy major roads, and the incidence of all kinds of traffic is high throughout the year. The division has one magistrates' court at Lesdon, and it ranks sixth for 'business' in this research.

Division F combines a small borough and a rural district. Rather surprisingly, however, it is the division with the highest proportion of Social Classes III, IV, and V: 79·6 per cent of occupied and retired males are in these classes. It contains several local authority housing estates and a large number of agricultural workers. Also in this division are the two wealthiest residential areas in the District, one of which has the highest proportion (11 per cent) of Social Class I in any division. There are three very busy major trunk roads passing through; they are much used by all kinds of traffic, but there is a big increase in the summer months owing to holiday makers. It should be mentioned that this division includes one of the worst 'black spots' for accidents in the District: a particularly acute bend. The division ranks third for activity in this research and it has two magistrates' courts at Sefford and Mesley which it shares with Division G.

Division G includes the largest of the boroughs in the District, and its population is well balanced sociologically, with about 76 per cent of occupied and retired males in Classes III, IV, and V. It has several local authority housing estates and caravan sites, but a substantial part is residential. It lies astride six major trunk roads with a very high density of traffic all the year round, and it contains one of the major bottlenecks for holiday traffic in Britain. There are two notoriously 'fast stretches' of major road which have more than a fair share of accidents and offences. The two courts of Sefford and Mesley, which it shares with Division F, are among the busiest in the whole District. County Police Headquarters is located in the division and also a depot of the mobile squad.

Division H is an area with a high proportion of working-class people living in council housing estates and on caravan sites. It is possible that the 1951 census estimate of nearly 79 per cent in Social Classes III, IV, and V is an underestimate, for there has since been a big influx of population under London's overspill schemes. The division contains an unusually large Service population because several garrisons and training establishments are located within it; it also borders on a big military centre. There is none the less a fairly high proportion of Social Classes I and II (21 per cent), owing to the number of retired and serving officers of the armed forces who live in the area. The division is mostly urban and built-up, with a high density of traffic of all kinds. A major trunk road passes through, and it is one of the busiest in Britain with much commuting and heavy goods traffic; it also has a bottleneck for holiday traffic, and long queues of traffic are frequent during bank holidays and throughout the summer. The division has two magistrates' courts at Frockton and Barling.

THE POLICE

At the time of the research (1958–60) the police force in the District consisted of just over 800 men and about 30 women; it was therefore just over 100 personnel short of the establishment considered appropriate by the Standing Joint Committee of the parent county. The regulars were supplemented by about 700 men and 20 women of the Special Constabulary, a part-time force whose training does not permit members to assume full responsibility for dealing with cases after apprehension, when it is usual for a regular officer to take over.

The force is controlled by the chief constable from police headquarters, where there are the usual specialized departments and sections, including the Traffic Section. The latter consists of a number of mobile units which were equipped with Austin A105 or Sunbeam Rapier saloon cars and solo motor cycles, all carrying radio providing two-way communication with headquarters operations centre and with divisions. The cars were based at two depots in Divisions A and G, and the motor cycles were attached to divisions; but the whole Traffic Section with its car or motor-cycle patrols really forms a self-contained element of the force having its own command and control structure. Its patrols cover the entire District, but when initiating charges its members work through the division in which the offence occurred.

The basic organization of the force is, however, the police division, of which there are eight as described above. Each division is controlled by a superintendent with a chief inspector as his deputy and second-in-command; administration is dealt with by the divisional office under a sergeant with a small staff. Also at divisional headquarters is a small CID section under a detective inspector, with its own clerical staff.

The divisions are divided into subdivisions controlled by an inspector who is responsible for a number of sections, each under a sergeant and consisting of a variable number of constables. In rural areas the section sergeant has a 24-hour responsibility for supervising his 'beats' (the beat of each constable), but in urban areas this responsibility is shared by a number of sergeants known as 'town sergeants'. The subdivisions may also have a detachment of the CID, and probably one or two women police officers. Mobility at subdivisional level is provided by one or more light utility vans and a few motor cycles, all fitted with two-way radio.

Regarding the state of efficiency of the regular force, it may be thought that the writer's indebtedness alone would inhibit criticism, so that any praise could be dismissed as mere politeness. But, if compliments were unjustified, it would be easy – and quite proper – to say nothing and leave it at that. So when it is said that the high state of efficiency and sound training of the force were impressive, the statement can be taken to be quite sincere. Indeed it was noticeable that nearly all the cases reviewed in this study reflected a praiseworthy discipline and attention to detail, and the standards expected of quite young and inexperienced officers by their superiors were exceedingly high. (No comment is made on the 'specials', because little or nothing was seen of them in action, and they figure hardly at all in the cases studied.)

The manner in which the police handle motoring cases has already been described in Chapter 4 above.

THE COURTS

It has been seen that each police division is under the jurisdiction of specific magistrates' courts, and that these do not change. Hence it is to be expected that a rather special relationship would grow between the divisional police and the bench. That this was a good relationship was manifest in every division; indeed it may lend some support to the idea among offenders that the police and the courts are a corporate institution and that they are 'in league' with each other. Such a conception is likely to be reinforced by the practice in this District whereby the police conduct prosecutions in many cases, and provide the court ushers; also, as in most places in England, the courts are often in the same enclosure as the police station and are sometimes even in the same building. Yet, as Hood (1962, p. 8) found in a study of sentencing in magistrates' courts: 'It would be a wrong impression . . . if the magistrates' courts were to be seen as servants of the police; for the position is quite the reverse.'

As to the treatment of offenders in court – apart from sentencing, which is dealt with in Chapter 9 below – only one thing was striking: the subtle distinction made between motoring offenders and other offenders, in that the former never occupied the dock, but sat on a chair placed specially in front of it. However, until called, the motoring offenders waited in the hall of the court with all the others, from whom, it must be said, it was not easy to pick them out.

But there was another rather interesting point about the motoring offenders that might be mentioned: the rather incongruous fact that so many of them apparently came to court in their cars, without anyone to drive them away if they were unlucky enough to be disqualified. One offender was in a particularly awkward predicament after disqualification because he had come in a loaded ten-ton lorry; yet he had been charged with what appeared to be a cut-and-dried case of dangerous driving, and it seems strange that the man did not expect to be disqualified. In another case a medical practitioner was charged with dangerous driving: he had hit a pedestrian after overtaking another car on a main road at a speed well in excess of the limit. He drove to court by himself, in an immaculate Jaguar, apparently confident that he would 'get off lightly'. Though it was hard to see why he should have been treated leniently, his conviction was reduced to exceeding the speed limit and he escaped with a fine. However, it could be that a defendant who so anticipates conviction and disqualification that he goes to court in a cab is making a tacit admission of guilt!

Generally speaking, nothing remarkable was found about the courts in the District, either from personal inspection or from hearsay; they seemed to be respected by the police and the public, though, as we shall see, some were reputed to be more severe than others.

SUMMARY

To summarize the characteristics of the District, it seems to be fairly well balanced from a sociological standpoint, and not as unrepresentative in terms of age, sex, and occupational distribution as had been expected. Although some of its areas are very popular for retirement, the numbers of elderly people who live there are offset by the very substantial population of young people in the council housing estates and overspill scheme areas, to say nothing of the considerable number of servicemen in military establishments. Also the social classes, in the occupational sense of the term, are quite well distributed. Urban and rural areas are represented without an undue proportion of the former, considering the proximity of the District to the London area. From a topographical standpoint the District is in no way unusual, being neither mountainous nor flat, and including in its 1,500 miles of road a high proportion of major trunk roads that are used by a great variety of traffic all the year round.

In the event, the choice of area proved to have been fortunate: it was a choice that was largely fortuitous and dependent on the interest and enthusiasm for the study of the chairman of the quarter sessions and the chief constable.

7

The Offences

INCIDENCE

The total number of cases analysed was 653, distributed among the eight divisions of the Police District as shown in *Table 27*. It is stressed that this is the total number of cases that came within the terms of reference of this research, and it will not cross-check with the statistics for prosecutions shown in the Home Office Returns of *Offences relating to Motor Vehicles*, or with the returns of convictions made by the police. This is because:

(*a*) It was necessary to rely on busy police clerks to find the cases in three divisional offices, and it may be that some were missed.

(*b*) The chronological basis for inclusion or exclusion was the date of conviction. Hence, offences that occurred within the period 1957–59 were not included unless the offenders were convicted within the period also.

(*c*) Offenders were counted only once in the category of the principal offence; e.g. an offender convicted for driving under the influence and for dangerous driving also, was counted once only: in this case under the former offence. (Where, as in this example, the offences were of nominally equal seriousness, the choice of one or other as the principal offence was made arbitrarily, according to the hierarchy in which the six offences are shown in *Table 27*.)

(*d*) Certain convicted offenders were excluded to avoid overloading the research (as explained on p. 56 above): *In cases of failing to stop, and failing to insure, aiders and abettors were excluded, and so were all those who lived outside the District; and, to reduce the amount of data, a random sample was taken of one in ten of the persons within the District convicted for failing to insure.* Moreover, insurance offences were not included where they were the 'automatic' consequence of another offence that was not within the scope of the research, e.g. taking and driving away a vehicle without the owner's consent.

It is not easy to explain the differences between the divisional totals for each of the six classes of offence. The reasons for the low incidence of driving while disqualified in Divisions B and F, and for the high incidence

Table 27

DISTRIBUTIONS OF OFFENCES BY DIVISIONS

Offence	Police Division								
	A	B	C	D	E	F	G	H	Total
Causing death by dangerous driving				2				3	5
Driving while disqualified	12	3	9	6	11	2	16	10	69
Driving under the influence of drink or drugs	23	12	8	6	8	15	16	16	104
Driving dangerously or recklessly	54	31	31	32	23	54	36	24	285
Failing to stop after, or to report, an accident	17	19	10	7	19	13	15	17	117
Failing to insure against third-party risks	13	7	7	7	9	6	15	9	73
Total	119	72	65	60	70	90	98	79	653

of drunken driving in Division A, are hard to give because there are so many variables that could be involved, e.g. population size, traffic density and type, number of public houses, and so on. But it is possible to say more about the differences in the numbers of dangerous driving cases, especially as between Divisions F and H.

Dangerous driving (285 cases) was by far the most frequent of the offences, and the unexpectedly high incidence of these cases in the supposedly quiet Division F was striking when compared with the more urban Divisions G and H. It was also surprising to find the number of cases in Division F to be as great as that in Division A in which the traffic density was metropolitan in character. But the most interesting contrast was between Divisions F and H because the latter, although one of the busiest and most built-up, had the lowest number of these cases of all except one of the divisions.

A possible explanation of these findings could be some difference in the interpretation of the term 'dangerous' as between the police divisions, and in particular between the superintendents who decide whether process shall be undertaken on dangerous driving, careless driving, or both. It was, in fact, noticeable, when examining the cases, that behaviour that was deemed to merit a charge of dangerous driving in Division F seemed to be no more 'dangerous' than behaviour charged as 'careless' in, for example, Division H. This is, of course, a matter of opinion, but some justification for the belief that a difference in interpretation existed between the responsible police officers in the several divisions was found by considering convictions for dangerous and careless driving in the aggregate for each division, in order to see if there were marked variations in the proportions of dangerous to careless driving. (All charges reduced from dangerous to careless driving were excluded from this calculation.) The results showed a substantial difference between Divisions F and H. In Division F convictions for dangerous driving formed 24·5 per cent of convictions for careless and dangerous driving combined (less 'reduced charges'), while in Division H the percentage was only 6·1. For comparison, the percentages were 19·8 in Division G and 21·6 in Division A. These figures confirm the subjective impression gained from reading the cases.

HOW THE OFFENCES CAME TO BE KNOWN

It seems to be widely believed that the majority of motoring offences, except those concerned with parking and lighting, arise from accidents. Moreover, as discussed above (p. 8), this belief implies a rather curious use of the term 'accident' – a traffic accident is said to have happened whenever vehicles do damage to persons or to property (or are damaged themselves). This is not quite the same thing as the true accident, which would appear to be a chance event that could not have been prevented or, to put it loosely, 'an act of God'.

If the first, rather distorted, meaning is used then it is true to say that 58·7 per cent of the 653 cases were derived from accidents. But 42·3 per cent or just under half, were not: i.e. no damage was caused at all and the offence came to notice because of the offender's behaviour in itself. However, a close inspection of the evidence in every one of the 653 cases suggests that the actual proportion of offences in which the contribution by the offender was debatable was very low indeed, and it could not possibly be said that more than 14 per cent were cases of 'bad luck' or genuine errors of judgement. And even this estimate is stretching many points in favour of the offender.

The more subtle definition of the term accident is pertinent to the hypothesis that assumes that personality factors do not enter into motoring offences to any appreciable extent; but this will be considered more fully in the next chapter. As this section is concerned mainly with how offences came to be known, the word will be employed according to common usage.

In all, 383 of the 653 offences arose from accidents with other vehicles, pedestrians, or some other obtruction. The details are presented in *Table 28*. It can be seen that where accidents occurred, about 85 per cent were collisions with other vehicles, most of which did not involve injury to anyone; 3·4 per cent involved pedestrians, of whom all were injured in some way; and the remainder were mostly cases in which the only damage was to the offender's vehicle, and to posts or walls, etc., with which it collided.

Table 28

SERIOUS MOTORING OFFENCES DERIVED FROM 'ACCIDENTS'

Offence	Other vehicles	Pedestrians	Other	Total of offences derived from accidents	Total of offences	% of offences derived from accidents
Causing death	4	1	0	5	5	100
Driving while disqualified	7	0	2	9	69	13
Driving under the influence	30	0	20	50	104	48
Driving dangerously	174	6	20	200	285	70
Failing to stop or report	109	5	3	117	117	100
Failing to insure	1	1	0	2	73	3
Total	325	13	45	383	653	59

Where accidents occurred, either the police were on the scene or they were notified of their occurrence. But it is of interest to examine the 270 cases in which there was no accident, and it was the offender's behaviour that was apparently his undoing.

Where the offence was driving while disqualified or failure to insure, only a very small proportion came from accidents, and the majority were apprehended by the police. Among the disqualified, 32 per cent were stopped by officers purely on suspicion; 19 per cent were seen driving by officers who knew them to be disqualified; and the remainder were caught while committing some other offence, usually taking a vehicle without consent. Of the uninsured, 30·5 per cent were noticed by officers because of other offences, mostly being without a road fund licence; the rest were stopped on suspicion – as the police usually put it, 'I had occasion to stop him'.

In the 54 cases of drunken driving in which no accident occurred, 39 were noticed and arrested by the police, 6 were reported by pedestrians and 9 by other motorists. In the 82 cases of dangerous driving where there was no accident and the reporting agent was recorded, 67 were seen by the police, 3 by pedestrians, and 13 by other motorists.

As expected, all the cases where the behaviour was reported by someone outside the police were bad ones, especially when the reporting agent was another driver. Yet it is surprising that such a small proportion were reported by other drivers and pedestrians; perhaps this is because motorists dislike reporting each other, but the more likely reason is that they have not the time to stop, telephone the police, give statements, and then possibly spend several days in court. And no doubt the same would apply to the non-motoring public also. Whatever the reasons, it seems clear that the public do not do much to report the offending driver; they tend to leave the whole matter to the police as they seem to in most other instances where the law is broken.

TYPES OF VEHICLE INVOLVED

Table 29 gives the numbers and percentages of the different types of vehicle driven by the 653 offenders. It appears that the drivers of private cars are the main offenders in all cases except those of failure to insure. In the latter motor cyclists are in the majority, and they are prominent also in the driving while disqualified group; it is, however, noteworthy that motor cyclists form such a small proportion of those concerned in driving under the influence and failing to stop, etc. Perhaps this is because motor cyclists are younger than most other drivers: if it can be assumed that the young are less likely to drink heavily. And the paucity of motor cyclists among the failing to stop cases may be explained by the fact that the rider who is involved in an accident is likely to be either unseated or forced to stop.

Goods drivers provide a steady proportion of offenders in all cases except those of driving while disqualified, to which theirs is the lowest contribution. It may be that goods drivers are less likely to be disqualified, since their jobs depend on their licences; or they may be less prepared to risk driving when disqualified; also it is difficult for a disqualified driver to get hold of a goods vehicle unless he owns it.

There are, however, two obvious reasons why the above distribution of cases among the various classes of vehicle might be very misleading. First, it should be remembered that the failing to insure group is only a one in ten

Table 29

DISTRIBUTION OF OFFENCES ACCORDING TO TYPE OF VEHICLE

Offence	Goods vehicles		Private cars		Motor cycles		Public-service vehicles	
	No.	%	No.	%	No.	%	No.	%
Causing death	1	20·0	4	80·0	0	0	0	—
Driving while disqualified	8	11·6	37	54·0	24	34·4	0	—
Driving under the influence	20	19·2	77	74·0	7	6·8	0	—
Driving dangerously	54	19·0	171	60·0	60	21·0	0	—
Failing to stop or report	20	17·0	90	77·0	7	6·0	0	—
Failing to insure	13	17·8	20	27·4	40	54·8	0	—
Total	116	17·7	399	61·1	138	21·2	0	

sample of offenders resident in the District; even with the limitation of residence, the real total for these offenders is ten times as large, i.e. about 730. Clearly this puts the motor cyclist well in the lead for this offence (400 instances), with the motor car second (200 cases), and the goods vehicle a poor third (perhaps, rather, a 'good' third!). Second, the relative proportions of vehicles of different classes on the roads, and therefore 'at risk', have not been taken into account. Let us now do this (*Table 30*), using the proportions calculated by Chandler and Tanner (1958).

It will be noted that the unrealistic *sample total* has been used in showing

Table 30

DISTRIBUTION OF CASES ACCORDING TO THE
ESTIMATED PROPORTIONS OF VEHICLES ON THE ROAD

Type of vehicle	Estimated proportion on roads	Expected distribution of cases	Actual distribution of cases
	%		
Motor cycles	8·2	53	138
Private cars and taxis	52·17	341	399
Goods vehicles	31·38	205	116
Public-service vehicles	8·24	54	0
Total		653	653

the actual distribution of cases, yet the motor cycle is still the most prominent, with just over 2½ times the expected frequency of occurrence; the private car slightly exceeds the expected total, perhaps more so, since the Chandler and Tanner figure includes taxis, of which there are only two among the offences; but the goods vehicle is well below expectation and shows up relatively well. And the public-service vehicle has the best record of all. The real situation is, therefore, almost certainly the same as that revealed by the analysis of the national statistics. When the relative numbers of the various classes of vehicle on the road are taken into account, it is the motor cyclist who is the most frequent offender, with the driver of the private car some way behind.

THE DATES AND TIMES OF THE OFFENCES

Table 31 shows that the majority of the 642 offences for which the date was given occurred during weekends: Saturday was the peak day, with Friday next, and Sunday in third place. So it would appear that weekend drivers contributed substantially to the incidence of these serious offences, though it is not clear how many drove mostly at weekends. Moreover, it should be noted that this conclusion is established without the inclusion of bank holidays.

Table 31

642 SERIOUS MOTORING OFFENCES: DAY OF OCCURRENCE

Offence	Day of the week excluding bank holidays							Bank holidays[1]	Total offences
	Mon	Tue	Wed	Thur	Fri	Sat	Sun		
Causing death	0	0	1	0	2	0	2	0	5
Driving while disqualified	8	3	6	11	9	14	10	1	62
Driving under the influence	8	10	5	11	17	27	12	11	101
Driving dangerously	24	21	30	35	41	62	55	17	285
Failing to stop or report	13	13	11	11	24	23	14	8	117
Failing to insure	8	13	3	6	16	13	9	4	72
Total	61	60	56	74	109	139	102	41	642

[1] Christmas Day, Boxing Day, Good Friday, Easter Monday, Whit Monday, August Monday.

The Offences

According to *Table 32*, the most active months for the offences were June, July, and September. The quietest period was from January to the end of February.

Table 32

647 SERIOUS MOTORING OFFENCES: MONTH OF OCCURRENCE

Offence	Jan	Feb	Mar	Apr	May	June	July	Aug	Sept	Oct	Nov	Dec	Total offences
Causing death	1	0	0	0	0	0	0	2	1	0	0	1	5
Driving while disqualified	5	4	6	3	5	9	4	4	7	7	7	4	65
Driving under the influence	5	2	10	6	9	8	12	6	9	9	6	22	104
Driving dangerously	9	12	15	21	26	38	39	26	36	26	17	20	285
Failing to stop or report	7	9	7	5	6	12	15	11	12	9	11	11	115
Failing to insure	5	4	5	5	10	12	5	4	7	8	7	1	73
Total	32	31	43	40	56	79	75	53	72	59	48	59	647

In *Table 33* it will be seen that the peak times for the 643 offences in which the time of occurrence was available were during the period 2 p.m. to midnight; the majority occurred between 2 p.m. and 6 p.m., then the numbers tapered off until midnight, after which things were quiet. In comparison with these periods, the morning rush hours between 7 a.m. and 9 a.m. produced very few cases, and the quietest time of all was from 2 a.m. to 6 a.m.

But to treat these cases in aggregate regardless of the type of offence is rather meaningless, since it is likely that there will be 'favourite' times and dates for each kind of offence.

This might be expected of drunken driving. And, indeed, 33 of the 104 offenders were arrested between 10 p.m. and midnight, 26 between 6 p.m. and 10 p.m., and almost the same number between 2 p.m. and 6 p.m. Compared with these times other periods were very quiet, though 12 offenders were arrested between midnight and 2 a.m. The peak days for drunken driving were, not surprisingly, Friday and Saturday; Wednesday was the low point in the middle of the week. As expected, December was the busy month for this offence, with July next.

For dangerous driving the peak hours were between 2 p.m. and 6 p.m.

The Documentary Study

Table 33

Offence	10 a.m.– noon	noon– 2 p.m.	2–6 p.m.	6–10 p.m.	10 p.m.– mid- night	Mid- night– 2 a.m.	2–6 a.m.	6–10 a.m.	Total offences
Causing death	0	0	4	0	1	0	0	0	5
Driving while disqualified	6	3	11	16	14	8	3	3	64
Driving under the influence	1	2	25	26	33	12	3	1	103
Driving dangerously	24	33	86	71	32	6	2	30	284
Failing to stop or report	18	16	36	21	9	3	2	11	116
Failing to insure	8	7	13	22	11	6	0	4	71
Total	57	61	175	156	100	35	10	49	643

with 86 cases; next was 6 p.m. to 10 p.m. with 71; hence 55 per cent of these cases occurred between 2 p.m. and 10 p.m., other times of day being relatively quiet. Again we find the Saturday and Sunday drivers the most frequent offenders, responsible for just over 40 per cent of all the cases; as before, this is exclusive of bank holidays. And, again as expected, we find these cases appearing most often in the summer months, June, July and September; but it is rather surprising to find August, October, and May with the same relatively low number of cases. It is, perhaps, significant that the lowest number of dangerous driving cases occurred in the worst winter months of January and February, when they were less than one-third of their number in the summer peak months. It would be attractive to say that this may be because drivers are more careful in the winter or because the weekend driver does not use his car in these bad months, leaving only the fairly experienced on the roads; but the truth may be that the density of traffic is much lower, and hence there are fewer people at risk.

Driving while disqualified seems to be a 'leisure hours' offence since its peaks were markedly in the 'after work' evening period from 6 p.m. to midnight. Friday and Saturday were, again, the most popular days, but apart from a peak in June the offences were spread throughout the months without any apparently significant pattern.

Failing to stop tended to be markedly a 'busy hours' offence with its peak between 2 p.m. and 6 p.m.; but it was nearly as frequently found between 10 a.m. and noon. Its incidence may not be unrelated to the fact that it was the offence in which women were found in the highest ratio to males in this research, for these are the times when wives are often driving the family car. Also it is noticeable that the offence tended to fall off in incidence after 10 p.m.

Failing to insure seems to follow much the same pattern as driving while disqualified, being a 'leisure hours' offence, committed mostly at weekends during the early summer months of May and June. Or perhaps it is that the police are more apt to 'notice' this offence at these times, for it is an offence that usually depends on the mobile policeman deciding to chase or to stop a suspicious-looking road user.

The cases of causing death by dangerous driving are too few in number to be commented on in this connection.

OTHER FEATURES OF THE OFFENCES

It is outside the scope of this research to conduct an analysis of the causes of accidents, which is done in other fields; hence it is not intended to deal with factors such as road and weather conditions unless they are of a gross nature. In any case, were the road and weather conditions the major feature in the circumstances surrounding an offence it is unlikely that there would be a prosecution, and even more unlikely that it would become a conviction. There were, however, a number of features about the cases which might be of interest in indicating some of the causal factors. An attempt was made to discern these in the various groups.

In the offences in which dangerous driving was alleged, i.e. causing death and dangerous driving, 34 per cent of the offenders appeared to have been driving at an excessive speed, given the circumstances; for example, one offender on a motor cycle capable of 100 mph passed another motor cyclist who admitted to 70 mph; when the offender came to a roundabout he was unable to turn, and drove right through the centre of it. And this was at 11 p.m. on an August Sunday night, in a built-up area, at the intersection of two major roads used intensively by holiday traffic. (The young man seems to have deserved his fine of £15 and twelve months' disqualification.) Of the others, 50 per cent were cases of overtaking other vehicles and 16 per cent were for driving in a selfish and aggressive manner.

An example of selfishness is one of the female offenders who, also in August, drove her car out of a side-turning straight across a busy holiday major road, causing oncoming drivers to brake violently, and creating a highly dangerous situation for them; when stopped by a patrol she was very abusive and accused the police of wasting her time in remonstrating with her. Another example is that of the offender (mentioned on p. 86 above) who became irritated at being held in a queue of traffic by a police pointsman; so he pulled out of line and drove his car up to the officer, blowing his horn and telling the officer to let him through. When told to get back into line he drove straight at the policeman who had to 'jump for it'.

Evidence of alcohol as a possible contributing factor appears in just over 8 per cent of all offences, excluding, of course, those of driving under the influence. This proportion, however, may be an understatement since the police are reluctant to mention drink, even in their files, unless it is intended to prosecute for one of the 'drink' offences.

There was, however, strong evidence that the offenders had been drinking in two of the five cases of causing death by dangerous driving, and in 8·4 per cent of the 285 cases of dangerous driving. The extent to which drink can be a major factor in dangerous driving, without leading to a charge of driving under the influence, will be evident from the following examples.

On a pleasant Saturday evening in August, a patrolman saw A's car swerving from side to side on a main road, preventing following traffic from overtaking. After watching him swerve into the path of an oncoming car and just avoid a collision, the patrol officer stopped A, who became abusive and claimed that it was perfectly safe for him to drive on the wrong side of the road since he knew what he was doing. A smelled of drink and his speech was slurred; moreover, his lady passenger was, according to the officer, very drunk. At the police station A did all the tests required of him satisfactorily, and when medically examined it was found that he suffered from a chronic complaint; so dangerous driving was the charge preferred. He was fined £5 and disqualified for one year.

On another Saturday evening in summer, a patrol car saw B's small family car swerving violently and occasionally mounting the kerb; B was then seen to drive round a roundabout in the wrong direction. When stopped he had 'clearly been drinking' and admitted as much at the police station. But the inspector did not think him 'drunk enough' to charge him with driving under the influence, and proceedings were taken on dangerous driving, for which he was fined £30 and disqualified for six months.

In the failing to stop group, drink was a possible contributor in 6·8 per cent of the cases; i.e. this was the proportion of cases in which it was mentioned. And here again there are borderline examples.

On an evening in July, C was seen by another motorist to 'blind straight out' of a side road onto a major road, and park in front of another car; in doing so, C reversed into the car behind him, damaging its wings and bumper. C then drove off, but a witness who saw his reactions formed the impression that he was very drunk. The motorist took C's number and reported him. C said later that he was very distressed because of 'an upset at the office', but since he had a previous conviction for driving under the influence, it is not improbable that the witness who thought him to be drunk was right.

It is interesting that drink was mentioned as a factor in 14 per cent of the driving while disqualified cases, and it may be that an offender is more likely to give in to the temptation to drive when under the influence of alcohol.

In the insurance cases, drink was a negligible factor, being mentioned in only one case.

Perhaps the only other factors worth mention at this point are instances of aggressive behaviour or of panic. One or the other, and sometimes both, were found in some of the dangerous driving cases, and also in cases of failing to stop after an accident. In this last offence panic is a dominant factor; an example was D, a young textile salesman who was driving his car for a quiet after-lunch 'spin round the area' on a Christmas Day. Dusk was closing in as he drove through the main street of a small town, and he did not see an elderly man cross the road in front of him until too late: 'I felt a bump and knew I'd hit him, but for some reason I can't explain I didn't stop . . . I was confused.' D then drove round the immediate neighbourhood for a few minutes, after which he returned to the scene. He got out of his car and walked over to look at the man lying on the pavement, where he was receiving attention from a passer-by; but D did not admit his involvement, he walked away and drove off. However, after a sleepless night, he reported his part in the affair to the police. At court two independent witnesses said that D had had no chance to avoid the pedestrian, and he was fined £10, there being no previous convictions.

This last example is an indication of the wide range of behaviour that occurs within each class of motoring offence; hence it is difficult to generalize about the offences *per se*, since no two incidents are alike in all respects.

As far as it is possible to generalize at all it would appear that most of the serious offences occurred at times when the offenders were at leisure; offence rates were especially high at weekends and on summer evenings, when many vehicles are being used for private pleasure. Moreover, the majority of offenders were using either motor cycles or private cars, and relatively few were driving goods vehicles. So it is possible that many serious motoring offences are off-duty occurrences which take place when the driver is relaxing or getting away from work; in other words, when he is most likely 'being himself'.

The link between the personality and the offence is indicated in the number of offences that did not arise from accidents or 'tricks of fate'. It has also been shown that deliberate overtaking at speed, and driving in a selfish manner contributed to a substantial number of offences.

Even so, as yet, there is only slender evidence pointing to the probability that the personal characteristics of the offender are relevant to the offence – though it may be enough to stimulate doubt as to whether the apparent tendency in motoring cases to expect the punishment to fit the crime rather than the criminal is justified by the facts. This is a question that can be answered only by concentrating on the offenders themselves, and it is the purpose of the next chapter to attempt to describe the kinds of individual who, generally speaking, commit the more serious motoring offences.

8

The Offenders

Of all the various sections of this research, the study of the offenders as a group was perhaps the most interesting. But it was not as easy as it might have been because the documentary evidence was concerned not so much with the characteristics of the offenders as with the events in which they were involved. There did not seem to be the interest in the offenders as people that might have been expected, and would almost certainly have been found, had these offenders been regarded as 'criminals' by the police. Where the latter are concerned, the recording of personal details, such as date of birth, way of life, background, and so on, is painstakingly thorough so that the task of tracing the offender, should he offend again, is made easier. With the motoring offender, even the serious one, this consideration does not seem to apply; he is treated with all the other traffic offenders as part of a group so large that time and patience preclude the recording of much detail. It was necessary, therefore, to make do with approximations about age and occupation, and to make numerous inferences from statements – a way of working which permits personal interpretations that may be open to question as such, and may not be the conclusions that other people would draw, looking at the matter from a different point of view.

Hence it might be best to begin the analysis of the offenders as a group with a category of information that admits of no confusion – distribution according to sex.

SEX DIFFERENCES AMONG OFFENDERS

The relative contributions of males and females to the 653 serious offences are shown in *Table 34*, and the proportions do not depart much from the expectations of the criminologist who has become used to finding males greatly predominant among criminal offenders. In the District the ratio is twelve males to every female convicted of the serious offences with which this study is concerned.

There is not a comparable ratio in the national statistics since it is not possible to isolate the six offences and show the sex of offenders. But, for all motoring offenders in England and Wales, the ratio is as high as 20:1,

The Documentary Study

Table 34

653 SERIOUS MOTORING OFFENDERS: DISTRIBUTION BY SEX

Offence	Males	Females	Total
Causing death	5	0	5
Driving while disqualified	69	0	69
Driving under the influence	97	7	104
Driving dangerously	279	6	285
Failing to stop or report	89	28	117
Failing to insure	63	10	73
Total	602	51	653

and for those convicted by the higher courts it is even higher at about 30:1. So the case goes against the male according to all the available statistics. The ratio of male to female among motoring offenders is, however, a provocative question, and one that is important in any study of personality factors. Hence it will be treated separately later in this chapter (p. 232 below).

AGE OF OFFENDERS

It is not usual for the police to record the date of birth of motoring offenders, and only an 'estimated age' is required. This is symptomatic of the general police approach to motoring offences since presumably they would never consider the accurate date of birth as unessential in dealing with an offender against property. In fact, however, the estimated age was adequate for following up additional offences through the Criminal Record Office (CRO), but the work would have been much easier had dates of birth been recorded.

Age is of interest for two reasons: first because we want to know which age groups are the most lawless, and second – and perhaps more important apropos of motoring offences – because it gives us some indication of the relationship between age, experience, and the tendency to offend. But here it is stressed that such an analysis can give only a speculative indication; since, for instance, a young driver who has driven more miles under more demanding conditions than an older one, will be more experienced as a driver. This is not often so, but it occurs frequently enough to make age a factor of doubtful use by itself.

Table 35 presents the age distribution of the 653 offenders. The most usual age for the 650 offenders whose age was recorded was 26; this tends to confirm the national statistics, which show the mode for the more serious motoring offenders as in the age group 21 to 30. The range among the 650 is, however, very wide, with the youngest offender aged 17 and the oldest aged 81; thirty-nine offenders were over 70 and three were 80.

Furthermore, as the table shows, there is a wide variation according to the type of offence committed. Drunken drivers and those who failed to stop are noticeably older than the others. (Stack and Walker (1959) and Munden (1962) made this same point with reference to drunken drivers.) The most usual age among the drunken drivers is about 46, and among the failing to stop group it is about 33. Also it is among the latter that the highest proportion of offenders aged 60 and over is found.

Table 35

653 SERIOUS MOTORING OFFENDERS: DISTRIBUTION BY AGE

Offence	14 and under 17	17 and under 21	21 and under 30	30 and under 40	40 and under 50	50 and under 60	60 and over	Age not recorded	Total
Causing death	0	0	0	3	1	1	0	0	5
Driving while disqualified	1	24	36	8	0	0	0	0	69
Driving under the influence	0	3	15	22	31	26	7	0	104
Driving dangerously	5	53	95	52	34	34	11	1	285
Failing to stop	0	7	22	24	20	22	20	2	117
Failing to insure	4	26	28	11	1	2	1	0	73
Total	10	113	196	120	87	85	39	3	653
% of 653 offenders	1·5	17·3	30·0	18·4	13·4	13·0	6·0		99·6

Among the dangerous drivers the ages are more widely distributed, ranging from 17 to 80 years of age; the modal age is, however, fairly young at just under 25. Of these offenders 54 per cent (including all the motor cyclists) were under 30.

Slightly younger were those convicted for driving while disqualified, with a mode of 23·4 years, and in this group also 88 per cent of the offenders were under 30 and none was over 40.

The Documentary Study

Youngest of all was the sample of insurance offenders whose modal age was 21·8 years. This was a 10 per cent sample of insurance offenders resident in the Police District, and if it were expanded tenfold it would make the mode for all the six offence groups just over 21, and 30 per cent of all offenders would be under 21. Such an expansion would not, however, yield a total comparable with the other groups, which (with the exception of those convicted of failing to stop or report) are not confined to residents in the District; it would still be an underestimate of the real total, and it is likely that the real modal age is not more than 21. This supports the evidence in the national statistics of a major contribution to the total of motoring offences by the young insurance offender.

OCCUPATION AND SOCIAL CLASS

Table 36 presents the occupational distribution of the 559 offenders whose occupations were recorded, according to a six-category scale. The latter was derived from a classification devised by Hall and Moser (1954), and offenders were allotted to it arbitrarily; but where doubtful cases arose as, for example, members of the armed forces, they were put in a higher rather than a lower category. Hence there should be a slight bias towards the higher groups (see pp. 44–5 above). Unfortunately, information concerning occupations was incomplete or incomprehensible in fifty-four of the cases; this figure includes a number of housewives designated as such, from whose cases it was impossible to infer the occupation of the husband. All these were omitted from the occupational analysis.

For reasons discussed in Chapter 2 above, it is hard to say whether any occupational group is under- or over-represented among these offenders, since there are no satisfactory census criteria for comparison. It is, however, possible to get some idea of the situation by comparing the occupational distribution of the offenders with the distribution of occupied heads of households in Britain in 1951, as calculated by Cole (1955, p. 153) from census data. This comparison is presented in *Table 37*.

These figures cast doubt on the belief that the serious motoring offender comes mostly from the white-collar classes, since the majority of the offenders in this study would be regarded as manual workers by almost any standard. Moreover, if Cole's proportions are reliable, it would seem that the two lowest occupational groups are over-represented among the offenders; the top group is over-represented too, but that is not surprising since it has been shown that there is a higher proportion of this class in the Police District than in the country overall. Perhaps the most instructive

Table 36

599 SERIOUS MOTORING OFFENDERS: OCCUPATIONAL DISTRIBUTION

Offence	Professional and higher admin.	Managerial and executive	Lower non-manual	Skilled manual	Semi-skilled manual	Unskilled manual	Total	% in manual occupations
Causing death	0	0	0	1	4	0	5	100
Driving while disqualified	1	0	3	11	17	37	69	94·0
Driving under the influence	13	17	26	26	17	5	104	46·0
Driving dangerously	26	26	44	31	80	18	225	57·7
Failing to stop or report	6	18	18	20	18	7	87	51·7
Failing to insure	1	1	12	7	23	25	69	80·0
Total	47	62	103	96	159	92	559	
% in each occupational group	8·4	11·1	18·4	17·2	28·5	16·4	100	62·1

The Documentary Study

Table 37

OCCUPATIONAL DISTRIBUTION: OFFENDERS COMPARED WITH
HEADS OF HOUSEHOLDS

Occupational group	No. of offenders	Percentage of offenders	Cole's percentage[1]
I. Professional and higher admin.	47	8·4	3·3
II. Managerial and executive	62	11·1	13·9
III. Lower non-manual	103	18·4	21·2
IV. Skilled manual	96	17·2	34·6
V. Semi-skilled manual	159	28·5	15·7
VI. Unskilled manual	92	16·4	11·3

[1] Cole's classification has been altered slightly to include farmers under Group II, and members of the armed services other than officers under Groups III or IV. It then corresponds more closely to the system used in the research.

indication is that the middle class, which might be considered to be Groups II, III, and IV above, is clearly under-represented among the offenders.

It will be evident that *Table 37* casts some doubt also on the original hypothesis that serious motoring offenders would be distributed widely over the Registrar-General's five classes rather than concentrated in the manual groups (as non-motoring offenders are thought to be). The Registrar-General's distribution at the 1951 census is compared with the distribution of offenders (*Table 38*), and it will be seen that the semi-skilled and unskilled manual groups among the latter exceed their proportions in the population at large. In this context, it is only realistic to consider Classes IV and V, since the Registrar-General's Class III includes a large number of non-manual workers who would be classified as lower non-manual or white collar according to the criteria used in allocating the motoring offenders.

However there is still the possibility that the proportion of manual workers may be lower, and that of white-collar workers higher, among motoring offenders than among offenders of other kinds. Unfortunately the evidence that is available about non-motoring offenders is too slight in this respect to permit any conclusion. As Wootton (1959, p. 48) has said: 'We are completely in the dark as to the contribution which particular social classes make to particular classes of crime.'

When the effects of the sampling procedure are taken into account, the proportion of offenders from the lower occupational groups becomes even higher: 80 per cent of the uninsured offenders were manual workers, so

Table 38

OFFENDERS: SOCIAL CLASS DISTRIBUTION

Social class	Percentage occupied males *1951* census	Percentage serious motoring offenders[1]
I. Professional, etc.	3	8
II. Intermediate	15	19
III. Skilled	53	17
IV. Partly skilled	16 } 29	28 } 44
V. Unskilled	13	16
	100	100

[1] Percentages are rounded and do not add up to 100.

even if they are restricted to residents in the District, their full number brings the total proportion of manual workers up to 72 per cent. The failing to stop group, however, would be unlikely to change the picture if the residential limitation were withdrawn, since just over half of them were manual workers.

The manual groups are almost completely dominant in three offences: causing death (100 per cent manual workers), driving while disqualified (94 per cent manual), and failing to insure (80 per cent manual). And they form just over half of the dangerous driving and failing to stop groups, and a surprisingly large proportion (46 per cent) of the drunken drivers. Here again it should be stressed that the number in the causing death group is perhaps too small to mean much, but the other proportions cannot be explained away so easily.

Particularly striking are the high proportions of manual workers among those convicted of driving while disqualified, and of driving without insurance. The reasons for this may be subcultural, in that manual workers may be less inclined than white-collar workers to think of either offence as being particularly heinous; or they may be financial, in that these people have less money than those in higher occupational groups and so are more likely to take risks to avoid what they may regard as the unnecessary expenses of using alternative transport (if they are disqualified) or of paying an insurance premium. It is also possible that manual workers may be more likely than non-manual workers to be caught driving while disqualified, because they are more likely to suffer disqualification for motoring offences in the first instance. Analysis shows that there is something in this possibility since 62 per cent of all the offenders in the manual occupational groups were disqualified compared with 55 per cent of those in the non-manual groups. This could be a contributory factor that may *help* to explain the preponderance of manual workers among those convicted of driving while disqualified and failing to insure, but the difference of 7 per cent between the two main groups is perhaps too small to be by any means a complete explanation.

It follows, then, that white-collar offenders are conspicuously few in the driving while disqualified and failing to insure groups. However, this may be because the police are less likely to stop persons from these groups on suspicion; moreover, they are unlikely to be people the police 'keep an eye on', and hence may more easily escape detection – a particular advantage when driving while disqualified. On the other hand, persons from these groups are more likely to have experience in understanding the intricacies of insurance, and are more likely also to appreciate both insurance cover and the consequences of driving while disqualified.

The highest proportions of non-manual offenders are found in the driving under the influence and the failing to stop groups. They are most heavily represented in the driving under the influence group (53·9 per cent) – the only offence in which more than half of the offenders are from non-manual occupations. Next comes failing to stop, with 48 per cent from white-collar occupations, but it must be stressed that a high proportion of the white-collar offenders in this group are women.

The variety of occupations found among the offenders is so great that it is neither possible nor justifiable to select any one group for detailed analysis. Perhaps the farthest one can go is to examine the extent to which offenders come from the ranks of professional drivers – those whose main job is driving a vehicle. To calculate the proportion of these 'professionals', those offenders who gave their occupation as 'driver', and those who were driving goods vehicles when they offended, were included in the category. All of these offenders were men and they formed 24·4 per cent of the total: a proportion that is interestingly close to the 25 per cent which Johnson and Garwood (1957) have stated to be the percentage of all vehicle insurance policies covering goods and commercial use (excluding the motor trade and commercial travelling). If 25 per cent can be taken as an approximation of the proportion of drivers who are professionals in the sense used above, then it would seem that they are neither under- nor over-represented among the offenders in this study. Incidentally it is noteworthy that there were no public-service vehicle drivers among the offenders, and only two taxi drivers.

Also, having said that servicemen might be over-represented in the Police District, it is useful to consider them briefly as a group. In fact it appears that they supplied only 7 per cent of all the offenders. They figure mostly in the driving while disqualified group, to which they contribute 28 per cent of the offenders; and in the 10 per cent sample of failing to insure cases, of which they form just over 8 per cent. It seems that the borrowing of cars and motor cycles is particularly common among servicemen, who do not make sure that they are covered by insurance to drive. Because they so often commit this offence and are so easily recognizable, they are often caught and are invariably disqualified as a result. Afterwards they are especially tempted to drive again to go on short leave or to get away from barracks when off duty, and it would appear that the proximity of London to the Police District offers a special temptation in this respect.

Enough has been said to warrant a reconsideration of the hypothesis that the majority of serious motoring offenders come from the ranks of the well-to-do, for it would seem to be beyond question that the facts do not support it. As for the original hypothesis that the offenders would be widely distributed over the Registrar-General's five occupational groups rather than concentrated in the manual occupations (as non-motoring offenders are believed to be), again the evidence does not substantiate it. However, it must be remembered that there may not be such a high percentage of manual workers among serious motoring offenders as there is among offenders of other kinds; hence there may be more middle-class people among motoring offenders than among offenders of other kinds. Even so, they do not form anything like the proportion needed to justify labelling the serious motoring offence as a 'white-collar crime'.

BEHAVIOUR IN COURT

In order to test the hypothesis that serious motoring offenders usually elect trial by jury when it is possible to do so, information was sought about pleas to charges; it was also the intention to record details about appeals against finding, sentence, or disqualification, to see if they could throw further light on the kind of individual the serious motoring offender might be.

In the event it was not easy to get accurate information about pleas from the records, because usually the only indication of a guilty plea was the cancellation of witnesses before the hearing; but this is not very reliable because offenders do change their minds and plead guilty after it is too late to cancel witnesses' attendance at court. However, enough information was available to give some idea of the proportion who pleaded guilty. Data concerning election of trial and appeals were, on the other hand, simple to record and should be accurate.

In calculating the proportion of guilty pleas, cases of failing to insure were omitted, since these are nearly all the result of guilty pleas; usually the facts in these cases are unarguable, and there is little point in defendants pleading otherwise. So, without the insurance offenders, it seems that about 14 per cent of the others pleaded guilty. Most of the guilty pleas were found in the drunken driving cases and in those of failing to stop or report: in both these groups about one-quarter of the offenders pleaded thus. The lowest proportions were for dangerous driving (7·4 per cent of the cases) and for driving while disqualified (13 per cent).

The percentage of offenders pleading guilty to drunken driving, or to failing to stop after or report an accident, was unexpectedly high, because it could be supposed that there would usually be some defence in these cases; hence one might speculate about their motives in so choosing. There seemed to be at least four possibilities. A guilty plea could be the result of ignorance, or of inability to afford legal advice as to the most sensible plea; or it could be because of police pressure or, finally, from the belief that it might lead to more lenient treatment. These points are examined in the interviews with offenders; but there is some indication in the documentary evidence about whether the guilty pleas are likely to have resulted from ignorance or from inability to afford advice. If they were to be explained thus, the majority of the offenders who pleaded guilty would be likely to be from the lower occupational groups – in fact, there were approximately equal numbers from the manual and the non-manual groups.

The low proportions of offenders pleading guilty to dangerous driving or to driving while disqualified are not hard to explain. In dangerous driving the outcome of the case usually depends on an intense conflict of opinion between prosecution and defence, which is undertaken with some gusto by both sides as a matter of 'principle'; hence guilty pleas are unlikely. The opposite is true of driving while disqualified, and it may be that the low proportion of guilty pleas in these cases is a false picture. This could be so because reliance was placed on the attendance of witnesses as an indication of the plea and, since driving while disqualified often accompanies other offences, it is uncertain whether the witnesses were brought to contest a plea of not guilty to the driving while disqualified or to the accompanying offence: most probably the latter. But, on the other hand, it is possible that offenders charged with an offence like driving while disqualified would be experienced in the ways of the law, and so more likely to plead not guilty as a matter of course.

Those who elected trial by jury were bound to be confined to those charged with drunken driving, dangerous driving, or both. Defendants charged with causing death have to go for trial at assizes, and there would be no option for the others but summary trial by magistrates.

Of the 104 drunken drivers, twenty-two elected to be tried by jury: a much smaller number than was expected. However it was no surprise that only five of these were manual workers. The cases tried by juries show no special features to distinguish them from those tried summarily; the main element seemed to be the defendant's hope that he would be acquitted by a jury. There was, of course, the risk of being punished on conviction more heavily in the higher courts than in the magistrates' courts, but in the event the risk was justified since none was given the maximum punishment or anything near it.

Of the 285 offenders convicted of dangerous driving, twelve appeared at higher courts: one was a young soldier who was committed for sentence (he was convicted additionally of taking a car without consent), another was committed on a charge of causing death that was later reduced to dangerous driving, and ten elected trial by jury. There was not much to distinguish the cases that went to the higher courts from those that did not; but it is noteworthy that all but two of the offenders who elected trial by jury were apparently well-to-do people. It should be mentioned also that five of the twelve cases contained substantial evidence that the defendant had been affected by drink. One such case was that of F, an executive in his late forties who was charged with dangerous driving, with failing to stop after an accident, *and* with failing to report it. He was traced after careful forensic work had shown that pieces of painted metal, which had been found near a man lying dead on a major road at night, had come from his car. Though a broadcast appeal for information did not yield any reply for some days, the defendant ultimately offered to help when he was told by a friend that the police were on to him. The evidence was that he had called at several inns on the night of the incident and had drunk as many as five double gins at one of them. But there were no witnesses of the incident or of the manner in which F was driving at the time, and it was only on his own admission, that he had been driving fast with sidelights only, that a charge of dangerous driving could be sustained. Adequate evidence of his condition was not available, but there was more than a suggestion that he was under the influence, and it would seem that there were good grounds for thinking so if only because of the numerous calls at public houses, which were substantiated. But calls at public houses, and evidence of consumption therein, are not evidence of drunkenness, and so the case went forward on a slender charge of dangerous driving and a more definite, though denied, charge of failing to stop or report (since the defendant denied knowledge of hitting anything). The result: conviction on all charges, with fines totalling £80, and one month's disqualification. Costs were charged to him but there was no record of the amount.

Another offender who elected trial by jury was G, an engineering consultant aged 42, who was followed for about a mile by another motorist who noticed that he was swerving from side to side of the road, once nearly causing a collision with an approaching car. When G stopped at a road junction, this motorist and his passenger (who happened to be a police officer from outside the District) got out of their car and went up to see if G was ill. They said in evidence that they noticed his glassy eyes and slurred speech, so they asked him to get out of his car, which he refused to do; whereupon they pulled him out. He was then said to have been unable to stand without support, and fell on his back onto the grass verge. When the police arrived G was quite cooperative and he continued to be so at the police station, though he hotly denied that he was drunk. At his trial he admitted that he had had only one piece of toast for breakfast and two pints of Guinness for lunch; he also admitted to a two-hour stay at a public house where he had five gins and tonics (two of them large ones) just before the incident leading to his arrest. It was, in fact, estimated from a urine test that he had consumed not less than the equivalent of $8\frac{1}{2}$ pints of beer at the time he was arrested. His defence was that a steering defect had caused his car to swerve, and that his behaviour was due to a chronic stomach disorder which made him feel unwell; moreover, he said that he was not influenced by the drink he had consumed because he had been in Africa for many years and 'knew how to drink' – he was 'used to it'. G was acquitted of driving under the influence of drink, but he was found guilty of driving dangerously, and was fined £25 plus £14 costs. This was nowhere near the maximum, and he was not disqualified, so it clearly paid G to elect trial.

Also of interest is the case of H, aged 25 and of independent means, who was seen, by several witnesses, driving at speed down a narrow road and over a narrow bridge, blowing his horn continually. Chased by other motorists whom he had 'baulked', he was seen to pull up outside a public house and get out of his car; when challenged, he denied that he was the driver but later admitted that he was. He also admitted that he had been drinking, but denied that he was drunk. He was not charged with drunken driving, but charges of dangerous driving and of failing to produce a driving licence and insurance were proved; he was fined a total of £32 plus £21 costs, with six months' disqualification.

Only five of the 653 offenders appealed against the findings or sentences in their cases: four succeeded in securing reductions in their sentence and one managed to get his conviction quashed.

Some of these appeal cases are of interest: for example the case of J, who was charged with and convicted of aiding and abetting his lady-friend in driving under the influence of drink, in driving dangerously, and in driving without insurance or a driving licence. She was fined a total of £100 and was disqualified for three years; but J was given a total of eleven months' imprisonment and fifteen years' disqualification. He appealed at once against his sentence, and his appeal was heard eleven days afterwards.

The circumstances were that, early one afternoon, a police superintendent who happened to be travelling behind them saw the appellant and his lady-friend pursuing an erratic course on a major road. When stopped in what turned out to be a hired car, the woman driver appeared to be drunk, and J – her passenger – also, though not so obviously. They were both quiet and cooperative, however, and admitted that, after leaving the hotel where they had lunched, they had been involved in a slight accident with another car, only a few minutes before they were stopped. No details of this accident could be produced because the other motorist refused to say anything; he had given his word that he would settle the matter out of court and he kept it, although the fault was not his. When summoned to appear at court, both J and his friend failed to do so and a warrant was issued for them; they were eventually arrested, living together under assumed names. At the trial it was said that J had been a bad influence on the woman, upon whose independent means he had been living for some years, and a life history was described which certainly lent substance to the view that he was an undesirable influence. It appeared that J was the son of a clerical officer in the Civil Service. He left school at 14, served for fifteen years in the army, and was discharged at the end of the war as a lance-corporal. After a few months as a civilian he re-enlisted, but was soon discharged 'on psychological grounds'. During the next nine years he committed five offences of false pretences, one offence of dangerous driving and failing to stop after or report an accident, and another offence a year later of driving without insurance; he was also convicted of assaulting his wife (for which he was sent to prison for twelve months). In all he had served three terms of imprisonment. The woman had no previous convictions, nor was she known to the police.

The appeal was based on the submission that the court had allowed J's criminal record to influence them unduly, and that this had been reflected in a very severe sentence. His appeal was successful to the extent of securing the substitution of fines totalling £106 for the imprisonment, and a reduction in the period of disqualification to just over three years. But the fines carried alternatives of imprisonment for six months and it is not known which he chose. However, the records show that he was back in prison within two years of the appeal, for stealing and false pretences; and the woman was committed to prison at about the same time for failure to pay her fines for the motoring offences described.

It will be seen that this case has some interesting features, in view of what has been discussed about attitudes to motoring offences and offenders. First, it was thought proper to mention J's non-motoring offences in court, even though these are usually held to be irrelevant; moreover, the court obviously took them into account when deciding the sentence.[1] Second, this was a case in which an aider and abettor was dealt with more severely than the principal offender – probably because the latter was a woman, and because of the relationship between her and J. These considerations, along with the failure to answer the summons to appear, can be assumed to have influenced the sentence too, but it seems reasonable to infer that the real weight of the sentence was imposed because of J's record – as a criminal, not as a motorist. Could it be that if a motoring offender has a record of non-motoring crime it is likely to be produced only if he upsets the police or the court by some incidental behaviour, like failing to answer a summons? There is no definite evidence to support this, but the inference is certainly possible from the experience of J and his friend.

Another case committed for trial is that of K, a national serviceman aged 21, convicted of driving while disqualified. K had a criminal record going back to the age of 10; it included three convictions for larceny and nine for various motoring offences. Of the latter three were for driving while disqualified. His first motoring offence was in September 1956, when he was convicted for driving a motor cycle without insurance, L plates, or road fund licence; for this he was fined, and disqualified for one year. But before his disqualification was completed he was caught driving; he then disappeared and was not brought before a court until April 1958,

---

[1] A striking contrast to this was a bad case of hit-and-run driving before the same court, in which the offender (a known criminal) had eight quite serious previous convictions for offences against property, and two motoring convictions—careless driving, and driving under the influence of drink. Only the two motoring convictions were produced in evidence before the court. The offender was sentenced to three months' imprisonment and three years' disqualification.

when he was sent to prison for one month and disqualified for two years. By September of that year he was back before the court for another offence of driving while disqualified and without insurance; this time he was given six months' imprisonment and was disqualified for a further five years. In the following June (nine months later) he was stopped in the Police District by a patrol, while riding a borrowed motor cycle; of course he could not produce either driving licence or insurance, but he gave the name of the owner of the machine (a 16-year-old boy) as his own, and undertook to produce insurance and licence at his nearest police station within five days. He was then on leave from the army, to which he returned without producing licence or insurance, and he absconded from his unit before the police could catch up with him. He was not heard of again until the police found out that he had appeared before another court outside the Police District, once again for driving while disqualified – this time in a van – and had received six months' imprisonment. He was then brought from prison to be tried for the offence on the borrowed motor cycle, and was given another six months in prison and a fine of £2 for giving a false address (with the alternative of a further four weeks in prison).

K appealed against this last sentence because he complained that a letter he had written to the magistrates was not read before sentence; he was believed by the Appeals Committee, and his sentence was reduced to four months' imprisonment. The letter K wrote is of some interest and it is produced uncorrected as Appendix D. Its writer was educated at a secondary modern school until he was 14, and he had many labouring jobs before being called up into the army, where his record was poor, with several entries for absence. By the time he was 21 he was married with three children, but he was living apart from his wife at the time of this conviction. Incidentally, his wife agreed with his mother that he was not worth a surety while awaiting trial, since they were sure he would abscond. The letter is a pathetic document from a man whose life is in the mess that is typical of the petty criminal. Here is the stuff of the recidivist motoring offender, committing repeated offences of driving while disqualified, regardless of the probability of prison sentences or of further disqualifications. Yet he is not an especially extreme example of the driving while disqualified group of offenders in this research.

The remaining three appeals were all against convictions for dangerous driving only.

L, a dealer aged 50, was driving his own lorry when he overtook another lorry as he was approaching the brow of a hill, thereby causing two oncoming cars to brake so suddenly that they ran into each other; L did not stop, and he succeeded in convincing the police that he was unaware of the incident. He was fined £20 and was disqualified for one year. On appeal his conviction was quashed; there were no previous convictions.

M, aged 40, whose occupation was not stated, also overtook when approaching the brow of a hill in his 1½-litre saloon, and collided with an approaching motor cycle combination. His defence was that he was forced onto his wrong side because the car he was overtaking pulled out to the centre of the road and accelerated, so that he could not regain his correct position. However, one is inclined to wonder why M should have thought it defensible to overtake while approaching a blind crest, and it may not be without significance that two other motorists had complained of his overtaking and cutting in prior to the incident. M was fined £25 and disqualified for one year. On appeal the fine was upheld, but the disqualification was halved. There were no previous convictions.

O, a professional driver aged 50, was fined £10 for turning his lorry suddenly to the right, in order to enter a side road from a main trunk route, across the path of an approaching car, the driver of which could not avoid a collision. On appeal, this sentence – an unusually light one for court G – was upheld.

It may be noted that in three out of the four appeals which were partially successful it was the disqualification that was modified. As will be seen later, disqualification seems to hurt offenders more than any other penalty except imprisonment, and it would not be surprising if most appeals were aimed at getting these orders reduced or quashed. In all the cases during which the writer was present it was the question of disqualification that called forth the greatest eloquence from the defence; the plea in mitigation was often the most powerful part of the case, and it was generally based on the extent to which the defendant used and depended upon his vehicle.

On the evidence present it seemed to pay an offender to appeal; but it is noticeable that none of the offenders except K had any additional convictions, which might have been a handicap in their appeals. It is possible that the next group to be considered would not have been so fortunate.

OFFENDERS WITH ADDITIONAL CONVICTIONS

Perhaps the most crucial part of this research from the criminological standpoint is that dealing with the criminal history of these serious motoring offenders. Is it true to say that there is no history of criminal activity in all but a tiny handful of cases?

Now, by 'criminal history' the police, and perhaps many laymen, mean a record of *non*-motoring offences for which it is not unusual to find offenders committed to prison, or – reverting to the previous criteria of crime – a record of offences that could be regarded as being intentional, harmful, or dishonest. This meaning of the term eliminates a large number of cases that are tried summarily, and also the large group of offences that are classified as administrative in this particular study, e.g. offences connected with licensing dogs and wireless sets, with the Sunday trading laws, with playing in the street, with maintenance orders, and so on (even though these offences are often antisocial).

The additional convictions and police records of all the 653 offenders were, therefore, checked; and here it should be explained that the category 'additional convictions' means those recorded in addition to, and exclusive of, the conviction that qualified the offender for inclusion in this study. So, wherever possible, it was decided to take into account not only convictions previous to this qualifying one, but also convictions that had occurred subsequently. (Information of this kind is likely to be more complete in respect of offenders convicted in 1957 and 1958 than it is for those convicted in 1959, since the research data do not go much beyond May 1960.)

The procedure of checking was easier for the 64 per cent of offenders who lived in the Police District than it was for the 36 per cent who did not, since the records held at the headquarters of the division in which the offender lived could be considered reliable. But the documents available in the Police District concerning offenders who lived elsewhere did not necessarily record their non-motoring convictions, because it is not the practice for other police forces to forward details of these when a person is prosecuted for a motoring offence only. It was to fill this gap that the Home Office Research Unit arranged for the entire list of offenders to be checked in the Criminal Record Office, which furnished full particulars of any convictions which were recorded there. Even this, however, could not be conclusive proof that all additional convictions were taken into account, because files are not opened at the CRO as a matter of routine for every offence that comes into the police category of 'criminal', but only where fingerprints are taken; so an offender might have quite a few convictions for petty crime without necessarily having a file at the CRO. Moreover, it could well be that an offender who was only a recent arrival as a resident had convictions for offences of a petty criminal nature, but that this information had not yet been sent on after him by the police authorities concerned to the police in his new locality. Hence the record of additional offences might be under-stated: it is very unlikely that it is over-stated.

After a somewhat ruthless elimination of the administrative offences, it was found from police records that 138 of the 653 offenders (21·13 per cent) had convictions for additional non-motoring offences; of these, fourteen were first offenders, and if they are excluded the percentage falls to 18·8 per cent (see *Table 39*).

Table 39

138 SERIOUS MOTORING OFFENDERS WHO ALSO HAD
CONVICTIONS FOR NON-MOTORING OFFENCES (EXCLUDING
ADMINISTRATIVE OFFENCES)

Offence group	No. of offenders in offence group	Number of additional non-motoring convictions per offender						Total convicted	
		1	2	3	4	5–10	over 10	No.	% of offence group
Causing death	5	1	0	0	1	2	0	4	80·0
Driving while disqualified	69	6	7	9	6	16	9	53	77·0
Driving under the influence	104	4	4	1	1	6	3	19	18·3
Driving dangerously	285	11	11	6	5	5	0	38	13·4
Failing to stop or report	117	4	0	1	0	0	1	6	5·1
Failing to insure	73	5	3	3	3	3	1	18	24·5
Total	653	31	25	20	16	32	14	138	21·13

If less rigorous standards are used we can add to the 138 offenders referred to above a further thirteen persons whose additional non-motoring offences were eliminated as administrative. Strictly speaking, these are criminal offences and they might be thought to indicate antisocial or possibly sociopathic attitudes: six of the offences were trivial, but the remaining seven included repeated failure to comply with maintenance orders, pavilion-breaking, exposing the person, etc. If these are taken into account, the total number of offenders who had additional non-motoring convictions becomes 151, or 23·2 per cent of the 653 offenders.

It should also be noted that there were some sixty offenders who were known to the police as notorious or suspected persons, although they had not been convicted of a non-motoring offence. This group is possibly rather more 'criminal' than the group of thirteen administrative offenders; hence it would not seem to be unfair or unrealistic to include them in the reckoning. This would bring the total number of persons in whom the police had cause to be interested for reasons unconnected with motoring to 211, or 32·3 per cent of the 653. These 62 suspects are shown in *Table 40*, together with the 119 offenders (18·2 per cent of the 653) who had files at the CRO.

Table 40

119 OFFENDERS WITH CRO FILES AND 62 OFFENDERS
KNOWN TO THE POLICE

Motoring offences	Offenders with CRO files	Offenders known to the police
Causing death	4	0
Driving while disqualified	51	3
Driving under the influence	15	8
Driving dangerously	31	19
Failing to stop or report	5	22
Failing to insure	13	10
Total	119	62
% of 653 offenders	18·2	9·2

However, to forestall any criticism of this work on the grounds that trivial offences have been included in order to make a sensational attack on the integrity of motorists, let us say that not more than 21·13 per cent of the 653 offenders can be regarded as having 'criminal' records. The next question is whether this proportion is higher than would be expected in a random sample of the population of England and Wales. We need to know, therefore, what percentage of the total population has been convicted for criminal offences other than trivia. Evidence on this point is difficult to get, but various estimates are available.

One figure, quoted by Hoskins (1961), was based on a survey carried out by Superintendent H. Battley, a former head of the Criminal Record and Fingerprint Department, of the records for England and Wales at his disposal. Apparently he eliminated first offenders and the files recording only one offence over a long period; he also ruled out those unlikely to be heard of again because of their age, length of sentence, or probable decease, and so reduced his files to the charted activities of a core of professional criminals. He estimated them as constituting about ·1 per cent of the population of England and Wales, i.e. one in every thousand persons.

Another figure that can be considered is the proportion of offenders aged 14 and over who committed non-traffic offences in any one year: in 1959 this was 1·12 per cent. But this proportion is based on the total numbers of offenders convicted of principal offences, as given in the *Criminal Statistics*, and these might include the same person several times over. In this research, however, the same individuals are not counted twice for any purpose; hence it is better to take for comparison the proportion of *different* persons who committed *indictable* offences in (say) 1959, which, as a ratio of the population aged 8 and over, is ·357 or nearly ·4 per cent.[1]

There is, then, a wide gap between the lowest comparable percentage of the 653 offenders, i.e. the 18·2 per cent who have CRO files, and any of the percentages given above; and even if the reader takes for comparison the relatively high estimate made by Emmett (1952) – that one in ten of the British population is likely to have been convicted by a criminal court during his lifetime – the proportion found among the 653 offenders is still markedly higher. And the difference is even more marked if we consider that 23·2 per cent might be a more realistic proportion of the offenders in this study, for purposes of this comparison.

Let us now take a closer look at *all* the additional convictions that were recorded, that is, for both motoring and non-motoring offences. They concerned 307 – or 47 per cent – of the 653 offenders. *Table 41* shows the numbers of additional convictions of all kinds, and *Tables 42* and *43* give the types of *offence*.

In *Table 41* the offenders are divided into three groups:

(*a*) Those with additional convictions for *non-motoring* offences only
(*b*) Those with additional convictions for *motoring* offences only
(*c*) Those with additional convictions for *both non-motoring and motoring* offences

For purposes of clarity, however, the analysis that follows deals with the offenders mainly as two groups: those offenders who also had non-motoring convictions; and those whose additional convictions were all for motoring offences.

---

[1] It should be noted that this is the proportion convicted in any single year; yet the percentage given for the serious motoring offenders (21·13 per cent) represents an aggregate for the number of years during which they were at risk. At a modal age of 26 they might be assumed to have been at risk for 19 years since the age of 8. Taking the same number of years at risk for the population at large, the proportion convicted of indictable offences would be ·357 × 19, or 6·78 per cent.

It will be seen from *Table 41* that the slightly larger group of the two is the one with additional motoring offences only – 156 (24 per cent) of the 653 offenders. Of the group with additional non-motoring offences 118 (18·1 per cent) have convictions for both motoring and non-motoring offences, and 33 (5·1 per cent) have convictions for non-motoring offences only. So there is not very much difference in numbers between the 156 motoring offenders 'pure and simple' and the 151 offenders with convictions for other kinds of offence (118 + 33 = 151). The 'motoring offence only' group is not, therefore, in the substantial majority that might have been expected; nevertheless, a detailed examination shows that there are clearly marked differences between the two groups.

As the 'motoring offence only' groups had no non-motoring convictions, ____ ____ group which had such convictions only on ____ ____ butions to motoring crime. The 156 ____ ing offences, of which most of the ____ driving, and speeding. The ____ motoring *and* non-motor- ____ g offences among them, ____ or failing to insure: a ____ the former group (*Table*

____ in the number of indi- ____ more times for motoring ____ to 41 (26 per cent) of the ____ ver, the number of first ____ ng offence only' offenders. ____ riminal of the two groups ____ ntribution to crime *of all* ____ re can be little doubt that ____ re the more criminal of ____ t) of the 151 had three or ____ g offences recorded against ____ e members of the other group ____ nders accounted for at least 610 ____ d only 13 of these could be cate-

gorized definitely as trivial; moreover this number is probably a considerable understatement because full details were not always available for those offenders who had not CRO files (*Table 42*).

OFFENDERS WITH ADDITIONAL CONVICTIONS (INCLUDING

Offence group		Number of offenders in offence group	Number of additional motoring convictions per offender						Total offenders with additional motoring convictions	
			1	*2*	*3*	*4*	*5–10*	*over 10*	Number	% of offence group
Causing death by dangerous driving	A		—	—	—	—	—	—	—	—
	B		0	0	0	0	0	0	0	
	C		1	0	1	0	1	0	3	
	Total	5	1	0	1	0	1	0	3	60·0
Driving while disqualified	A		—	—	—	—	—	—	—	—
	B		8	2	1	2	1	1	15	
	C		4	11	11	7	16	5	54	
	Total	69	12	13	12	9	17	6	69	100·0
Driving under the influence of drink or drugs	A		—	—	—	—	—	—	—	—
	B		10	9	3	3	1	0	26	
	C		2	2	2	6	1	2	15	
	Total	104	12	11	5	9	2	2	41	39·4
Driving dangerously	A		—	—	—	—	—	—	—	—
	B		42	14	12	5	3	0	76	
	C		4	6	5	3	6	2	26	
	Total	285	46	20	17	8	9	2	102	35·8
Failing to stop or report	A		—	—	—	—	—	—	—	—
	B		11	11	2	1	3	1	29	
	C		3	1	0	2	0	1	7	
	Total	117	14	12	2	3	3	2	36	30·8
Failing to insure	A		—	—	—	—	—	—	—	—
	B		4	4	0	1	1	0	10	
	C		3	2	3	0	3	2	13	
	Total	73	7	6	3	1	4	2	23	31·5
Grand total	A		—	—	—	—	—	—	—	—
	B		75	40	18	12	9	2	156	23·9
	C		17	22	22	18	27	12	118	18·0
		653	92	62	40	30	36	14	274	
% of offence group		100	14·1	9·5	6·1	4·6	5·5	2·1	41·9	

A – Those with additional convictions for non-motoring offences only.
B – Those with additional convictions for motoring offences only.
C – Those with additional convictions for both non-motoring and motoring offences.

41

THOSE FOR ADMINISTRATIVE OFFENCES)

Number of additional non-motoring convictions per offender						Total offenders with additional non-motoring convictions		Offenders with additional convictions A + B + C	
1	*2*	*3*	*4*	*5–10*	*over 10*	*Number*	*% of offence group*	*Number*	*% of offence group*
1	0	0	0	0	0	1		1	
								0	
0	0	0	0	1	2	3		3	
1	0	0	0	1	2	4	80·0	4	80·0
0	0	0	0	0	0	0		0	
								15	
7	8	8	6	16	9	54		54	
7	8	8	6	16	9	54	78·6	69	100·0
1	1	1	0	2	1	6		6	
								26	
4	3	1	1	4	2	15		15	
5	4	2	1	6	3	21	20·2	47	45·2
7	5	2	0	2	1	17		17	
								76	
9	6	4	4	2	1	26		26	
16	11	6	4	4	2	43	15·1	119	41·7
3	0	1	0	0	0	4		4	
								29	
4	1	0	0	2	0	7		7	
7	1	1	0	2	0	11	9·4	40	34·2
2	1	1	1	0	0	5		5	
								10	
3	2	2	2	4	0	13		13	
5	3	3	3	4	0	18	24·7	28	38·4
14	7	5	1	4	2	33		33	
								156	
27	20	15	14	30	12	118	18·1	118	
41	27	20	15	34	14	151		307	
6·3	4·1	3·2	2·3	5·2	2·1	23·2		47·1	

The Documentary Study

Table 42

ANALYSIS OF ADDITIONAL NON-MOTORING CONVICTIONS
SHOWING TYPE OF OFFENCE

Offence group	Offences against property	Sex offences	Taking vehicles without consent	Other non-motoring offences	Total non-motoring offences	Number of offenders concerned
Causing death	14	0	0	2	16	4
Driving while disqualified	184	5	62	41	292	54
Driving under the influence	74	1	8	21	104	21
Driving dangerously	83	8	2	27	120	43
Failing to stop or report	14	0	2	11	27	11
Failing to insure	30	5	4	12	51	18
Total	399	19	78	114	610	151

Offenders with Additional Non-motoring Convictions

Having found that the offenders who also had non-motoring convictions are more criminal than the 'motoring offence only' group, in that they perpetrated a higher proportion of motoring offences too, let us now arrange the six offences in a hierarchy according to the proportion of offenders in each group who had additional non-motoring convictions (*Tables 41* and *42*).

The first two places in such a hierarchy are not hard to fill. Four of the five offenders convicted of causing death by dangerous driving had convictions for offences against property, and three for motoring offences – mostly for speeding. Thus, despite the small number in the group, this offence ranks first. A possible explanation could be that the authorities are more inclined to bring this charge against offenders who already have non-motoring convictions than against other offenders, who are allowed to escape with the lesser alternative of dangerous driving (even though a death has occurred in the incident). There was no evidence to support this view; nevertheless, the possibility cannot be dismissed out of hand since there was only one case of dangerous driving in which a fatality occurred.

Next come the offenders convicted of driving while disqualified who, because of their numbers, seem to be the least law-abiding of the six groups. No less than 54 (78·6 per cent) of the 69 offenders had additional non-motoring convictions, and they contributed the highest *number* of non-motoring offences also. The most characteristic offences were those against property, and taking vehicles without consent (*Table 42*). Moreover, the frequency with which they 'take and drive away without consent' is reflected in the fact that their contribution to the purely motoring offences is the greatest of the six offence groups; their most frequent motoring offences were failing to insure (which inevitably accompanies taking without consent) and additional offences of driving while disqualified. However, they seemed to commit fewer of the 'driving' offences (dangerous or careless driving, driving under the influence, or failing to stop, etc.) than the offenders in the other offence groups. This supports Gibbens's view (1958) that joy-riders and car thieves are not necessarily dangerous drivers: probably because they have much to lose by drawing attention to themselves.

As there seems to be some association between driving while disqualified and the insurance offences, it is not surprising to find the latter in a prominent position in the hierarchy. Even as a 10 per cent sample of residents these offenders achieve third place, and they would easily head the other five offence groups if they were expanded to their full population. Of the sample of 73 insurance offenders, nearly 25 per cent had additional convictions for non-motoring offences; the majority were for offences against property, and about 8 per cent were for taking vehicles without consent. Most of the motoring offences were breaches of the law regarding insurance or licensing, and the inference is that these individuals save a lot of money by taking a chance on being caught without insurance, driving licence, or excise licence.

Fourth in this somewhat doubtful order of merit are the drunken drivers. Of the 104 offenders, 21 (20·2 per cent) had committed additional non-motoring offences, mainly against property; and it is worth noting that in this group there was a fairly high incidence of taking vehicles without consent. Their additional motoring convictions were mostly for driving dangerously or carelessly, or for speeding; but this group also contained the highest number (11) of additional convictions for drunken driving in any of the six groups, though it is of passing interest that only four of these people had convictions for being drunk and disorderly or for simple drunkenness.

Following the drunken drivers are the dangerous drivers: 43 (15·1 per cent) of the 285 offenders in this group had additional non-motoring convictions. Of the latter, 69 per cent were for offences against property; there were also eight sex offences, the highest number found in any of the

215

Table 43

OFFENDERS WITH ADDITIONAL MOTORING CONVICTIONS

Offence group		No. of offenders with additional motoring offences	NUMBER AND TYPE OF ADDITIONAL MOTORING OFFENCE								Total additional motoring offences
			Causing death	Driving while disqualified	Driving under the influence	Driving dangerously or carelessly	Failing to stop or report	Failing to insure	Speeding	Other motoring offences	
Causing death	B	0	0	0	0	0	0	0	0	0	0
	C	3	0	0	0	0	0	0	4	5	9
	Total	3	0	0	0	0	0	0	4	5	9
Driving while disqualified	B	15	0	3	1	1	0	12	3	27	47
	C	54	1	34	1	5	1	108	9	126	285
	Total	69	1	37	2	6	1	120	12	153	332
Driving under the influence	B	26	0	0	6	13	2	2	9	25	57
	C	15	0	3	5	13	2	6	7	31	67
	Total	41	0	3	11	26	4	8	16	56	124
Driving dangerously	B	76	0	0	0	17	4	6	38	85	150
	C	26	0	1	4	6	4	10	19	34	78
	Total	102	0	1	4	23	8	16	57	119	228
Failing to stop or report	B	29	0	0	3	7	3	2	17	41	73
	C	7	0	0	0	2	2	3	1	25	33
	Total	36	0	0	3	9	5	5	18	66	106
Failing to insure	B	10	0	1	0	0	1	4	4	14	24
	C	13	0	0	0	0	1	19	2	55	77
	Total	23	0	1	0	0	2	23	6	69	101
Total	B	156	0	4	10	38	10	26	71	192	351
Total	C	118	1	38	10	26	10	146	42	276	549
Grand total		274	1	42	20	64	20	172	113	468	900

B – Those with additional motoring convictions only.

six motoring offence groups. Their additional motoring convictions were mostly for speeding and failing to insure; only six of the 78 additional motoring offences committed by this group were cases of dangerous or careless driving, and there were only four cases of failing to stop after or to report an accident: a rather different picture from what had been expected.

Finally, there is the group convicted of failing to stop after or to report an accident; it must be remembered that this was a sample confined to residents in the Police District, and it is not possible to say what proportion it represents of all such offenders, whether resident or not. Of the 117 people in the sample, 11 or 9·4 per cent had non-motoring convictions: about half were for offences against property and only two were for taking vehicles without consent. The additional motoring convictions were mostly for insurance and licensing offences; the number of 'driving' offences was negligible, an unexpected finding that is not repeated when the records of their 'opposite numbers' in the motoring offence only group are considered below. Having regard to the nature of this offence it was not anticipated that its perpetrators would be last in the hierarchy; but it may be because there were so many women and middle-class people among them.

The order of the offence groups is unchanged when they are ranked according to the proportion of offenders in each group who had three or more additional convictions for non-motoring offences (*Table 44*).

Table 44

OFFENDERS WITH THREE OR MORE NON-MOTORING
CONVICTIONS

Offence group	*Percentage of group with 3 or more non-motoring convictions*
Causing death	60
Driving while disqualified	57
Failing to insure	14
Driving under the influence	12
Driving dangerously	6
Failing to stop or report	3

These offenders who had non-motoring convictions were responsible for a substantial number of motoring offences also: 79 of the 151 offenders (51 per cent) had three or more additional convictions for motoring offences, and many seemed to alternate frequently between the two kinds of offence. An example is the case of P.

P was a car salesman, aged 42. He was found late one night, sitting in his car, which had its wheels in a ditch and was blocking a main road. He was convicted of driving under the influence of drink and was sent to prison for four months; he was also disqualified for ten years. This man had had quite a reasonable start in life, and at 21 had gone into business with his brother in a garage which they ran for three years; he then left the firm to become a car salesman, and began a series of criminal offences that was broken only by a period of service in the second world war. When he came to notice in this research he had twenty-six previous convictions, fourteen for motoring offences and twelve for non-motoring offences. Of the latter nine were for stealing and two for taking cars without consent; and there were also convictions for car theft, fraud, and false pretences. The motoring offences included one previous conviction for drunken driving, two for dangerous driving, and one for driving while disqualified. He had served eight prison sentences, the longest for eighteen months, and there were two previous disqualifications from driving.

In this particular case it is interesting that many of the criminal offences were concerned with cars; e.g. cars were stolen or taken without permission, the offender perpetrated a fraud or stole to acquire a car, and so on. Thus, rather than being *merely the means* of committing criminal offences – which cars are usually assumed to be – the car is *itself the focus* of a constellation of criminal offences. This is obvious in cases of 'taking vehicles without consent', as Gibbens (1958) has shown.

Another offender whose criminal activities embraced motoring and non-motoring offences is Q, a 32-year-old builder's foreman. At about midnight his car, which was without lights, was seen by the police, swerving from side to side of a main road. When stopped he was found to be drunk, and urine tests showed that he had consumed the equivalent of $5\frac{1}{4}$ pints of beer. At the police station he was truculent and abusive, and it was said that the woman passenger in his car was clearly terrified of him. Inquiries revealed that he was the man wanted for knocking a youth off his bicycle a month earlier and driving away without stopping; also he had stolen petrol from a filling station. He was fined a total of £65, and was disqualified for five years for all these offences.

Q's criminal record is interesting. It began at the age of 13 with a finding of guilt for wilful damage and, with a break during the war, he went on to amass twelve convictions for offences against property (mostly breaking in and burglary). and seventeen for motoring offences, including two for driving without due care and attention. After the conviction that brought him into this research, he drove while disqualified and was concerned in another accident which he failed to report (for obvious reasons); he was convicted also of driving without care and attention and of failing to insure against third-party risks. He was sent to prison for three months and disqualified for a further ten years. Then, within days, he appeared again at another court for burglary and stealing, and was sent to prison for three years.

Yet another example is that of R, aged 36 and unemployed, who was stopped on his motor cycle by a suspicious policeman. He had no driving licence or insurance to show, and undertook to produce them at his local police station later – but did not do so. It took nearly four months to get him to court, but failures to appear and applications for adjournments prolonged his trial until six months after his offences. Eventually he was sent to prison for three months and fined £5, but he was not disqualified despite a criminal record that began at 16 with the same offence – driving uninsured. From that he went on to accumulate seventeen motoring offences, including six for driving uninsured and four for driving while disqualified. Alternating with these were eleven non-motoring offences, including larceny, receiving, fraud, and taking a vehicle without the owner's consent. Like P he had served eight prison sentences, but none was for more than nine months – and none had deterred him from offending again.

R's life history was typical of the petty criminal. He left school at 15 and drifted from job to job, mostly in the motor trade, until he was called up for army service. After one year's war service he was discharged with an indifferent character. He then went into an aircraft factory, where he was soon rated lazy and an all-round nuisance. For the ten years prior to the offence which qualified him for the study, he had been 'self-employed', working casually as a motor mechanic, and only three of the ten years seem to have been without a court appearance for something.

It may be noticed that these three offenders were all over 30, a fact that may give a misleading impression, since 70 per cent of the offenders with criminal records were under 30, with the mode in the group aged 21 and under 30 years. The preponderance of young people is almost certainly explained by the high proportion of offenders who were convicted of driving while disqualified.

Occupationally, the people with records were concentrated rather heavily in the manual groups, from which 78 per cent of them came. Most of these were semi-skilled and unskilled workers, and only a handful professed some kind of skilled trade. Only 5·4 per cent were of occupational status above 'lower non-manual', and these were marginal, with none in the highest occupational group (i.e. professional and higher administrative).

Offenders with Additional Motoring Convictions only

When the offenders who also had non-motoring convictions are excluded, and the offence groups are ranked according to the proportions in each group who had additional convictions for motoring offences only, a very different order of 'merit' emerges.

Now the dangerous drivers head the list, with 76 (26·6 per cent) of the 285 offenders having additional motoring convictions. They were responsible for 150 offences, of which the majority were similar ones of dangerous or careless driving, or speeding. None had additional convictions for drunken driving or for driving while disqualified.

Next come the drunken drivers: 26 (25 per cent) of the 104 offenders had additional motoring convictions, mostly for speeding or for dangerous driving, but it is notable that this group accounted for six additional offences of the same kind.

The drunken drivers are followed closely by the failing to stop group, of whom 29 (24 per cent) had additional motoring convictions. They contributed 73 offences, of which most were 'moving' offences, i.e. speeding, and dangerous or careless driving.

The next group, the disqualifieds, are surprisingly low in this order: 15 (21·8 per cent) of the 69 offenders had additional convictions for motoring offences only. (This percentage contrasts with the 78 per cent of their counterparts who had additional convictions for both non-motoring and motoring offences.) These offenders committed a total of 47 additional motoring offences (their opposite numbers committed 285); most were insurance or licensing offences and there were also a number of cases of failure to carry L plates.

As none of the causing death by dangerous driving group had additional motoring convictions only, the last of the offence groups is the insurance offenders. In this 10 per cent sample 10 (13·6 per cent) had additional motoring convictions only, and 2 had three or more. The group committed 24 offences in all, of which the majority were licensing and L plate offences. But it should not be thought that this is a group of innocent 'technical' offenders: five of them were not bad cases, but the remaining five were notable in respect of false addresses, difficulty in getting the offender to court, and deliberate evasion. Looking through these latter five cases, it seemed that most of the offenders had their feet on the first rung of the ladder leading to repeated offences.

The Offenders

As far as the writer is aware, the term 'recidivist' has never been applied to motoring offenders in respect of motoring offences. Yet among this group of 653 serious offenders there are 120 (18·3 per cent) who have three or more additional motoring convictions recorded against them. The offenders who also have non-motoring convictions include a much higher proportion of 'repeaters' than the motoring offence only group: 52 per cent of the former had three or more additional motoring convictions compared with 26 per cent of the latter.

Moreover, it can be seen from *Table 45* that 134 (20·5 per cent) of the 653 offenders were repeaters, not only because they had more than one additional conviction, but also in that they had committed the same offence (or another that might be regarded as equally serious) more than once. It is especially noticeable that nearly one-third of the 'disqualifieds' had committed the same offence more than once, and so had about 10 per cent of the drunken drivers.

Table 45

134 SERIOUS MOTORING OFFENDERS WITH ADDITIONAL
CONVICTIONS FOR THE SAME OR A SIMILAR OFFENCE

Offence group	Offenders with additional convictions for the same or a similar motoring offence		Total
	Same offence	Similar offence	
Causing death	0	0	0
Driving while disqualified	22	40	62
Driving under the influence	10	14	24
Driving dangerously	17	14	31
Failing to stop	3	7	10
Failing to insure	7	0	7
Total	59	75	134

Such people would seem to constitute a hard core of serious motoring offenders, and the following examples should cast considerable doubt on the validity of the hypothesis that the serious motoring offender does not repeat his offence – although, it must be admitted, we are discussing a minority.

The Documentary Study

The first example is not, strictly speaking, a motoring offence repeater as defined above, since he had only two additional motoring convictions, and one of these (taking a vehicle without consent) is more an offence against property than a motoring offence. But the other was the gravest motoring offence possible: motor manslaughter.

S, a young soldier, was stopped by a suspicious policeman on a summer evening, when he was driving a borrowed motor cycle along a busy trunk road. He could not produce his licence or insurance certificate, but offered to bring them to the nearest police station within the statutory five days; he failed to do so and had to be traced to his unit, where he produced another soldier's licence and insurance certificate as his own. It was then found that he was in fact disqualified, having been sentenced two years earlier to concurrent sentences of twelve and eighteen months' imprisonment, with twenty years' disqualification, for the manslaughter of his accomplice, which had occurred when S was driving a vehicle that they had taken without permission. For driving while disqualified he was sent to prison for six months, plus a further three months for driving without insurance.

S had been punished severely in court and he had lost his friend, yet he was not deterred from committing these further offences. In fact it would seem that disqualification *per se* does not keep people such as S off the roads; they take the risk and drive again, and the interviews with offenders (see Chapter 10 below) suggest that cases of this kind are not unusual. In the light of these findings, then, is it always wise to disqualify serious offenders for very long periods? For a young man of 18, a twenty-year disqualification might as well be disqualification for life, and he may develop a 'might as well be hung for a sheep as a lamb' attitude, knowing that he will be unable to withstand temptation for twenty years, though he might have done so for one or two. Indeed, very long periods of disqualification may bring about more crimes than they prevent – a view that will be taken up again later in this study.

More typical of the 'recidivists' is T, an 18-year-old labourer who managed to achieve no less than twenty-four convictions for motoring offences in twenty-one months (*Table 46*). This is a formidable list: though none of the offences is really serious, except driving while disqualified, they suggest a wholesale disrespect for the law. It should be said in fairness that a few of the offences could have arisen out of a single journey as the offender drove from one division to another; but this is unlikely, and it is more probable that these are in fact a succession of unconnected offences.

The Offenders

Table 46

OFFENDER T – RECORD OF ADDITIONAL CONVICTIONS

Date	Court	Charge	Sentence Fine	Other
1957				
3 Jan	Outside District	Speeding No lights	£2 10s.	
2 May	Treeford	Failure to produce insurance Learner, no L plates	£1 £2	
13 June	Treeford	Learner, no L plates	£5	Disqualified 3 months
11 July	Treeford	No rear lights (2 offences) Failure to stop on police signal Learner with unqualified passenger	£1 £1 £10	Disqualified 1 year
12 July	Treeford	No lights, pedal-cycle	£1	
5 Dec	Treeford	Driving while disqualified No insurance		Detention centre, 4 months Probation order, 2 years
1959				
7 May	Treeford	Failure to stop on police signal Learner, no L plates (4 offences)	£3 £10 on each offence	
13 May	Opsley	No driving licence No road fund licence	£3 £5	
28 May	Batwick	Learner, no L plates Learner with unqualified passenger	£2 £2	
15 July	Batwick	Speeding Learner, no L plates	£5 £4	
21 Sept 23 Oct	Elston	Failure to obey traffic signal Appealed: disqualification removed	£10	Disqualified 2 years

This kind of thing could be illustrated equally well from the histories of another thirteen offenders with ten or more motoring convictions each, and there are a further thirty-six offenders with between five and ten convictions each who could match T's record quite closely.

Another typical repeater problem is U, a 19-year-old labourer who came to notice on his conviction for eighteen motoring offences at a single hearing. They were the ones usually found in the repeaters' histories – insurance offences, using vehicles in a dangerous condition, speeding, and driving either without L plates or without a driving licence or an excise licence. Time after time these individuals commit such offences until they are eventually disqualified; next comes the almost inevitable charge for driving while disqualified, with the equally inevitable committal to prison or the equivalent. U was no exception, and the court had little option on the occasion mentioned above but to send him to prison, since he had already been fined fourteen times, and disqualified twice, for fourteen previous motoring offences, besides having been twice committed to a detention centre for property offences. Though U's overt occupation was reported as 'labourer', his main line was the purchase, renovation, and sale of rather decrepit cars, and it was while driving them in the course of his transactions that he seems to have been caught for most of his offences. It would be wrong, however, to give the impression that U was the victim of bad luck; he was well known to the local police as a young criminal whose undetected activities were probably more impressive than those which were found out. Needless to say, the prognosis by the police was not a good one.

It might be expected that these repeater offenders, or motoring recidivists, would be criminals who used vehicles in connection with non-motoring crime and were caught while so doing. But this is not supported by the evidence, and only one case could be attributed directly to the commission of other crime – in this instance, shopbreaking; in none of the others is there any reason to suppose that the offenders' business (apart from their driving conduct) was anything but lawful. Rather does their motoring behaviour reflect a general disrespect for the provisions of law, an attitude that is with them whatever they are doing. The cases of V and W are examples in point: while not qualifying yet for classification as repeaters or recidivists, they seem well on the way to becoming eligible.

V, another 19-year-old labourer, had a string of property violations going back to his thirteenth year. He lived with his mother and stepfather in a council house, but had spent most of his youth in 'very poor circumstances' in a Nissen hut. His stepfather was unable to control him 'because of the difference in their heights', and he was known as an aggressive youth with several convictions for wilful damage, and one for grievous bodily harm. He was mentally backward also. In June 1958 he approached a garage near his home, and found among the cars displayed for sale on the forecourt an unlocked car with ignition key in place; it had been left by one of the salesmen who had gone for lunch. V took the car, and drove five miles to a nearby town where he had to report to his probation officer. He duly reported, drove back to the garage, returned the car to where it had been – and was caught in the act. For that escapade he was sent to a detention centre for three months (his second spell of restraint, having been committed to an approved school at 14 for housebreaking) and disqualified for two years. Yet, six months after discharge from the detention centre, he committed an almost identical offence: he took another car from the same garage car park, where it had been left with ignition key in place by the same salesman. V then collected a party of friends from the local pub and drove them all to Brighton. On the way back in the small hours V and his party were halted by a level-crossing – and by a policeman who happened to be standing by. His suspicions were aroused when V could not produce either driving licence or insurance, and gave an expensive London address which was not in accord with his appearance. At the police station V admitted everything, and on conviction he was sent to prison for three months and disqualified for four years.

But perhaps W, a 20-year-old army private, would be a good example of an incipient recidivist with whom to conclude this section. In February 1959 he was convicted for taking a van without the owner's consent and for driving it without either a driving licence or insurance; on that occasion he received a very lenient sentence – a fine of £4 10s. and one year's disqualification. Three days after this conviction he took a small car from the drive of a private house near his camp, to absent himself without leave and go home; but this time he was sent to prison for three months, fined £3, and disqualified for three years. Significantly his army conduct was said to be 'poor', and he was suspected of many other offences of 'taking and driving away' in the area.

It is a pity that the documents available did not give more information about these repeaters, especially about their social backgrounds and personality characteristics. If only because this small problem group of offenders give the police and the courts so much trouble, they would repay investigation on a serious scale, and could be compared, on a variety of tests, with control groups of non-motoring offenders and of non-offending motorists.

PATHOLOGICAL PERSONALITY TRAITS

In seeking to answer one of the main questions behind this research – namely, whether the data lend any support to the view of Tillmann and

Hobbs (1949) that an individual drives as he lives – an attempt was made to discover whether a significant proportion of the 653 subjects showed evidence of pathological personality traits which might be associated with their offences. In the event, the extraction of such information proved to be very difficult because it is one of the faults of non-medical documentary material of this kind that it tends to be very subjective, based as most of it is on the judgements of persons without psychological or psychiatric training. The available evidence was, therefore, highly impressionistic, and it tended to be biased according to the amount of cooperation offered by the offender to the police; the traits of the uncooperative seemed to be 'played up' in reports, and those of the cooperative were relatively ignored. The extent to which an offender cooperated with the police could not, in itself, be accepted as any indication of an offender's personality since refusal to cooperate could often mean reluctance to say anything lest it should be incriminating; and – especially in drunken driving cases – it often meant that the offender refused to undergo any tests. Such responses are to be expected from any accused person who does not intend to plead guilty from the outset; they do not signify that he is uncooperative and awkward.

Even so, only about one-third of the 653 offenders were said specifically to have been uncooperative, and there is no doubt that they included some who went beyond mere reluctance to make statements or undergo tests. Some definitely obstructed by the most blatant lying and subterfuge the entire course of the police investigations: e.g. Mrs AB, who drove on after hitting a pedestrian who, without looking, had stepped off the pavement in front of her car. Witnesses saw her car and she was traced, but she denied being near the scene at the time until faced with evidence connecting paintwork from her car with the clothing of the injured man. She then admitted that she had been in the area and had hit what she thought to be a pile of rubbish in the road, so she had driven on without concern – a strange story for a lady who had previous convictions for failing to stop after an accident, failing to stop for a school crossing, careless driving, and obstruction. Though the police files remarked on her 'very bad driving', she had not been disqualified for any of these previous offences, and for the offence described above she 'got off lightly' with a £10 fine.

Information of this nature is not, however, sufficient to justify inferences about the presence of pathological traits in an offender's personality. More specific evidence is required, such as might be found in an offender's criminal record, in the remarks of medical witnesses, or in behaviour of an extreme kind at the scene of the offence or immediately afterwards.

The Offenders

There was such evidence, indicative of unusual traits, in 165 cases (25·3 per cent of the 653). These offenders were roughly classified into three categories: the aggressive or ruthless, the neurotic, and the remainder who could not be placed in either category.

For the ruthless and aggressive classification, the criteria were previous convictions for violence against persons or property, or specific evidence of violence or aggression in the case under study: 77 offenders (11·8 per cent of the 653) were placed in this group.

In the neurotic category were the offenders who exhibited hysterical, depressive, or compulsive behaviour; or whose histories contained evidence of instability, e.g. broken marriages, inability to settle in employment, drunkenness, and convictions for sexual offences: 75 offenders (11·6 per cent of the 653) were thus categorized.

Finally there were 13 offenders (2 per cent of the 653) who could not be placed in either category, but who seemed to display features that suggested a personality disturbance: for example, offenders with very long records of crime, and those whose behaviour could not be envisaged as normal in any sense of the word. There was the offender T who, although he had been disqualified on the evidence of the local policeman, drove past the officer's house twice in daylight when the policeman was in his front garden and an obvious spectator. Or the army corporal: he was driving back to camp late at night with two other soldiers with whom he had been drinking; he hit two pedestrians on the kerbless road, killing one and seriously injuring the other, but did not stop. When traced he was charged with causing death by dangerous driving, on evidence that he had cornered much too fast and had hit the pedestrians when out of control. He denied knowledge of any collision with pedestrians, and said he returned to the scene when one of his passengers told him there had been an accident. The passengers' story was rather different: they said that he not only was aware of the accident but resisted the urging of his companions to turn back for some time. In the event he was convicted of the lesser charge of driving dangerously, fined £25, and disqualified for ten years. He had two previous convictions earlier in the same year: one for failing to conform to a traffic light, and another for speeding in a built-up area, for which small fines were imposed. There is, however, a Dickensian coincidence to end this account, for one of the offenders interviewed in the final stages of this research (also a soldier) said that he had been given away to the police for driving uninsured by this same NCO, who was now in charge of the regimental police and had a reputation for 'getting' anyone he could on the slightest pretext. Perhaps a slender constellation of circumstantial evidence

227

for putting this man in the pathological group, but his inclusion seems justified, at least to a certain extent.

The 'aggressive' personalities were the easiest to classify, for the evidence was clear cut in most of the 77 cases that were placed in this group. Two of the worst were somewhat unusual. On one occasion a motorist, an elderly man, was driving along a country road with his wife, when he noticed a posse of eight black-clad motor cyclists behind him. Two of these came abreast of his car on either side, and the one on the offside abused him for his slow and bad driving, calling on him to stop and fight. When he ignored this and drove on, the rider who had abused him reached through the open window of the car and struck him in the face, knocking off his spectacles; the rest of the group then hemmed in the still moving car by driving two behind, two in front, and two on either side of it. These incidents were witnessed by the driver of a small van who was following with his wife and small baby; he overtook the group in order to seek assistance, and stopped at a road junction where there was a special constable on point duty. When waved down to stop the motor cyclists and their quarry drew into the kerb where the former dismounted and jostled the drivers of both vehicles, ignoring the policeman and (it was alleged) attempting also to overturn the van with the woman and baby inside. When the policeman said he was going to get assistance the party made off, but they were traced through their registration numbers. Tried for dangerous driving, their defence was that the motorist had impeded them earlier and was drunk; they had merely been trying to teach him a lesson. But it appeared that this was not the only instance of motorists being 'roughed up' on the main roads of southern England, and there seemed no doubt that this was a gang of young men out to make trouble when they could. Very properly the magistrates called it a case of 'real hooliganism on the roads', and they sentenced the ringleader, a 25-year-old plumber's mate, to three months' imprisonment and three years' disqualification. There were three previous convictions: one for stealing and two for speeding.

The second incident occurred on a summer evening when a Mr C was driving his family in their saloon down the A25 main road; there was light traffic moving in the same direction but a steady stream coming the other way. Mr C saw a large sports tourer pull out from the forecourt of a garage across the front of the approaching traffic, and move in his direction with the evident intention of cutting in front of him. Mr C pulled into his near-side to avoid a collision and passed the other car on its nearside; he was then followed by the driver of this vehicle, who was 'hooting furiously'. When Mr C pulled into the side of the road to see what was the matter the other driver was alleged to have driven deliberately into the back of Mr C's car, reversed away, and then driven off at speed. Mr C was quite sure that he had been rammed. A penitent driver reported the incident to the police three days later, saying that he felt guilty for a foolish act. The accused driver, a sub-postmaster aged 37, said he did not stop after the incident because he did not want his wife to know that he had been involved in an accident; he was very sorry for himself, and he gave this impression at the trial also. He pleaded guilty to careless driving and failing to stop or report, having begged the police not to charge him with dangerous driving, this being his first offence (he did not mention that he had two previous motoring convictions of which, unfortunately, there was no record). However, the punishment reflected his admitted guilt of a serious and dangerous piece of aggressive driving: he was fined £40 for careless driving, and the maximum of £20 on each charge of failing to stop after and failing to report an accident. There was, however, no disqualification, presumably because the defendant pleaded dependence on driving in his business.[1]

The majority of the cases of aggressive conduct were in the dangerous driving group, which accounted for no less than 62 per cent of them. The neurotics, on the other hand, were mostly to be found among the drunken drivers, who provided 70 out of the total of 75 offenders thus categorized. Many of these defendants broke down and wept hysterically when taken to the police station; realizing their predicament, some lost control of their motions and soiled themselves with urine, faeces, or vomit, presenting a wretched and pitiable sight. Others were in a state of hysterical happiness and could not grasp the significance of their position at all: they talked happily away about how much they had drunk and how fast they had driven – some even readily saying not only that they were drunk, but that they wanted to drive their cars away, thus furnishing the police with a cut-and-dried case. One actually challenged his captors to a race.

It was noticeable in many of these cases of driving under the influence that offenders talked a great deal at the police station after apprehension, and much of what was said was used as evidence of their condition. Some of this material was probably a good indication of disturbance, as in the case of some offenders who indulged in homosexual banter: e.g. one extremely aggressive and violent man who suddenly said to the police surgeon, 'you've a lovely face, I'd like to play kiss in the ring with you'; and another who told the station sergeant that he was 'a really lovely boy'. Much other conversation 'under the influence' showed domestic and

[1] This case was, in fact, deleted from the statistics, because the offender turned out not to be a resident of the Police District.

business stress, and it seemed unfortunate and unfair that so much of it was put into statements for the prosecution. It was more embarrassing than relevant, since the test of drunkenness (in so far as fitness to drive is concerned) would seem to be the *behaviour* of the accused rather than what he says.

It is worth remarking on the number of cases in this offence group in which the drinking had clearly not been done at a party or for amusement; it seemed mostly to be the behaviour of people who were under considerable stress, and having trouble with some aspect of their lives. An example was X, a middle-aged businessman, whose large fast saloon car charged into an approaching car, knocking it off the road and into a cyclist, injuring several people. The defendant was so drunk that he could not stand, and in so wretched a condition at the police station that he urinated in the middle of the charge-room. When sent for trial it emerged that his wife had left him and become pregnant by another man; as a result he had suffered a nervous breakdown, and after two weeks in hospital had gone away for a holiday with his two young sons. On his way back he had drunk too much at lunch and hence his predicament. He was sent to prison for three months and disqualified for twenty years, though there was full medical support for his story and also to the effect that he was suffering from arthritis. There were four previous convictions: two for drunken driving ten years and thirteen years before, one for speeding, and one for a parking offence.

The domestic theme was apparent also in the case of Y, a professional man in his fifties, whose regular appearance on the suburban railway station, impeccably groomed and apparently in the best of health, concealed a propensity to indulge in very heavy bouts of drinking which seemed to be related to his marital relations. This was certainly the case when his large car was seen by a mobile patrol, shortly after 10 pm on a Saturday evening, being driven erratically and mounting the pavement in a built-up area, just missing some pedestrians. On arrival at the police station he was recognized as an old acquaintance whose heavy drinking and frequent domestic quarrels were well known; he was very voluble: 'I'm gloriously pissed. My wife's driven me to it. How (to the inspector) would you like to be the co-respondent? I'd like to thrash her but I'm not big enough.' In the end he got thrashed himself with a fine of £60 plus costs, and a year's disqualification, which he soon sought unsuccessfully to have removed without having made any apparent attempt to change his habits.

It should be emphasized, however, that the police do not much like the business of dealing with drunken drivers. One can see why from the case of

Z, for instance, an advertising consultant aged 48, who was seen driving erratically early one evening by a police mobile patrol. When stopped he refused to leave his car and had to be got out by force. At the police station he was extremely abusive and aggressive, trying to assault the police doctor who eventually gave up attempting to examine him. He became so violent that the doctor had to ring his wife to see if there was any history of mental illness (there was not). According to the doctor: 'This man must have been a most dangerous driver who was capable of killing anyone who crossed his path.' Z was fined £50 and disqualified for one year; there was only one previous conviction for a lighting offence.

A strange incident that might be mentioned concerned a 44-year-old professional man: he was driving his small family car along a main road at about 6.30 p.m. just before Christmas, when he suddenly swerved into the path of an approaching motor coach, and collided head-on with it. According to four witnesses, the defendant appeared to charge the coach, and no explanation could be offered for the behaviour by them or by the defendant himself. He could remember nothing about the incident, and there was no evidence of any illness that might have been responsible. The road was straight, there was lighting, and the centre line was marked with cat's eye reflectors. This offender was fined £10 and disqualified for twelve months, but the disqualification was removed on application after seven months only. There was only one previous conviction for obstruction, otherwise nothing was known of the defendant. (It is interesting to consider this case in the light of Culpin's remarks (1937) on impulses to charge oncoming vehicles, which he described as an obsessional symptom.)

Finally, all the offenders were studied from the point of view of their reactions to their offences. Broadly speaking, it was possible to make a rough classification, from the comments of the police and the witnesses, according to whether the offender was ruthless in his driving behaviour, or violent and aggressive after the offence; whether he was indifferent to the whole business and showed no contrition; or whether he seemed to be genuinely concerned about what he had done. The offenders were grouped in the three categories as follows:

(*a*) The ruthless, shameless, or violent offender, who has little apparent concern for the needs or the safety of others, and seems to be quite indifferent to social or legal sanctions. About 11 per cent of the 653 were of this type.

(*b*) The driver who is neither ruthless nor violent, but who seems prepared to break the motoring law whenever it is expedient and sees nothing wrong in doing so 'if one can get away with it'. About 75 per cent of the 653 were in this group.

(c) The definitely law-conscious driver, who appears to be upset and conscience-stricken about breaking the law, especially when he has caused damage. About 14 per cent were in this category.

When the 151 offenders who had additional convictions for non-motoring offences are classified in this way, and compared with the remainder, as in *Table 47*, the former tend to show a more antisocial attitude.

Table 47

ATTITUDES OF OFFENDERS AS SHOWN IN POLICE AND
PRESS REPORTS

Attitudes of offenders	*151 offenders with non-motoring convictions*	*502 offenders with additional motoring convictions only or with no additional convictions*
	%	%
Ruthless, shameless, or aggressive	16	10
Indifferent	79	73
Contrite	5	17
	100	100

Since only about 14 per cent of the cases reviewed in this study can be called 'accidents' in the true sense (p. 180 above), in 86 per cent of the cases there may have been something in the offender himself that contributed to his offence.[1] In other words, it is highly probable that traits of personality are reflected in driving behaviour. It could be said, perhaps, that the vehicle gets the driver into trouble; but it is much more likely that the vehicle is merely an extension of the driver's self: he gets himself into trouble.

THE FEMALE MOTORING OFFENDERS

The sex distribution of the 653 offenders was presented earlier in this chapter and it will be remembered that the number of females was very

[1] Although this proportion is the same as the proportion of offenders who were contrite, it does not consist of the same people. It is true, however, that offenders whose behaviour seemed to have been inadvertent often showed contrition: perhaps this is a reaction typical of the conscientious person.

small – only 51, or just under 8 per cent of the total. Hence it was decided to deal with them as a separate group, but the foregoing calculations (totals and percentages, etc.) do not exclude them.

Perhaps the most striking thing about the women is the manner in which the six offences are distributed among them. None was convicted for either causing death or driving while disqualified, and they formed but a trivial proportion of the offenders in all groups except failing to stop after or to report an accident, to which they contributed 28 of the 117 offenders (24 per cent). Of all the female offenders, 55 per cent were convicted for this offence. By comparison we find 19·6 per cent convicted for driving uninsured, 13·7 per cent for driving under the influence of drink or drugs, and 11·7 per cent for dangerous driving (see *Table 34*).

Seventy-one per cent of the women were married, excluding three widows. The modal age of the female group was much higher than that of the 653 offenders as a whole – it was 54·4 years, in contrast to 26 for the males and females combined. In occupational distribution, too, the female offenders differ from the whole group, in that 94 per cent of those whose occupational status can be inferred are from the non-manual classes, compared with only 38·2 per cent of all the offenders.

If additional convictions are an indication, there is little doubt that the females live more closely to the stereotype of the 'upright, law-abiding citizen' than do their male counterparts, for only 17·6 per cent of them had additional convictions for motoring offences, and only two had more than two motoring offences to their discredit. The non-motoring offender is even more conspicuous by her absence in this group, since only one woman had a record for 'other offences', and with the doubtful exception of wilful damage, these were essentially administrative offences.

Of the two women whose cases aroused suspicion that they might live unstable lives, one was responsible for seven of the offences counted against the female group as a whole. This lady, in her late thirties, was found, late on a Saturday night, in a small van which was crumpled against a telegraph pole; she had a broken collar bone. At the hospital she was found to be the worse for drink, and it was recorded also that she had left her two-year-old baby alone in a caravan (in which the two of them lived) while she went out to a party. When charged with driving under the influence of drink her defence was that she had not been driving the van; the driver, she said, was a man to whom she had given a lift, but he had disappeared after the crash. She elected trial, but the jury disagreed after an ably conducted defence; however she was convicted on re-trial, and was fined £7 with disqualification for life. It is interesting that while waiting for her re-trial she was tried elsewhere by jury for a similar offence; this jury disagreed also, but in this case her re-trial resulted in acquittal. She had four previous motoring convictions and a conviction for wilful damage; one of the former was for drunken driving four years earlier.

The other lady whose background seemed to be markedly unstable was the one associated with the male offender J; as reported above, he was convicted for aiding and abetting her in driving under the influence of drink.

Study of the facts attending each case in which the offender was a woman driver does not suggest that women are any more likely than men to offend through incompetent or foolish driving. Really bad and incompetent driving was found most often in the group charged with dangerous driving, of whom only six were females; this is a proportion of only 1·7 per cent of the 653 offenders, and it is surely well below the proportion of female to male drivers on the roads (estimated by the treasurer of the Police District's parent county as one female to every three males). It is thus more than likely that females are really under-represented in the group of 653 serious offenders, and it is certainly so of drivers convicted of dangerous or drunken driving.

The same cannot be said, however, of the proportion of women among those convicted of failing to stop after, or to report, an accident. In this group they appear to be unusually well represented. Why this is so is not clear from the facts, but it would seem to be relevant that seventeen of the twenty-eight women convicted for failing to stop were married; perhaps they wished to avoid being involved in a traffic affair because they thought they would be blamed by their husbands for damaging the family car and someone else's also. Moreover, they could incur some displeasure for being responsible for the often considerable expense of fines, costs, repairs, and loss of the no-claim insurance bonus. It may be also that females are more likely than males to take fright at the prospect of an altercation with an irate injured party; they may panic more easily, having less experience of such matters. This was evident in the case of a pregnant woman who collided with a parked van when driving on her wrong side of the road; she damaged it badly but did not stop, although she heard 'the tinkle of glass', because she 'didn't want to see the damage done to the car' – *whose* car is not clear.

It is rather out of character, it may be thought, for a woman to run over a child's bicycle and drive off without stopping, especially when she could afford to pay for the damage done. This occurred in two of the twenty-eight cases, and in both of them the offenders were educated middle-class women who clearly knew that they had done the damage.

Another rather typical case was that of Mrs BB, 'a highly reputable resident whose honesty and integrity are beyond doubt' (according to the police officer investigating the case). A witness following her sports car saw it strike a parked car in pulling out to overtake, damaging its wing badly. She stopped some fifty yards farther on, looked over her own car, and then drove off. Her number was reported by an onlooker, and she was traced; she admitted the collision but said that no damage had been caused to her car so she did nothing about it; moreover she said she was forced into the parked car by an overtaking van (which no witness saw). She was fined £1.

Less typical, but illustrative of some of the defence mechanisms that may underlie the reactions of offenders in these cases, is the affair of two elderly ladies in their sixties, one of whom, Miss CC, was driving their small saloon on a summer evening. She was seen by witnesses to be holding up a stream of traffic on a major road while she reversed into it from a side-turning into which she had driven (apparently) in error. She was then said to have 'jerked off', swerving from side to side of the road (according to another two witnesses), sometimes mounting the kerb until, just before rounding a bend, she swerved over the white line onto her wrong side and collided with an approaching motor cyclist and pillion passenger, injuring both. She did not stop until she reached the gate of her house, where a witness who had followed saw her get out and stagger; he said that her speech was slurred and that she seemed to be in a 'paralytic state'. He called the police, who saw the defendant at home some forty-five minutes later, but they could bring no charge of drunken driving in the circumstances, and there was no mention of drink in the case since no police witness saw her when she was actually 'in charge'. For dangerous driving she was fined £25 and disqualified for one year, and for failing to stop she was fined £4; costs were about £7. Clearly this matter could have arisen for a multitude of reasons: she might have been drunk, or she might have been an incompetent driver confused by a sequence of events over which she had little or no control, or she might have been ill; and finally, her age might have had something to do with her behaviour. From the court's point of view, however, the question was a simple one of the manner in which she drove – at least that issue was clear cut.

From both a psychological and a criminological standpoint the group of female offenders was most interesting. They seem to typify the peculiar difficulty of judging the criminality of the motoring offence; the motives behind their behaviour are very hard even to infer, but the conclusion is inescapable that the most outwardly respectable and blameless citizens are prone to break the statute and the moral law when their personal convenience is impeded and they are in a hurry. By most standards, the offence of failing to stop and settle the consequences of either mistaken, foolish, or just bad driving is reprehensible and inconsiderate. What is surprising, then, is the comparative leniency accorded to this kind of behaviour.

Another point of interest is the concentration of these offenders in the higher occupational strata. Is it true to say that the female driver is still as predominantly from the middle and upper social classes as her male counterpart was once thought to be? If so, why is it that women have taken so long to become emancipated in this field? A digression, perhaps, from criminology – but an interesting one none the less.

FURTHER DISCUSSION

Let us now, in concluding this chapter, take another look at some of the hypotheses that this research is trying to test, and see whether the evidence so far presented is relevant.

First, the hypothesis that the 'serious motoring offender, unlike the majority of other offenders found guilty of criminal offences, e.g. offenders against property, is a respectable citizen whose behaviour apart from his offence is reasonably in accord with the requirements of law and order'. Even if the offenders are given the benefit of the doubt wherever possible, nearly 19 per cent of those studied do not conform to this hypothesis. And by more objective standards – less favourable from the offenders' viewpoint but perhaps fairer from the point of view of the public – nearly 33 per cent of them just do not measure up to it. Hence, by the rules of science, the hypothesis cannot stand as it is.

Second, the hypothesis that the majority of serious motoring offences arise from accidents and that there is nothing in the offender's personality or background which predisposes him to break the law. From the evidence so far there seems to be very little to support this assumption if the term 'accident' is defined as a chance event which happens so quickly that nobody could have prevented it. Only 14 per cent of the 653 offences at the very most could be put in the category of 'bad luck', and in the majority of the other cases the offence was undeniably brought about by the offender's own behaviour in consciously taking a risk. Enough should have emerged in this chapter about the characteristics of some offenders to question theories that look upon motoring offences as 'acts of God'. Morcover, those whose thinking has been influenced by psycho-analysis might feel that many of these offences are the logical outcome of antisocial drives which are characteristic of the offender's real personality.

Third, the hypothesis that serious motoring offenders come mostly from the white-collar classes, and its alternative form that they are likely to be considerably different from other kinds of serious offender in respect of occupational distribution. The facts certainly refute the first of these propositions and they go a long way to refute the second, alternative one also. The manual working groups are unquestionably in the majority among the offenders in this particular Police District where they constitute a smaller proportion of the population than in the country overall. And, where the really serious and incorrigible offenders are concerned, there is no doubt that the lower occupational strata predominate.

Fourth, the view that motoring offenders are not concentrated in any particular age group. If the six serious offences are taken in aggregate, then there is something to be said against this hypothesis too: there is a marked concentration of offenders in the age group aged 21 and under 30, with a mode of 26. But it may not be realistic to 'lump' all the offences together in this way; and if they are taken separately, then undoubtedly the ages are spread very widely, with the youngsters mostly among the driving while disqualified and failing to insure offenders, and their elders among the drunken drivers and those who do not stop after, or report, accidents. We have also seen that on average the females tend to be much older than the men.

Fifth, 'having been found guilty and punished for one offence of a serious nature the motoring offender does not repeat the offence'. Again, the facts do not support this assumption, whichever group of offenders is considered. Especially is it untrue of those who drive when disqualified or fail to insure against third-party risks, many of whom fall almost into the extreme category of repeaters or recidivists.

Sixth, it seems that the facts also discount the belief that serious motoring offenders will elect trial by jury if given the opportunity to do so. Only 8 per cent of those eligible adopted this course. The reasons for not electing trial were rarely apparent from the documents, and must be left to speculation, but it seems likely that most people wanted to avoid delay and to 'get it all over'. Financial considerations would also be important, and it should not be forgotten that the scale of fines imposed in the magistrates' courts did not keep pace with the inflation that obtained during the period under review.

To conclude, it is worth considering again the characteristics of the offenders as indicated by the reactions that they showed towards their offences: it was estimated that only some 14 per cent of the 653 were at all contrite or unduly concerned about what they had done. Furthermore, it was found that some differences in attitude could be distinguished between the offenders who also had convictions for non-motoring offences, and those who had additional convictions for motoring offences only or no additional convictions at all: there was some evidence for the view that the former group were the more antisocial.

It is stressed again that the deductions presented above are based on documentary sources which are subjective in nature and therefore open to several interpretations, of which this is but one. This limitation should be remembered, particularly when it is necessary to go beyond matters of fact, such as age and sex, to establish criteria that are much less definite – for example, those relating to behaviour or personality. Much more work is needed before conclusions of this kind can be drawn with certainty, and it is the purpose of this pioneering study to indicate lines upon which further investigations might proceed.

9

Treatment by the Courts

Earlier in this study it was shown that the British courts have been subjected to much criticism for their leniency in dealing with motoring offenders. Moreover, behind these criticisms lies the inference made by Wootton (1957) that motoring offenders are favoured because they are usually white-collar offenders, and people with whom benches can easily identify.

These issues were discussed tentatively in the analysis of the national statistics in Chapter 5, but the official data do not permit any sound conclusions to be drawn about leniency or the influence of social class as a factor in sentencing. It is impossible to tell from the statistics alone to what extent the courts were justified in sentencing as they did, nor can one compare one court with another.

Much more information can be gleaned, however, from the data that are available in this research. As *Table 48* shows, the majority of the 653 offenders were sentenced by the eleven magistrates' courts serving the Police District, and these courts can be compared. Also, it is possible to observe something of the operation of the class factor, since occupations (one index of social class) are known in most cases. The number of cases tried by the higher courts is rather too few for comparative study, but an analysis of them may throw at least some light on the advantages and disadvantages of electing trial, and on the treatment of persons causing death by dangerous driving.

Hence it is the aim of this chapter to examine the sentencing of the courts concerned with the 653 offenders studied, and to attempt an answer to the following questions:

(a) Are there any marked differences between the magistrates' courts in respect of sentencing, especially with regard to severity?

(b) Do the sentences of the courts have any apparent effect on the subsequent incidence of motoring offences of a similar kind in the locality in which the cases might be reported in the press?

(c) Are there any discernible differences in the manner in which the courts sentence offenders in the different occupational groups, with particular reference to professional drivers?

SENTENCES AND DISQUALIFICATION ORD

653 SERIOUS MOTORI

Offence and sentence		Opsley		Batwick		Treeford		Elston		Barchet		Seabridge		Le
		No.	%	No.	%	No.	%	No.	%	No.	%	No.	%	No.
Causing death by dangerous driving	Prison	—		—		—		—		—		—		—
	Fine	—		—		—		—		—		—		—
	Other	—		—		—		—		—		—		—
	Total	—		—		—		—		—		—		—
	% Disq.		—		—		—		—		—		—	
Driving while disqualified	Prison	12	100	2	100	1	50	8	100	1	100	4	80	8
	Fine	—		—		1	50	—		—		1	20	2
	Other	—		—										
	Total	12	100	2	100	2	100	8	100	1	100	5	100	10
	% Disq.		83		100		50		75		—		40	
Driving under the influence	Prison	—		1	12	—		1	20	—		—		—
	Fine	18	100	7	88	3	100	4	80	—		3	100	7
	Other	—		—								—		
	Total	18	100	8	100	3	100	5	100	—		3	100	7
	% Disq.		95		100		100		80		—		100	
Driving dangerously	Prison	—		—		—		—		—		—		1
	Fine	52	100	32	100	6	100	21	100	6	100	25	100	22
	Other	—		—		—		—		—		—		—
	Total	52	100	32	100	6	100	21	100	6	100	25	100	23
	% Disq.		54		44		50		43		50		12	
Failing to stop	Prison	—		—		—		—		—		—		—
	Fine	16	94	16	100	5	100	8	100	2	100	5	100	19
	Other	1	6	—		—		—		—		—		—
	Total	17	100	16	100	5	100	8	100	2	100	5	100	19
	% Disq		—		—		—		—		—		—	
Failing to insure	Prison	—		—		—		—		—		—		—
	Fine	13	100	5	100	3	100	6	100	1	100	6	100	9
	Other	—		—		—		—		—		—		—
	Total	13	100	5	100	3	100	6	100	1	100	6	100	9
	% Disq.		62		40		—		50		—		50	
Total all offences		112		63		19		48		10		44		68
% of 653 offences			17·1		9·7		2·9		7·4		1·5		6·7	

POSED BY COURTS IN THE POLICE DISTRICT
FENCES

efford No.	%	Mesley No.	%	Barling No.	%	Frockton No.	%	Qr Sessions A No.	%	Qr Sessions B No.	%	Assizes No.	%	Totals No.	%
—	—	—	—	—	—	—	—	—	—	—		1	20	1	20
—	—	—	—	—	—	—	—	—	—	—		4	80	4	80
—	—	—	—	—	—	—	—	—	—	—					
—	—	—	—	—	—	—	—	—	—	—		5	100	5	100
													100		100
2	50	11	79	3	60	2	100	4	100	—		—		58	84
1	25	2	14	2	40	—		—		—		—		9	13
1	25	1	7	—		—		—		—		—		2	3
4	100	14	100	5	100	2	100	4	100	—		—		69	100
	75		79		60		100		25	—					65
2	13	—		—		—		3	16	—		—		7	6
3	87	10	100	5	100	8	100	16	84	3	100	—		97	94
5	100	10	100	5	100	8	100	19	100	3	100	—		104	100
	87		90		100		100		90		100	—			93
1	1	1	4	—		—		—		—		—		3	1
4	99	25	93	8	100	12	100	10	100	1	100	—		281	98·7
		1	4	—		—		—		—		—		1	0·3
2	100	27	100	8	100	12	100	10	100	1	100	—		285	100
	61		45		37		75		100		—			—	52
3	100	10	100	5	100	12	100	—		—		—		116	99
								—		—		—		1	1
3	100	10	100	5	100	12	100	—		—		—		117	100
				—		—		—		—		—		—	—
		1	8	—		1	11	—		—		—		2	2·5
3	89	11	92	—		8	89	—		—		—		70	96·0
4	11	—		—		—		—		—		—		1	1·5
9	100	12	100	—		9	100	—		—		—		73	100
	45		42	—			89	—		—		—			53·5
3		73		23		43		33		4		5		653	
	16·6		11·2		3·5		6·6		5·0		0·6		0·8		100

(*d*) Do the courts make adequate and justified use of the powers vested in them, especially in regard to disqualification and the ordering of further driving tests?

To deal with these questions it is necessary to consider separately the handling of each of the six classes of offence, thus building up a general impression of sentencing in the District, which can be compared with the data available for England and Wales as a whole.

Causing death by dangerous driving is dealt with first, since it is the one offence the treatment of which cannot be the subject of comparison between the different courts in the Police District. It has to be tried by a court higher than quarter sessions, and in fact all five cases were tried by the assizes. As there are so few cases it is not possible to make any useful generalizations, but they can be looked at in greater detail than the more numerous cases in the other classes of offence.

CAUSING DEATH BY DANGEROUS DRIVING

(*Five years' imprisonment.*)[1]

The disposal by assizes of the five cases studied is shown in *Table 49*.

Table 49

CAUSING DEATH BY DANGEROUS DRIVING: DISPOSAL OF CASES

| Case number | Date | *PENALTY* | | |
		Fine	Prison sentence	Period of disqualification (years)
I	1957		9 months	2
2	1958	£75		7
3	1958	£50		7
4	1959	£50		10
5	1959	£1		3

The offender in Case I was the first to be convicted in the Police District for this offence which, it will be remembered, was introduced as a specific offence in 1956, only a year before this case occurred. He was also the only

[1] For ease of reference, the *maximum* penalties for each class of offence, as laid down by the Road Traffic Acts, 1930 and 1956, which were current at the time, are given briefly in parenthesis following the heading for the offence under discussion.

242

offender to be sent to prison – and one is inclined to wonder whether his offence was worse than the others, or whether he was just unfortunate in appearing in court at a time when the judges were uncertain as to how these cases should be sentenced and so began with severity.

The facts were that the defendant was driving with his family in his six-cylinder saloon early on a winter Sunday afternoon. He was on a main road, when he overtook a bus as it was approaching a bend, and came into a head-on collision with a sports car, the driver of which was killed outright.

The evidence was that the defendant was not travelling fast when he overtook and, indeed, had he used the power and speed of which his car was capable, it was said that he might have avoided the collision to some extent, if not entirely. His defence was that the sports car was being driven at an excessive speed and the driver lost control; but witnesses asserted that it was in fact travelling at a very moderate speed (a witness who was said to be a car enthusiast noticed it because it *was* travelling at such a moderate speed) and on its correct side of the road. Incidentally, it appeared that the 21-year-old deceased was using his father's car without consent, and was not insured.

The background of the defendant is of interest. He had no previous convictions, had an 'exemplary' army record as a tradesman senior NCO, and was a respected and competent skilled tradesman in the employ of a public authority. A married man, aged 50, he had driven for twenty-five years without any recorded incident; his only connection with a motoring offence was as a parent, when his eight-year-old son had been knocked down and killed by a lorry some years before.

From what has been said about this case there seemed to be no special justification for imposing a prison sentence rather than a heavy fine, and it may be, as suggested above, that the defendant was unlucky in that the judge did not want to create the impression that it was intended to treat this new offence less seriously than manslaughter, for which it is a euphemism. There is some support for this suggestion in the trend of the statistics for England and Wales for the period, which show a reduction in the proportions of offenders committed to prison for this offence from 1957 to 1959. It is, however, improper to make such an inference without first considering the facts in the other four cases.

In Case 2 the defendant was a 30-year-old car breaker. He had two lady passengers in his private saloon car, and was driving along a minor road just before midnight on a summer evening. Overtaking another private car at a point from which he could not have seen approaching traffic, he was well on his offside of the road when he met a solo motor cycle in a head-on collision; the young rider was killed and his pillion passenger injured.

According to the driver of the vehicle overtaken, the defendant's speed was about 40 mph or just over, and that of the approaching motor cycle was not 'unreasonable' (the pillion passenger endorsed this view, but the speedometer of the motor cycle was jammed at 58 mph; it had been travelling downhill and the deceased youth was a learner driver who had only recently failed his test). It appeared that the accused had spent the evening in a working men's club where he had met the two ladies who accepted his offer to drive them home; as it was a 'nice night' they had gone for a 'run round' before the passengers were dropped, and it was while on this 'run' that the incident occurred. One might infer from the facts that the accused had been drinking, and that he had been 'showing off' to the two women; anyhow, the judge said that the defendant was convicted 'on the clearest evidence'.

This offender was a married man with four children. His work record was not impressive, including many unskilled and semi-skilled jobs, of which he had lost at least two for unsatisfactory work. He had four previous convictions for stealing and receiving, spanning a period of nineteen years, during which he had been to prison once; and three convictions for motoring offences, including one for speeding. By comparison with the offender in Case 1, it would seem that this defendant was lucky to escape a second prison sentence.

Case 3 has already been mentioned (see p. 95 above). The facts were that the accused man was driving his very old saloon car along a major road on the outskirts of a busy town, in a long line of traffic during the late afternoon of a summer weekday. According to witnesses he 'suddenly veered to his offside', and his car struck the rear of a lorry which was passing in the opposite direction; the lorry was being followed by a motor cyclist who was just overtaking it when the collision occurred. The motor cycle ran straight into the defendant's car with fatal consequences for its rider, and causing serious injuries to his pillion passenger. The evidence was that all the vehicles concerned were moving quite slowly at the time of the incident because of the density of the traffic but the defendant had been seen to be driving with one hand and holding his head with the other, and there was a suspicion (not mentioned by the prosecution) that his driving may have been influenced by drink since there was a half-bottle of gin in the car. However, he was not seen by the police until several hours after the incident, because he had complained of concussion when it occurred, and was driven

244

off to hospital with the motor cyclists. Both the defendant and the deceased were provisional licence holders, and neither was displaying L plates.

The defendant, a married man with two children, was in his late thirties and had been employed as a waiter. He came to Britain from a foreign country during the second world war, and not much was known of his record to the age of about 19; however, as far as could be ascertained, his early conduct had been good. Since the war he had had several jobs as a waiter and an electrician, but between 1954 and 1958 he had been convicted six times for non-motoring offences (stealing a car, stealing a motor cycle, false pretences, and fraud), and there were also five motoring convictions: two for speeding and three for driving on a provisional licence without a qualified passenger or L plates. At the time of the conviction reported in this study he seemed to be unemployed, but he was given eighteen months to pay a fine of £50, or an alternative of six months' imprisonment; whether the fine was paid is not known.

Case 4 derived from another Sunday afternoon ride, after which the defendant was hurrying along a main road in his family saloon in order to get his two boy passengers back to an approved school on time. His haste was such that he appeared to hit the verge on his nearside when passing a long line of summer holiday traffic moving in the opposite direction; then, so witnesses said, he lost control, and his car 'bounced' off the verge into the line of traffic on his offside, cannoning first into a motor cycle combination and then into a car which was following it. The impact killed the rider of the motor cycle and his young daughter who was on the pillion; his wife and two other children in the sidecar were injured, as well as the occupants of the following car (one of whom had just been collected from hospital after a traffic accident). In the defendant's car, his mother was killed and all his passengers were injured, making a total of three killed and eleven injured in the incident. The defendant was so badly shocked that he could not remember what had happened, except that 'his clutch seemed to slip'; but it appears that he was another inexperienced provisional licence holder, driving a new car which he had not really got used to, and he lost control. He, like the defendant in Case 3, was driving without L plates or a qualified driver.

This man was a caretaker in his late thirties, with a good service and civilian employment record in unskilled and semi-skilled jobs. There was only one previous conviction, for housebreaking and larceny some twenty years earlier, for which he had been bound over.

The last case, No. 5, arose from an incident in which the driver's mate of a coal merchant's lorry was hit and killed outright by another lorry; he was standing in the centre of a main road trying to halt oncoming traffic while his driver backed the coal lorry into a driveway. According to witnesses, the defendant was driving 'fast' before the impact, and had been seen to overtake another vehicle in such a manner that he had only just missed hitting a child cyclist riding in the opposite direction. The defendant (though in a restricted area in which he should not have been exceeding 30 mph) was travelling too fast to stop, though other vehicles were apparently able to do so in time.

On the defendant's behalf it was submitted that the deceased had 'asked for trouble' by standing as he did in the middle of a busy main road when dusk was falling on a winter afternoon. In any case, it was evident that the driver of the coal lorry had chosen a very dangerous spot in which to turn; hence the two men were possibly exposing themselves and others to some degree of danger, and would not appear to have been blameless.

The defendant in this case was a professional driver in his forties, a married man separated from his wife; there were no children. He had emigrated at an early age and spent his adolescence abroad, returning to Britain when old enough to enlist as a regular soldier. After a short engagement he went back to civilian life and unskilled work until he was recalled to the Colours on the outbreak of war. His war service included four convictions by Field General Court Martial: the first in 1942 for absence without leave and insubordination; and three more convictions towards the end of the war for desertion, robbery and larceny, and losing equipment by neglect, for which he received sentences of penal servitude totalling fourteen years. His only civilian conviction was for speeding in 1956, though he had been cautioned on three different occasions, in 1957 and 1958. Since the war he had been employed in various semi-skilled jobs, and had apparently given satisfaction.

An interesting point about these two cases, 4 and 5, is that in both there was a slight difference of opinion between the Director of Public Prosecutions and the police authority. In Case 4 the police were doubtful whether the driving of the accused was sufficiently reckless to secure a conviction on the charge, but the DPP thought, correctly, that it was. In Case 5 the opposite occurred: the DPP was doubtful if a conviction could be secured because of the danger to which the deceased had exposed himself, but the police took the other view, and this time *they* were right – though the rather nominal fine of £1 and the short period of disqualification (three years would seem to be short in this instance, by comparison with Cases 2, 3, and 4) would suggest that the judge did not regard it as a bad case of this particular class of offence.

This brief account of only five cases shows the wide range of driving behaviour that can constitute an offence under this head because it involves a fatality. On the facts adduced there seems to be no doubt that the driving of all five offenders could be considered dangerous and, with the possible exception of Case 5, that it caused the deaths of the deceased. It is, however, tempting to speculate as to what would have been the outcome in these cases had the victims not been killed. This is a hypothetical question and to some extent an illegitimate one in a study of this kind; nevertheless, it seems probable that the consequences would not have been much different for anyone except, perhaps, offender No. 1, who might not have gone to prison. It is, however, more difficult to say that the outcome would have been the same in some of the cases of dangerous driving that came into this research, if they had involved a fatality. For example, there is the case of an offender who was convicted for dangerous driving and fined £30 without disqualification: he was driving his Ford Zodiac in a built-up area, and overtook a long line of traffic at such speed that drivers in the queue said their cars were 'rocked' as he went by; he then hit a lady cyclist who was turning right from the line after giving a signal. She was able to throw herself clear but her cycle was completely crushed. The skid marks made by the defendant's car indicated a speed of at least 65 mph in a 30 mph limited area. Had the cyclist been killed the penalty would almost certainly have been a heavy one, and the driver's behaviour was as bad as any described in Cases 1 to 5 above. Another example is that of the driver of a sports car who overtook a line of cars at speed while approaching a crest; another vehicle came over it with which he collided head-on – a case not vastly different from Case 1 – but nobody was hurt. The defendant was fined £30 without disqualification, and it could be that, in this instance, the defendant had only the stoutness of the body on the other vehicle to thank for the fact that he avoided the severe penalty that a conviction for causing death by dangerous driving would have entailed.

Hence it seems to be largely chance that determines whether an offender whose driving has been dangerous appears on the serious charge of causing death or on the less serious charge of driving dangerously, or even of driving without due care and attention. An example of this phenomenon was reported in the national press recently when an 80-year-old baronet was fined £10 for careless driving, although he had been involved in an incident in which two cyclists were killed and a number of others injured. It appeared that he was driving his elderly family saloon along a wet road, when he skidded while rounding a bend and collided with a group of oncoming cyclists. This case shows once more the fallacy and the injustice of having to distinguish arbitrarily between 'dangerous' and 'careless' driving. On the evidence it would seem that careless driving was the correct charge, if there were to be one at all, and nobody would have questioned it had there been only the alternatives of either manslaughter or reckless driving; but, as the law now stands, the case excited controversy, and it carried inferences that the unfortunate defendant's social position might not have been uninfluential apropos of the charge, though there is no reason to think that these had any foundation.

Before leaving the specific discussion of these homicide cases it is interesting to note that the victims in all the cases except No. 4 were themselves committing offences when the fatalities occurred.

DRIVING WHILE DISQUALIFIED

(Six months' imprisonment or, in special circumstances, a fine or £50, or both. May disqualify.)

Sixty-nine offenders were convicted for this offence by the magistrates' courts, of whom four were committed to quarter sessions for sentence. The sentences are summarized in *Table 50*, which also shows (in parentheses) the percentages of comparable sentences passed by the courts of England and Wales as a whole.

Perhaps the most striking aspect of these sentences is the apparently high proportion of offenders sent to prison by the District magistrates: 83 per cent, by comparison with 58 per cent for the magistrates' courts of the

Table 50

DRIVING WHILE DISQUALIFIED: SUMMARY OF SENTENCES

Sentence	Quarter sessions Police District No.	Quarter sessions Police District % (rounded)	Quarter sessions England and Wales[1] %	Magistrates' courts Police District No.	Magistrates' courts Police District % (rounded)	Magistrates' courts England and Wales %
Prison and disqualified	1	25	—	36	55·4	
Prison only	3	75	—	18	27·7	(58)
Fined and disqualified				9	13·8	(23)
Probation and disqualified				2	3·0	
Total	4	100·0		65	100·0	

[1] No percentages can be estimated for the higher courts.

country as a whole. The District magistrates also seem to be more severe in imposing disqualification upon 72 per cent of their offenders, in contrast to the 32 per cent who were disqualified by the courts of England and Wales (Home Office Returns of *Offences relating to Motor Vehicles*, 1957, 1958, and 1959).

The majority of offenders sent to prison were given a three-month sentence, but the range of sentence was from one to six months with a mean of 3·7 and standard deviation (SD) of ·6. The orders of disqualification were distributed over a wide range from nine months to ten years; the mean period was two years and four months (SD 9·9 months), but the most usual order was five years, showing how severely this offence tends to be punished.

Table 51 compares the eleven magistrates' courts in the District in respect of, first, the percentages of offenders sent to prison for six months, and second, the percentages disqualified for two years or more. It will be seen that, in general, the courts that sentence the highest proportions of offenders to imprisonment are often severe in imposing long periods of disqualification. In statistical terms, however, there is no significant rank correlation between the courts when they are arranged in two hierarchies: one according to the proportions sent to prison, and the other according to the proportions disqualified for two or more years. If a prison sentence of at least six months is taken as a criterion of severity, Barling ranks first, having sentenced three of its five offenders thus. Next come three courts of equal rank, Lesdon, Frockton, and Sefford, of which only Lesdon with ten cases had any appreciable number to deal with.

A study of the class factor is not very rewarding, in that nearly all the offenders were manual workers, and 91 per cent of these were sent to prison. Of the four non-manual workers only one was imprisoned, and he was an offender with over ten convictions for non-motoring offences. Another non-manual offender was a young officer in a distinguished regiment, who was fined a total of £70 with five years' disqualification for a second offence of driving while disqualified.

Analysis of the eleven cases in which the offenders were not sent to prison shows extenuating circumstances in only one instance, where there was doubt about the intelligence of the accused being sufficient to grasp the significance of his offence. All the others were brash and 'glaring' instances of this class of offence with nothing to excuse them, and it is hard to see how the offenders escaped prison; it must be said in fairness, however, that these lenient sentences were distributed among the courts and no particular bench can be singled out in this respect.

Table 51

DRIVING WHILE DISQUALIFIED: RANK ORDER OF SEVERITY OF MAGISTRATES' COURTS

Court	% sent to prison for 6 months	Rank	% disqualified for 2 years or more	Rank
Opsley	42	6	100	3
Batwick	0	10	0	10·5
Treeford	0	10	100	3
Elston	25	7·5	60	8
Barchet	0	10	0	10·5
Seabridge	25	7·5	100	3
Lesdon	50	3	57	9
Sefford	50	3	100	3
Mesley	45	5	91	6
Barling	60	1	67	7
Frockton	50	3	100	3

$$r = \cdot 31 \ (p > \cdot 1)$$

Finally, 58 per cent of those who were convicted of this offence had been disqualified previously for periods exceeding twelve months. Again, the data prompt the question whether long periods of disqualification do not defeat their purpose by over-taxing a driver's powers of self-discipline. Clearly long periods are necessary where it is in the interests of public safety that an unfit or incompetent driver should be forbidden to drive; but where disqualification orders appear to be intended to have only a deterrent or retributive effect, it is doubtful whether any useful purpose is served by extending them beyond the minimum period necessary to achieve this. How long such a period should be is, of course, a matter of opinion; but possibly twelve months would be more than sufficient.

DRIVING UNDER THE INFLUENCE OF DRINK OR DRUGS

(First offence: £100 fine and/or four months' imprisonment; disqualification for at least twelve months. Second and subsequent offence: £100 fine and/or six months' imprisonment; disqualification for any period. May order re-test.)

Of the 104 offenders who were convicted of this offence in the Police District, twenty-two elected trial by jury and the remainder were dealt with summarily. Their sentences are listed in *Table 52*, with comparable percentages (in parentheses) of sentences passed by the courts of England and Wales for this category of offence.

Table 52

DRIVING UNDER THE INFLUENCE OF DRINK OR DRUGS:
SUMMARY OF SENTENCES

Sentence	Quarter sessions			Magistrates' courts		
	Police District No.	England % (rounded)	and Wales %	Police District No.	England % (rounded)	and Wales %
Prison and disqualified	2	9·1 } (6·5)		4	5·0 } (4·7)	
Prison only	1	4·5		0	90·0	
Fined and disqualified	17	77·3 } (81·0)		75	91·0 } (95·0)	
Fined only	2	9·1		3	4·0	
Total	22	100·0		82	100·0	

From the above figures it would seem that there is little or no difference between the sentencing policy of the courts in the District and that of the country as a whole. This is certainly true of the magistrates' courts, but not necessarily of the higher courts, since the national statistics do not include all those sent to prison or fined by the higher courts: it is the practice in the Home Office Returns to group disposals under the heading 'no separate punishment' where the offender has been convicted of additional offences. However, it is likely that the percentages shown for the national higher courts are an underestimation, and that the real proportions are closer to those of the District.

In the magistrates' courts the average fine was about £30, ranging from £2 for an offender on a moped to £200 for two offences by a lady under the influence of drugs; the SD of 17·6 shows the variety of sentences. The most frequently occurring fine was about £25 – which corresponds approximately to the national average calculated from the Home Office Returns for the period, and also to averages of between £10 and £30 calculated by Stack and Walker (1959) from a sample of 300 drunken drivers in 1957.

Ninety-three per cent of the 104 offenders were disqualified, exactly the same proportion as in the courts of England and Wales during the period. The average period imposed was thirty months (SD 21·0); the mode was one year, a finding that also agrees with the study by Stack and Walker (1959, p. 6).

251

In the higher courts the treatment was more severe. The average fine was about £40, but the range was wide, from £5 – coupled with disqualification for life – to £75 (SD 17·9). The mode was about £50. Disqualification again covered a wide range, from life to one year; the average was about three years (SD 1·5), and the most usual period was one year. These figures lend some slight support to the belief that there are disadvantages in electing trial if conviction results.

Unfortunately, no consistent record of costs was kept. Where they were recorded, the highest in the magistrates' courts amounted to £24, and the majority were about £5; in the higher courts, however, costs of £50 were not unusual, and in most cases seemed to be about £25 – a sizeable addition to the penalty paid by an offender.

When the magistrates' courts are ranked according to the proportions of offenders fined £30 or more, and again according to the proportions disqualified for two years or over (*Table 53*), there is a positive degree of correlation ($r = ·73$, $p < ·02$). In this case, again, the courts that are severe with their fines tend also to be severe with their disqualification orders, and it is noticeable that Sefford, Opsley, Batwick, and Mesley rate consistently high in both respects.

With regard to the class factor in sentencing, it does not seem that the non-manual groups fared any better than the others; rather worse, in fact.

Table 53

DRIVING UNDER THE INFLUENCE OF DRINK OR DRUGS: RANK
ORDER OF SEVERITY OF MAGISTRATES' COURTS

Court	% fined £30 or more	Rank	% disqualified for 2 years or more	Rank
Opsley	50	2	35	5
Batwick	48	3	63	3
Treeford	0	8·5	0	9
Elston	25	5	75	1
Barchet	No cases	—	—	—
Seabridge	0	8·5	0	9
Lesdon	0	8·5	29	6
Sefford	62	1	64	2
Mesley	30	4	40	4
Barling	20	6·5	0	9
Frockton	0	8·5	25	7

$r = ·73$ $(p < ·02)$

Of the seven offenders sent to prison, three were from non-manual occupations (non-manual workers formed about 54 per cent of the total offenders convicted for this offence), and so were twenty-seven of the thirty-seven offenders who were fined over £30. With one exception, all the offenders disqualified for periods of over five years were from white-collar groups.

DRIVING DANGEROUSLY

(*First offence: £100 fine and/or four months' imprisonment; disqualification for any period. Second and subsequent offence: £100 fine and/or six months' imprisonment; disqualification for a minimum period of nine months, unless more than three years have elapsed since last conviction. May order re-test.*)

Of the 285 offenders convicted for this offence, ten elected trial by jury, one was sent to quarter sessions for sentence, one was found guilty at assizes of dangerous driving rather than of causing death by dangerous driving, and the remaining 273 were dealt with summarily. The disposal is shown in *Table 54*, with the relevant proportions for the courts of England and Wales given for comparison (in parentheses); for convenience the one case heard at assizes is included under quarter sessions.

Table 54

DRIVING DANGEROUSLY: SUMMARY OF SENTENCES

Sentence	Quarter sessions Police District No.	Quarter sessions % (rounded)	Quarter sessions England and Wales %	Magistrates' courts Police District No.	Magistrates' courts % (rounded)	Magistrates' courts England and Wales %
Prison and disqualified	0	0	(7·9)	3	1	(1·9)
Fined and disqualified	11	92 }	(97·5)	138	51 }	(97·5)
Fined	1	8 }		131	48 }	
Probation and disqualified	0	0		1	·3	
Total	12	100		273	100	

With regard to the higher courts, it would seem that the District's higher courts were rather less severe than those of the country as a whole, as far as the proportions of offenders sent to prison are concerned. It is not, unfortunately, possible to compare these courts in respect of sentences of disqualification, since details are not available for the higher courts of

England and Wales. The District's magistrates' courts compare very closely with those of England and Wales in the percentages of fines and sentences of imprisonment, but they are much more severe when it comes to disqualification: the magistrates' courts of England and Wales disqualified about 42 per cent of their offenders during the period in contrast to the 52 per cent disqualified in the District. But that is not to say that there were no striking examples of leniency in this respect.

One example is that of a 24-year-old lorry driver who was out for an evening run with his girl-friend in a private car. About 10.45 p.m. a police officer cycling along a main road in an urban area noticed the defendant looking backward as he drove along, and took his number purely on the suspicion that he might have been concerned in an accident. Cycling farther on he came across an injured man lying in the road, and witnesses said that the defendant had been seen to round a bend at speed, lose control, and swerve on to the offside pavement where he hit the injured man who was walking along with a friend; the pedestrian was carried on the bonnet of the defendant's car for 'several yards' and severe lacerations to the head were caused. The defendant did not stop and, when traced, explained a smashed headlamp (bits of it were found at the scene of the incident) as the result of his having hit a tree; he denied all knowledge of the incident and so did his girl, who said her eyes were closed when they were driving along that particular road, although she did remember the defendant saying later, 'What have I done?' He was charged with driving in a manner dangerous to the public, having no road fund licence, and failing to stop after or to report an accident: on the first charge he was fined £10, on the second £2; his licence was endorsed and he was ordered to pay costs of £8. The remaining charges were dismissed, and there was no disqualification. Here one must agree with a police superintendent's comment that it was 'a shocking case which could have been due to drink'. Had the injured man died, the similarities between this case and *Andrews v. DPP* [1937] (see p. 82 above) would have been striking.

It is also noteworthy that five of the offenders who were fined, but not disqualified or ordered to take a re-test, were over 65 years of age, including two septuagenarians, and on the evidence available in respect of each it is hard to say that their driving could have been other than atrocious. At the other end of the age range were five offenders aged 18 and under, including one of 16 whose obvious lack of experience would seem to have justified at least an order to take another driving test before being let loose on the roads without the label of 'learner'. In fact, re-tests were ordered in only four of the 285 cases: all were elderly persons.

Treatment by the Courts

In the magistrates' courts the most usual fine for this offence was £25, with a mean of £23 (SD 12·2) and a range of from £2 to £75. The only figure that can be derived for England and Wales is an average calculated from the Home Office Returns which, for the three years under review, was about £15; but it is not very much help, since the standard deviation and the range are not known. The data on disqualifications in England and Wales must also go unchecked, but for the District's magistrates' courts the mean period was 13·7 months (SD 3·4) and the most usual period was twelve months, with a range of from one month to ten years. At quarter sessions the average fine and the average period of disqualification were roughly the same as those in the magistrates' courts; the main risk in electing trial appeared to be an increased likelihood of being disqualified.

When ranked according to the proportions of offenders fined £20 and over, and again according to the proportions disqualified for one year or more (*Table 55*), the magistrates' courts show no correlation (r = ·03). So there is no general tendency for courts that impose heavy fines to disqualify for long periods also; nor does a heavy fine necessarily mean a shorter disqualification. Mesley, Sefford, and Batwick were the most severe for fines, and the first two courts were severe for disqualification also. Sefford ranked second for both fines and disqualification, and is an exception to the general rule.

Table 55

DRIVING DANGEROUSLY: RANK ORDER OF SEVERITY OF
MAGISTRATES' COURTS

Court	% fined £20 or more	Rank	% disqualified for one year or more	Rank
Opsley	58	4	28	8
Batwick	72	3	23	9
Trecford	33	6	0	10·5
Elston	53	5	33	6·5
Barchet	16	11	33	6·5
Seabridge	32	7	0	10·5
Lesdon	18	10	44	5
Sefford	82	2	58	2
Mesley	84	1	50	4
Barling	25	8·5	67	1
Frockton	25	8·5	55	3

r = ·03

The Documentary Study

Here again the class factor does not appear to influence the sentencing behaviour of the courts to any discernible degree; the only noteworthy observation is that all sixteen of the offenders who were fined over £40 came from the non-manual groups; disqualifications were roughly proportionate in each occupational group, though offenders from the semi-skilled and unskilled groups tended to be disqualified for longer periods than others. There was a clear reluctance to disqualify professional drivers for long periods, and only one of the seventeen who were disqualified was suspended for more than one year.

Of the offenders sent to prison, two were known criminals with CRO records; the third was the leader of a gang of motor cyclists whose pleasure was to harass motorists and pick fights with them (see p. 228 above for a description of one such case).

FAILING TO STOP AFTER, OR TO REPORT, AN ACCIDENT

(First offence: fine not exceeding £20. Second or subsequent offence: £50 fine or three months' imprisonment.)[1]

The cases studied under this head were a sample, it will be remembered, of offenders who were resident in the Police District, and therefore the data may not be fully representative. Of the 117 offenders convicted of this offence, all but one – who was discharged absolutely – were fined in respect of it. But for offences which accompanied failure to stop or report, one offender was sent to prison and five more were disqualified. This is one of the ways in which this analysis of penalties may be distorted, since just under one-third of the 653 offenders were convicted of motoring offences additional to the ones which brought them into the scope of this study; in such cases it is not known how much the courts were influenced by a particular offence or group of offences when deciding how the penalties should be distributed.

For this offence, the sentences imposed by the District courts have not been compared with those passed by the courts of England and Wales as a whole, because the fine is so usual. In this connection the national statistics are puzzling in that they show disqualifications for this offence: according to Wilkinson (1960, p. 128), these would be illegal.

The average fine imposed was £4 10s. (SD 4) with a range of from 10s.

[1] According to Wilkinson (1960, p. 127), it is debatable whether an offender charged with failing to stop *and* failing to report can be punished for *two* offences. This was done in one of the cases studied; there was no appeal (see p. 229 above).

256

to the maximum of £20; the most usual fine was £3. But the high standard deviation is an expression of the considerable differences in the nature of the cases that came into this category. At one extreme is the case of a lorry driver who was struck by a woman driver as he was turning right; she reported the incident and he did not, and there were doubts as to whether he had made signals before turning – he was fined 10s. At the other extreme is the case described on p. 189 above, of the young man who hit a pedestrian on the afternoon of a Christmas Day, killing him; though the accident was held to have been the pedestrian's fault, the defendant did not stop or report the accident, of which he was admittedly aware. Yet he was fined only £10: half the maximum.

That the penalties possible under this head are somewhat inadequate is demonstrated by another case, that of an 81-year-old man, who drove his car from a minor road into a main road in the path of an approaching Green Line bus, which had to swerve onto a pavement to avoid a major collision. The accused, who did not stop, was fined £4 but, considering the damage and injury that *might* have been caused had there been other traffic about, and the age of the offender, it is unfortunate that it was not possible to disqualify or to order a re-test; had the charge been preferred under 'without due care' – which it could have been – then either restriction could have been imposed.

The impression that the courts tend to treat this offence rather leniently is reinforced by the results of three cases in which the offenders had previous convictions for the same offence. Two of them were women. The first was aged 80, and, like the old man in the case mentioned above, she turned her private car out of a minor road into the path of another car approaching on a major trunk road; the driver was forced to swerve and brake violently to avoid her, and he later overtook her and stopped in front to rebuke her. The accused ran into the rear of the other car, reversed away, and drove off. When seen later that day by the police she 'seemed confused' and said that she wished she had a chauffeur. A charge of careless driving in this case was dismissed, and she was fined £1 for failure to stop after, or to report, an accident. The case of the other woman driver was described above (p. 226) – she drove on after hitting and seriously injuring a pedestrian who stepped off the pavement into her path; she was fined £10. A £10 fine was also imposed on the third offender, a man who was returning from a rugby match at 10.30 p.m. on a Saturday night, when he struck a motor cyclist and unseated him; he did not stop but reported the incident next day, because the damage to his car suggested that he had hit something, though he could not remember having done so.

The ranking of the courts according to the proportions of offenders fined £5 or over shows Sefford and Mesley to be far the most severe (*Table 56*) The court with the most offenders recorded is Lesdon, yet this appears to be among the most lenient; so it cannot be that severity is proportionate to the number of cases brought before the particular court.

Table 56

FAILING TO STOP AFTER, OR TO REPORT, AN
ACCIDENT: RANK ORDER OF SEVERITY OF
MAGISTRATES' COURTS

Court	% fined £5 or more	Rank
Opsley	19	5·5
Batwick	19	5·5
Treeford	0	10
Elston	25	3
Barchet	0	10
Seabridge	0	10
Lesdon	10	7
Sefford	85	1
Mesley	50	2
Barling	20	4
Frockton	8	8

Classification of the offenders by occupational groups does not suggest any marked class bias in the treatment of this offence, though it might perhaps be noted that four of the six offenders who were fined £10 or more came from the non-manual groups.

FAILING TO INSURE AGAINST THIRD-PARTY RISKS

(*£50 fine and/or three months' imprisonment. May disqualify.*)

The 73 offenders convicted for this offence are also a sample – 10 per cent of the offenders resident in the District; they were all dealt with summarily and their sentences are given in *Table 57* (with comparable percentages for England and Wales in parentheses). It would seem that the District's courts were rather less inclined to impose sentences of imprisonment for this offence than were those of the country as a whole. But they appear to have used disqualification more readily, since 53·5 per cent of their offenders were so dealt with, in contrast to only 36·5 per cent for England and Wales over the same period.

Table 57

FAILING TO INSURE AGAINST THIRD-PARTY RISKS: SUMMARY
OF SENTENCES

	Magistrates' courts		
Sentence	*Police District*		*England and Wales*
	No.	*% (rounded)*	*%*
Prison and disqualified	2	2·5	(4·4)
Fined and disqualified	37	51·0 ⎫	(88·9)
Fined	33	45·0 ⎭	
Conditionally discharged	1	1·5	(3·9)
Total	73	100·0	

The average fine was just over £6 with a range of from £1 to £25. (SD 4·06), and the most usual fine was between £3 and £5, with six or twelve months' disqualification. The range of disqualifications imposed was from one to 120 months (mean 10·5, SD 7·2).

It is, perhaps, worth mentioning that there seemed to be nothing very unusual about the offences of the two defendants who were sentenced far more severely than any others in the sample. The one who was fined £25 was stopped by a police patrol when he was driving a van for which he had cancelled the insurance two months previously; it was a blatant one, but no more so than others for which the fines did not exceed £10. It could be that the fine was particularly heavy because there was no disqualification. The other case was also one in which the defendant was stopped by the police while he was driving an uninsured van; there was a fine of £2 with disqualification for ten years. In neither case had there been previous convictions for insurance offences: the first man had a clean record, but the second had four non-motoring convictions and one motoring conviction recorded against him – probably one of those cases in which the non-motoring offences *were* taken into account!

When the courts are ranked according to the proportions of offenders fined £5 or over, and again according to the proportions disqualified for one year and over, Mesley and Sefford are found to be the most severe (the Barchet court – which ranks first in fines – had only one offender). Moreover, both Mesley and Sefford show a tendency to impose relatively high fines together with long periods of disqualification; this association does not hold for the other courts, and the rank correlation coefficient for all courts is only ·19 (*Table 58*).

Table 58

FAILING TO INSURE AGAINST THIRD-PARTY RISKS: RANK
ORDER OF SEVERITY OF MAGISTRATES' COURTS

Court	% fined £5 or more	Rank	% disqualified for one year or more	Rank
Opsley	69	4	25	6·5
Batwick	20	9	33	4·5
Treeford	0	10	0	9·5
Elston	50	6	33	4·5
Barchet	100	1	0	9·5
Seabridge	67	5	100	1
Lesdon	44	7	20	8
Sefford	75	3	50	3
Mesley	83	2	80	2
Barling	No cases	—	—	—
Frockton	25	8	25	6·5

$r = ·19$

When the sentences are considered from the point of view of the occupational classification of the offenders, there is a possibility that manual workers were treated more severely than others. The two offenders with the highest fine (£25) and the longest disqualification (ten years) were both manual workers; yet the only two white-collar offenders received £10 fines and escaped disqualification. Also, the evidence suggested that excuses of ignorance or forgetfulness were more likely to be accepted from white-collar offenders than from others.

GENERAL IMPRESSIONS

After this brief analysis of the manner in which the courts dealt with the six classes of offence, let us return to the questions posed at the beginning of this chapter.

First, are there any marked differences between the courts in respect of sentencing, especially with regard to severity?

Table 59 consolidates the ranking of the courts for severity that has been carried out for the offence groups separately (*Tables 51, 53, 55, 56,* and *58* above). It will be seen that each court is given a rank relative to the others for each of the five classes of offence taken into account (causing death is, of course, excluded as it is not dealt with by magistrates); and when the ranks are added together, each court can be given a score represented by the sum of the ranks. The courts who rank highest for severity will have the lowest scores, since their ranks will tend to be four or less; the more lenient courts will have high scores. For example, Sefford is ranked as follows in contrast to Lesdon:

	Driving while disqualified	Driving under the influence	Driving dangerously	Failing to stop	Failing to insure	Total ranks	Score
Lesdon							
Fines	3	8·5	10	7	7	35·5	
						+	=63·5
Disqualifications	9	6	5	0	8	28	
Sefford							
Fines	3	1	2	1	3	10	
						+	=20
Disqualifications	3	2	2	0	3	10	

Table 59 shows that the most severe penalties were imposed by the courts at Sefford and Mesley, and the least severe by those at Lesdon and Seabridge. Although Treeford appears to be the least severe court, it takes only a small proportion of cases from the Police District and is not comparable with the courts that serve the District exclusively.

As regards consistency of sentencing in motoring cases, the only courts which can be said to be predictable are the severe courts of Sefford and Mesley and the lenient court of Lesdon. Among the others the sentences cover a very wide range, as is evident from the large standard deviations for fines and disqualifications for each class of offence (except for driving while disqualified).

Where comparisons with the other magistrates' courts in England and Wales have been made, it seems that the District's courts do not depart markedly from the national norms, except perhaps in their greater tendency to pass sentences of imprisonment for driving while disqualified. Comparisons between the District quarter sessions and the higher courts of England and Wales are difficult to make, owing to the manner in which the

Table 59

FIVE CLASSES OF OFFENCE: CONSOLIDATED RANKING OF
MAGISTRATES' COURTS FOR SEVERITY

Court	CLASS OF OFFENCE AND RANK					Total ranks	Total score
	Driving while disqualified	Driving under the influence	Driving dangerously	Failing to stop	Failing to insure		
Opsley							
Fines	6¹	2	4	5·5	4	21·5	44
Disqualifications	3	5	8	—	6·5	22·5	
Batwick							
Fines	10¹	3	3	5·5	9	30·5	57·5
Disqualifications	10·5	3	9	-	4·5	27	
Treeford							
Fines	10¹	8·5	6	10	10	44·5	76·5
Disqualifications	3	9	10·5	—	9·5	32	
Elston							
Fines	7·5¹	5	5	3	6	26·5	46·5
Disqualifications	8	1	6·5	-	4·5	20	
Barchet							
Fines	10¹	No	11	10	1	32	58·5
Disqualifications	10·5	cases	6·5	—	9·5	26·5	
Seabridge							
Fines	7·5¹	8·5	7	10	5	38	61·5
Disqualifications	3	9	10·5	—	1	23·5	
Lesdon							
Fines	3¹	8·5	10	7	7	35·5	63·5
Disqualifications	9	6	5	—	8	28	
Sefford							
Fines	3¹	1	2	1	3	10	20
Disqualifications	3	2	2	—	3	10	
Mesley							
Fines	5¹	4	1	2	2	14	30
Disqualifications	6	4	4	—	2	16	
Barling							
Fines	1¹	6	8·5	4	No	19·5	36·5
Disqualifications	7	9	1	—	cases	17	
Frockton							
Fines	3¹	8·5	8·5	8	8	36	55·5
Disqualifications	3	7	3	—	6·5	19·5	

¹ Rank order for sentences of imprisonment, not fines.

national statistics are presented for these courts in the Home Office Returns of *Offences relating to Motor Vehicles*.

It should be noted again that any attempt to assess the sentencing policy of the courts is hindered by the fact that in a large proportion of motoring cases several motoring offences are committed at the same time; although separate penalties are shown against each offence, there is no way of knowing which of the offences was most influential in determining the aggregate sentence. This is true especially of the penalty of disqualification, in cases where a charge of failing to insure has accompanied other motoring offences for which the court cannot disqualify; the ultimate period imposed is very likely to take these other offences into account.

Second, do the sentences passed by the courts have any apparent effect on the subsequent incidence of offences? This is a difficult question to answer because the period under review is short: only three years. It would be necessary to follow up the incidence of convictions for each class of offence for a longer period in order to obtain a valid impression, but time and resources did not permit this. Moreover, an increase or decrease in convictions can be influenced by many factors other than the reputation of the court: e.g. number of licence holders, greater holiday traffic, increased or decreased police activity, and so on.

However, for what it is worth, it would seem that the incidence of convictions in the divisions served by the severe courts of Mesley and Sefford did not go down. For the five classes of offence under review, total convictions increased in all the police divisions between 1957 and 1959 (*Table 60*).

Table 60

PERCENTAGE INCREASES IN CONVICTIONS FOR 5 CLASSES
OF OFFENCE 1957–59

Police division	*Courts*	*% difference in total convictions for driving while disqualified, driving under the influence, driving dangerously, failing to stop, and failing to insure, 1957 to 1959 inclusive*
A	Opsley	+42%
B	Batwick; Treeford	+19%
C	Elston; Batwick	+52%
D	Barchet; Seabridge	+58%
E	Lesdon	+53%
F	Sefford; Mesley	+51%
G	Sefford; Mesley	+38%
H	Barling; Frockton	+ 8%

It will be seen that in Division F, where the majority of offenders were dealt with by the more severe Sefford court, the percentage increase is fairly high relatively to the other divisions; this is not so true of Division G, in which a few cases were handled by this court and the other severe court of Mesley, but a rise of 38 per cent is quite substantial none the less. Moreover, the increases in both Divisions F and G are higher than those in Divisions H and B, in which the courts tend to be among the more lenient; and Division E, which is served by the most consistently lenient court at Lesdon, has not a noticeably greater increase in convictions than Division F.

It could, of course, be said that an increase in the incidence of convictions might be expected in divisions where the courts are severe, if conviction itself is taken to be the criterion of severity. Indeed it may be that this analysis is deficient in taking as a criterion of severity the sentence passed rather than the percentage of convictions out of the offenders prosecuted, or a combination of the two. However, even if all the bench lists were examined again to get these data, it is questionable whether they would yield results from which any valid conclusions could be drawn. Let us suppose, for example, that one court convicted a higher proportion of offenders prosecuted than another: this could be because the court's attitude was more severe, but equally it could be because the cases for prosecution were selected more stringently by the police. However, in the final analysis, the criterion of severity should be reflected in the sentence, not in the finding of guilt, which ought to depend on the facts of the case and not upon the attitude of the court. But the practice is often so different from the ideal, that a statement of this kind cannot be made without reservations. Clearly, more skilled and detailed research on these aspects is required.

The third question was whether any differences could be discerned in the manner in which the courts sentenced offenders in the various occupational groups, with special reference to professional drivers.

Perhaps the most striking difference between the classes is in the proportions of offenders sent to prison: unquestionably it is those in the manual group who are most often sentenced in this way, since they supplied 94 per cent of the offenders imprisoned. Most of these (81 per cent) were in the driving while disqualified group, for whom prison is, more or less, the rule; nevertheless, there are reasons for supposing that weight was given to social class, as in the case of the young army officer who was fined after a particularly blatant second offence of this kind. However, it is difficult to allege any such bias without having been at the hearing.

A more definite bias was occasionally revealed against offenders who had several previous non-motoring convictions; in some of these cases prison sentences were given, although the offences did not seem to be especially heinous in comparison with others.

It was noticeable also that rather heavier fines were imposed on those in the top half of the occupational scale than on those in the lower half, as might be expected. But the latter tended to be disqualified more often (62 per cent of the manual workers were disqualified, compared with 55 per cent of the non-manual); this tendency, however, may be related to the proportion of manual workers in the driving while disqualified group.

Otherwise there is no evidence to suggest that any occupational group was treated much differently from another. The only discrimination that was shown in respect of professional drivers was that the courts tended to refrain from imposing on them long periods of disqualification. An exception to this consideration was in drunken driving, when the professionals fared no better than other offenders.

The final question was whether the courts made full and justifiable use of their powers, especially their powers to disqualify and to order offenders to take a further driving test.

It is, of course, very difficult to say just what constitutes 'full use' of a court's powers, and it is perhaps equally difficult to say whether the powers were used justifiably without having been present at the hearings. However, it might be reasonable to assume that powers were not being fully used if the majority of the sentences were concentrated in the lowest quarter of the permitted sentencing range – a range which many people might consider lenient in any case. On the question of justifiable use of powers, the recorded evidence provides some indication of practice, but inferences drawn from it should be treated with reserve.

In one class of offence the powers of the court were certainly used flexibly and without much restraint: in dealing with cases of driving while disqualified, the magistrates' courts of the District proved much more severe than the courts of England and Wales generally, especially in committing offenders to prison. Since prison is mandatory for this offence unless there are 'special reasons', it could be that the magistrates of the District were more in sympathy with the law than most others; on the other hand, it was sometimes difficult to see what the 'special reasons' could have been for not committing an offender to prison when an alternative course was decided upon.

Of the other offence groups it is not possible to say the same: in these cases the majority of the sentences passed were in the lowest quarter of the range prescribed. However, there is no reason to suppose that there was any marked departure from the national norms in this respect.

Although they did not seem prepared to use the upper ranges of their sentencing powers, the District courts tended to compensate for this apparent leniency by their use of disqualification orders, which they imposed in a higher proportion of cases than did the magistrates of England and Wales. At the time of the research, magistrates could disqualify for four of the serious offences under review – drunken driving, dangerous driving, driving while disqualified, and failing to insure; the District magistrates disqualified in 51·5 per cent of these cases in the period 1957 to 1959 inclusive, in contrast to the magistrates' courts of England and Wales as a whole, which disqualified in only 41·2 per cent of comparable cases. Even so, the impression is that the majority of the serious offenders studied who escaped disqualification were very lucky to do so, since their cases were no less heinous than those in which this penalty was imposed. On the other hand, in many cases the length of the disqualification period seemed to bear little relation to the offence, which raises the issue of the criteria by which benches decide the matter. The effectiveness of long periods of disqualification has already been questioned, as a result of some of the findings in this study.

The Divisional Court has ruled (*R. v. Appeals Committee of Surrey Quarter Sessions ex parte Commissioner of Police for the Metropolis*, [1963] I Q. B. 990), that disqualification is not a sentence. What, then, is its aim? If it is a punishment, does it fall into the category of a retributive, a preventive, a deterrent, or a reformative measure, and are the relevant principles taken into account when orders are being made? Clearly disqualification is not regarded as a reformative measure since, if it were, it would probably be linked with an order for the offender to undergo another driving test. Orders for re-tests were made in only six of the 653 cases, all of them elderly drivers; yet it appears that they could have been applied more often and more widely with profit, adding an essentially constructive element to disqualification, and giving some incentive to the offender to improve his behaviour. They seem especially appropriate in cases where the offender is old or incompetent. At the time that this research was done, an order for a further test could be made only in cases of drunken, dangerous, or careless driving; under the Road Traffic Act, 1962, the measure can now be applied over a considerably wider field.

Two further points will conclude this chapter. First, it is important to note the complete inadequacy of the power possessed by the courts at the time of the research to deal with the offence of failing to stop after, or to report, an accident. Recent legislation has increased the courts' power in this respect too, and with justification, since this charge can cover very serious misbehaviour and irresponsibility. Previously, the maximum sentence permitted was a fine not exceeding £20 for the first offence.

Finally, prolonged study of the facts in these 653 cases leaves an inescapable impression that sentencing is very much a matter of chance. It is virtually impossible for the observer, and perhaps for the offender also, to see why one person is fined £25 and another £20 for seemingly identical offences, or why one is disqualified for one year and another for two. No coherent policy based on definite criteria is evident, nor does there seem to be any attempt to follow up sentencing practice by statistical methods in order to discover its effects.

This criticism has often been made, of course, with regard to sentencing policy in general, and it has stimulated a good deal of research, notably in the development of prediction techniques to assist justices to discharge their sentencing functions (see Mannheim and Wilkins, 1955). Research of this kind needs to be extended to the courts' treatment of motoring offenders, since they constitute a formidable problem which is not being dealt with effectively by present methods. Some of the measures employed in the United States for the treatment of traffic offenders have been discussed (see pp. 22 ff. above). A study of these suggests that it may no longer be to anyone's benefit to continue with the hit-and miss methods that appear to be the rule in British courts for dealing with motoring offenders.

PART THREE

The Interview Study

SOME OFFENDERS AND THEIR ATTITUDES

10

Interviews with Forty-three Offenders

This chapter presents the impressions gained from interviews with forty-three people who had been convicted of one of the offences with which this study is concerned. The planning of this section of the research, and the procedures used, are described in detail in Chapter 2 above.

Altogether fifty persons were approached: four in court after conviction, and the remainder at home, having been chosen at random as their names appeared in two specified local newspapers. The offences for which they had been convicted are given below; seven of the fifty refused to be interviewed.

Driving while disqualified	1 (who refused interview)
Driving under the influence	12 (1 refused interview)
Driving dangerously	15 (2 refused interview)
Failing to stop or report	9 (2 refused interview)
Failing to insure	13 (1 refused interview)
	50

In the event no case of causing death by dangerous driving occurred in the District during the period available for interview; and there was only one case of driving while disqualified, in which the offender refused to be interviewed. The absence of offenders in the causing death group is a deficiency from the research point of view, because it would have been valuable to compare them with offenders convicted of, say, dangerous driving, since it has been inferred that there are many imponderables in the decision to prosecute, let alone convict, for the latter offence. For instance, do the personality and social characteristics of the offender have any bearing on the decision made in a particular case? The omission of offenders convicted of driving while disqualified is perhaps less serious, since they appear to be a group more or less indistinguishable from the criminal offenders who are the usual subjects of criminological research, and it is unlikely that interviews would have uncovered anything new.

Interview Refusals

As is usual in this kind of situation, those who refused to participate were as interesting as those who agreed to do so. Three of the seven refusals

271

resulted from the initial attempt to secure an interview by attending the hearing and approaching the offender afterwards, a procedure that was undertaken with very little confidence that it would be successful and with a strong feeling that it was in breach of good taste.

The first person approached in this way was a young man of 17 who had been convicted of an inexcusable offence of driving a motor cycle while disqualified; seen in the hall of the court before going in for trial he was very polite and pleasant, and readily agreed to talk about the case, whatever the outcome. He was put on probation – largely because the probation officer and his father spoke so well of him – and after the hearing his father asked if his son could be left alone, since the whole trial had upset him; it was impossible, therefore, to persist. In this case there were several previous convictions.

The second court refusal was by a female offender who had been convicted of driving without due care, and of failing to stop after an accident. This was a particularly blatant case: the defendant's family saloon had hit a parked vehicle on her offside, when she overtook (at speed, it was said) a lorry where the road was too narrow. She denied knowledge of the incident and claimed that she had heard nothing, although the owner of the parked car heard the impact from inside a house and others 'threw up their windows to see what had happened'. She was fined a total of £45 and disqualified for one month. This defendant also appeared to be in some distress after sentence, so an approach was made to her husband who thought she would agree to an interview if an appointment were made by telephone. Two telephone calls were made, preceded by an explanatory letter, but it was impossible to contact the offender who was clearly taking avoiding action. There were no previous convictions.

The third court refusal was rather similar. The offender was an airline pilot convicted of driving under the influence of drink, for which he was fined heavily and disqualified for two years. In order to spare the feelings of the defendant, who was clearly embarrassed and shaken by the proceedings, his solicitor was approached; he asked that his client should not be included in the study because of certain facts 'which should not be probed'. (These had to do with the offender's occupation, which was not revealed in court or in the press.) However, since it was entirely a matter for the offender himself to decide, an approach was made to him by letter; as expected, there was no reply. No previous convictions were recorded.

The remaining four refusals were from offenders who were visited at home. One was a middle-class alien who was most polite, but said that his application for naturalization papers was pending and he did not wish to take part in anything that might hinder it; he may have thought that the police or security services had something to do with the matter. A suspected connection with the police might also have accounted for the rather strange behaviour of a young working-class man, who answered the door of his council house, listened politely to what the visit was for, excused himself to go and finish his dinner, and then left the house – and the interviewer standing. The next refusal was from a van driver convicted for failing to stop after an accident; three attempts were unsuccessful in finding him at home, and it became obvious from his wife's demeanour that she was acting on instructions. In this case the fact that another member of the family was involved in a charge of wounding a man with intent to murder by stabbing may have had something to do with the adoption of a defensive attitude. Finally, another offender visited at home made a further appointment, then failed to keep it.

It is tempting to speculate as to why people refuse to take part in research interviews and to suggest complex reasons for their behaviour, when, in fact, they may simply have a perfectly natural wish not to disclose matters which they regard as personal and closed; moreover, they probably do not wish to give up the time. Indeed it was surprising that the great majority of the offenders approached cooperated to such a degree: most of them were busy people who were called upon without warning, when they had, no doubt, other things to do, yet in all cases they were courteous and interested. In the event, what had been regarded as a forbidding aspect of the research turned out to be most pleasant.

AGE AND OCCUPATION OF INTERVIEWEES

Forty men and three women agreed to be interviewed. Their ages and occupations are presented in *Tables 61* and *62*. They were, generally speaking, a young group of offenders: the most usual age was 20 (for the 650 offenders whose ages were recorded it was 26). The youngest was just 19 and the oldest was 70. Two of the women were aged 20 and in the lower non-manual occupational group; the third was aged about 33 and in the semi-skilled manual group.

From an occupational/social-class standpoint the offenders who were interviewed did not differ much from the 653 offenders in the documentary study: 60 per cent were in manual occupations. A more accurate assessment was practicable in the case of the interviewers, since they were seen at their homes, and this confirmed the occupational grouping as a satisfactory index

The Interview Study

Table 61

43 OFFENDERS: DISTRIBUTION BY AGE

Age	Driving under the influence	Driving dangerously	Failing to stop or report	Failing to insure	Total
17 and under 21		6	1	7	14
21 and under 30	3	6	1	3	13
30 and under 40			3	2	5
40 and under 50	3	1	1		5
50 and under 60	3				3
60 and over	2		1		3
Total	11	13	7	12	43

Table 62

43 OFFENDERS: OCCUPATIONAL DISTRIBUTION

Occupational group	Driving under the influence	Driving dangerously	Failing to stop or report	Failing to insure	Total
Professional and higher administrative	5	1			6
Managerial and executive	2		1		3
Lower non-manual	2		1	4	7
Skilled manual	1	2	2		5
Semi-skilled manual	1	8	3	4	16
Unskilled manual		2		4	6
Total	11	13	7	12	43

of social class. The equivalent social classes are listed below, and they were found to be appropriate for the offenders.

Occupational group	Social class
Professional and higher administrative	Upper middle
Managerial and executive	Upper middle and middle
Lower non-manual	Middle and lower-middle
Manual	Working

274

Interviews with Forty-three Offenders

Experience and knowledge of driving varied enormously among the interviewees, ranging from forty-seven years to a few months; but on the whole the respondents were not an inexperienced group, since only six of the forty-three had been licence holders for less than two years, and only three of these were holding provisional licences. The most experienced drivers were in the group convicted of driving under the influence of drink: ten of the eleven offenders in this category had been driving for over five years. Of the dangerous driving offenders, only one had driven for less than two years. Five of the offenders could be called 'professional' drivers (two had driven when drunk, two were dangerous drivers, and one had failed to stop after an accident).

A surprisingly large number had not taken a civilian driving test (seventeen of the forty-three), but nine of these were older men (mostly among the drink cases) who had obtained licences before tests were required; one motorist, aged 20, had held a provisional licence for four years without 'bothering' to take a test. Eight offenders had had to take more than one test before passing successfully, and all but two of these were in the dangerous driving and failing to stop groups.

In the course of conversation with the offenders, and when looking at their vehicles, it was possible to obtain some idea of whether they were interested in motoring for its own sake, and the enthusiast was not hard to diagnose. Nineteen of the men seemed to be quite genuine enthusiasts, with enough knowledge to do most of their own maintenance and to talk about their vehicles in technical terms; they spoke with familiarity of either Brands Hatch or Silverstone or both, and were readers of the motoring press. Perhaps the keenest of the group were the young motor cyclists – nine of the forty-three – who were all apparently devotees of motor cycling, and who appeared to have few other interests; a genuine interest and enthusiasm were easy to discern when performance and different makes were discussed, and five of them were deeply involved in oil and grease when visited.

In so far as it is possible to give an opinion, it seems that the typical offence for the enthusiast among these offenders was driving dangerously, with failing to stop or to insure as poor seconds; only three of the drinking drivers could be called enthusiasts, and most of them used their cars only as a means of transport.

Even so, enthusiasm is not a measure of competence, and it was virtually impossible to gain any idea of how good or bad the individuals were as drivers. If their own opinions are anything to go by, they could be presumed to be of at least average standard, since no fewer than eighteen of the forty-three considered themselves to be better drivers than most others on the roads today, and only four graded themselves as below the average. The former group included the oldest offender of all, and also one of the youngest – a confident young lady; but most of the 'experts' were among the older drivers convicted of driving under the influence or of dangerous driving. The four who rated themselves as 'poor' did so on self-assessed grounds of poor eyesight, excessive caution, and – in the case of two provisional licence holders who had been learning when they were apprehended without insurance – sheer inexperience. It was noticeable that the drinking drivers who considered themselves above the average made the point, in defence of their innocence of the charge, that they could not have been incapable of handling their vehicles. The remainder rated themselves 'as good as most others'.

EDUCATIONAL BACKGROUND AND INTELLIGENCE

The main point in considering educational background was to use it as a criterion of intelligence but, in the event, there was no specific questioning on the matter, lest it should make the subjects suspect that there would be some probing into personality factors. It was, however, possible to infer from interview the type of education the subject had received: it appeared that eighteen of the forty-three had been to secondary modern schools or the equivalent, and fifteen had been to either public or grammar schools; three of the latter were graduates.

However, as an index of intelligence this information did not help very much, nor did the interview, at which it was possible to gain only a superficial impression of the subject's quickness in understanding and responding to questions. From these very inadequate indications, only four of the offenders could perhaps be considered to be below average in intelligence; the majority were alert, responsive people who seemed able to discuss their offences and see the implications of them. Hence there is here a slender piece of evidence to suggest that the serious motoring offender is not, generally speaking, a stupid individual. But no more than this can be said, and there is certainly not enough evidence to test the hypothesis that it was hoped to examine when the research was being planned: namely, that motoring offenders as a group do not include an undue proportion of those with the minimum standards of education.

PERSONALITY

Very much the same kind of reservations hold with regard to any attempt to assess the personality characteristics of the offenders. The sample is very small, no personality inventory was given, and the interviews were rarely of more than an hour's duration; moreover, the interviewer was without psychiatric qualifications. On the other hand, the offenders were seen mostly in their home surroundings, and they seemed prepared to talk quite naturally and uninhibitedly, so that some impressions were formed. These will be discussed at the end of this chapter, after all the evidence from the interviews has been presented.

ATTITUDES TO THE OFFENCES

One of the original hypotheses was the statement that 'the offender convicted of a serious motoring offence does not regard himself as a criminal, nor does he think himself to be regarded as such by the rest of society'. Here again the limitations of the small sample preclude any proper testing of this hypothesis, and permit only a few observations that might be suggestive for future research into the attitudes of motoring offenders.

Generally speaking, the majority of respondents did not think of themselves as criminals, and many objected to mixing with criminal types and with sex offenders when in court; nor did they think of their offences, or of most motoring offences, as crimes. However, they had difficulty, as expected, in keeping these distinctions when they were asked to define the terms 'crime' and 'criminal'. Most respondents were obsessed with criteria of dishonesty or of causing bodily harm of some kind, and they could not see that motoring offences could involve either. Another requirement of criminal behaviour was a substantial degree of intention on the part of the offender, whereas frequent comments on motoring offenders were: 'They don't mean to hurt anyone'; 'They aren't dishonest'; 'It's just one of those things that happens on the spur of the moment and you don't think'; and the inevitable 'It could easily happen to anyone'.

There were, however, some exceptions: nineteen of the forty-three respondents defined some motoring offences as crimes, and their perpetrators as criminals. These offences were driving under the influence of drink, and failing to stop or report if there was any question of injury to a person. Antagonism to the drunken driver was very noticeable among the younger respondents, who expressed condemnation without apparent hesitation. It was in their attitude towards offences, more especially

277

towards their own, that the most marked distinction was found between the male and female respondents, although there were unfortunately only three of the latter. All three females appeared to have a strong sense of guilt about their offences, and to have been very upset about being involved in 'a court case'; in this respect they were in contrast to the majority of the men, who were relatively unconcerned.

However, there were twelve men, in addition to the three women, who showed some contrition about their offences, and a surprisingly high proportion of them were among those convicted of driving while uninsured. It seemed that the implications of the offence, had anything happened to a third party, were appreciated now though they had not been appreciated before conviction. It was also surprising to find some of the dangerous drivers contrite: three out of the thirteen realized that they had endangered lives – two were young working-class motor cyclists, arrested for riding at an alleged 80 mph on a busy urban road. The remaining ten in this category were, on the contrary, quite indifferent about their offences, and considered that they had been victimized. Of the drunken drivers, only three were in any way contrite, and these were all upper-middle-class men who seemed genuinely to think that their conduct had been highly irresponsible – 'even criminal', they said. But the majority were quite without remorse or any great concern, except for the inconvenience of disqualification, and they also felt that they had been unlucky to be caught for something that most people do or have done; perhaps 'It was just my bad luck to be caught' is the most apt of the comments from those who realized that the finding of guilt was justified. (Two offenders vehemently believed that they were not drunk at all when arrested.) Among the failing to stop cases, one woman and two men expressed contrition about their behaviour; all had hit other cars, the woman in parking (she was also uninsured and unlicensed), and the men while overtaking other vehicles. In all three instances there was an admission of panic and flight from the scene of the incident; for example, one man said that he had taken fright on hearing the impact with the other car, and had then turned off his lights and accelerated away into the darkness. In another four cases in which collisions with vehicles had occurred, the offenders denied knowledge of the incident and, as far as one could tell, it was one person's word against another's.

Thus there were in all twenty-eight respondents who were relatively indifferent about their offences, including fifteen who did not think that they had done anything wrong at all. The attitudes of the offenders who were interviewed are compared with those that were inferred for the 653 offenders in the documentary study (*Table 63*). It is possible that the interviews revealed much more positive information at the extremes of 'shame-lessness' or 'contrition'. In the documentary study the offenders' responses were to the police, which could have inhibited 'shamelessness' to some extent; moreover, a considerable number of the 653 cases had to be con-signed to the 'indifferent' category, because the evidence was rather vague.

Table 63

ATTITUDES OF THE TWO GROUPS OF OFFENDERS

	Ruthless, shameless, or aggressive	Indifferent	Contrite
	%	%	%
43 offenders	21·0	44·0	35·0
653 offenders	11·5	74·5	14·0

ATTITUDES TO THE POLICE

So it is not surprising to find that only the fifteen respondents who seemed to be genuinely contrite looked with any favour upon the police; the others appeared to think that the police were 'all right until they had a chance to charge you, and then they did not spare themselves to get you if they could'. It was almost unanimously believed, even by the contrite, that police officers had to achieve a certain quota of arrests in order to avoid stricture and to have some chance of promotion; indeed, four respondents who had relations in the police force were particularly emphatic about this. Thirty-five respondents thought that over-zealousness on the part of the police was the main reason for the increase in road traffic offences since 1955, and only eight blamed the greater volume of traffic or the condition of the roads.

There was no marked occupational or class distinction between those who were favourably disposed towards the police and those who were not; about half of the former were working-class people, including two young motor cyclists who might at first have been thought to be typical teddy boys. Both these young men looked on their cases with insight, and praised the police for being fair and helpful despite their wrongdoing: 'We asked for it,' they said.

On the other hand, eighteen of the respondents were definitely hostile to the police. In five cases the hostility seemed to be based on a belief that the offender had been charged for something he had not done; in the case of the others it was more deep-seated. For example, six young motor cyclists, three of whom had non-motoring convictions, believed that the police had declared war on the young working-class boy with a motor bike and were going all out to 'hound him off the roads'. Four offenders were convinced that the charges brought against them were the outcome of personal vendettas by policemen who lived near by and who knew them; one officer was alleged to spend much of his off-duty time around the housing estate, lurking behind hedges to catch residents parking without lights, pushing motor cycles when uninsured, and so on; he was also alleged to be very ambitious, with his heart set on becoming an inspector within a few years. However ridiculous these statements may appear in cold print, there was no doubt that the respondents concerned believed them – and so, apparently, did their parents.

It was, however, rather unexpected to find hostility of a more rational kind among five of the white-collar offenders, including a doctor who had clearly had a lot to do with the police in his professional capacity. Allegations were made of motorists bribing the police, especially to escape prosecution for minor traffic offences in London, and of police being over-zealous in charging motorists so as to stand well in the eyes of superiors; and it was also alleged that the police were not averse to 'roughing up' any suspect who proved intractable. As the doctor put it: 'They are all right until they get you with your trousers down, and then they really take it out of you; they know the public look down on them, and when they can get their own back they do.' Most of this was hearsay, and it was almost impossible to pin the respondents down to quoting specific instances of ill treatment that they themselves had received from policemen; often their antagonism seemed to derive from the belief that the police had been unreasonable in handling their cases, especially when the offender had pleaded guilty.

Twenty-eight of the offenders had pleaded guilty, and eight also asserted that they had been advised to do so by the police in order to avoid adjournment of their cases and a long wait for trial, and in some instances in order to obtain a more lenient sentence than they might get if they argued about the facts. Three of these people had driven under the influence of drink, three were dangerous drivers, and two were offenders who failed to stop after an accident. The three drunken drivers were quite bitter about the business and felt that they had been tricked into a situation over which they had no control.

A particular example was a case that was dealt with outside the Police District by another force. The respondent, who had no previous convictions, was found guilty of driving under the influence. He was a chargehand in his early fifties, who had attended a works party where he had, he said, very little to drink. He was quite sober when he drove some of his work-mates home; however, he lost his way after dropping them, and was off his route when he stopped at some traffic lights about 11 p.m. When moving off he veered slightly to his left, because he had stopped with a slight pull to the left on his steering, and he scraped the side of a sports car whose driver was abusive; both drivers then moved to a side road, and the respondent telephoned for the police who, on arrival, told him that he was drunk and took him to the station. He thought they formed this impression because of an impediment in his speech which occurs when he is distressed or excited; and he explained that this had been caused by plastic surgery to his face and throat after a serious accident five years before when he ran into a lorry on his motor cycle. At the police station he was questioned in the charge-room under a bright light – a stimulus which had caused him great distress ever since his previous accident and which induced in him an urge to shout at the top of his voice – if he could not shout, tension mounted and his behaviour became very distressed; but the police would not believe him and put his behaviour down to drink. When the police doctor arrived the respondent was kept under the bright light for examination despite his protests, and he said that the doctor refused to believe his story and became very aggressive when he stuck to it. When he told the doctor that he was impelled to shout, the doctor gave instructions that he should be put in a cell and kept there, and he refused to reconsider the matter, though the respondent complained that his distress was increased by confined spaces. After a 'miserable night waiting' he was let out at 5 a.m. and given a cup of tea, and when the inspector gave him back his possessions in the charge-room he was told that he would be charged with drunken driving; he said that the inspector then told him that if he pleaded guilty he would 'speak for him' and he would only be fined a few pounds and lose his licence for about twelve months. The inspector was very nice to him and so he agreed to cooperate, after the inspector had also pointed out that there might otherwise be a long delay while witnesses were obtained, and that there would certainly be heavy costs and a heavy penalty.

This man felt that he had been tricked into pleading guilty by the police who had taken advantage of his confusion and distress; he also felt that he had been at their mercy since his own doctor could not (or maybe would not, since his doctor did not seem to be too sympathetic from what the offender said) come out at that time of night, and it did not occur to him to ask for a solicitor to attend him. Moreover, he did not see any point in contesting the issue at court because he realized that he had compromised himself by agreeing to cooperate and to plead guilty.

This case has been referred to already (see p. 115 above), and it has a disquieting aspect. Although the respondent appeared to be somewhat disturbed and neurotic, his account suggests that the 'highly strung' motorist who is rather apt to panic might easily convict himself unnecessarily and unjustifiably when subjected to the stress and pressure of arrest with nobody to take his part.

Other respondents, most of whom had also been convicted of drunken driving, felt that the police had acted in breach of faith by producing in court evidence that was not thought by the offenders to be required once a plea of guilty had been entered. For example, in many cases accounts were given of what defendants had said at the police station after apprehension; evidence of this kind could be damaging to a defendant's reputation without necessarily affecting the outcome of the charge, and he had no opportunity to contest it. Four respondents stated: 'Had I known what the police were going to say, I would not have pleaded guilty.' One offender made remarks on arrest which could have indicated the presence of an embarrassing sexual perversion, and these were reported in remorseless detail both in court and in the local press. On the other hand, another respondent was grateful to the police for not revealing what had been said at the police station on his arrest; it had apparently been agreed that this should not be disclosed if there were to be a guilty plea. The offender said that the arrangement had been made by his solicitor and counsel. Incidentally, the latter had advised the offender to elect trial by jury because he was convinced that an acquittal could have been secured; but, like at least three other respondents, this man was unwilling to risk the additional publicity of trial at quarter sessions, which would, he thought, have been harmful to him professionally.

It is, of course, probable that far from attempting to trick offenders into pleading guilty, the police officers concerned were in fact trying to help them to 'get off lightly', and there was no evidence adduced to prove that this was not so. Indeed, in one case a woman had been charged with failing to stop after or to report an accident; she had torn the bumper from another car while parking her small saloon which she had not driven for several years. She had no licence and was therefore not insured, but she had taken the car on impulse to get to the shops before they closed, in order to buy some special food for an invalid husband; after the incident she had 'waited to see if anyone came', and then driven off. (Acquaintance with the offender suggested that this rather timid and self-conscious woman might have become frightened or panic-stricken.) A police officer, 'who was well known and liked about the district', advised a plea of guilty, on the grounds that any other plea was pointless and would be likely to alienate the considerable sympathy that the bench might have. The offender thought that the officer's advice was wise – and it probably was; moreover, it was manifest that the police chose to ignore the quite serious offence of driving while uninsured, which would have led to a bigger fine and perhaps disqualification also. There were no previous convictions in this case.

It will be seen that no clear-cut picture of the police has emerged from the interviews. Less than half of the respondents were hostile in their attitude towards the police; the remainder either were favourably disposed or – and this was the majority – they could not find anything in particular to criticize, e.g. 'Well, I suppose they have their job to do, and that's that' (from an uninsured motor cyclist).

ATTITUDES TO THE COURTS

All the respondents were asked how they thought they had been treated by the courts: fourteen said that they were satisfied in this respect, and twenty-nine that they had not been treated fairly. The highest proportions of complainants were among the dangerous drivers and those convicted for failing to stop; of the drunken drivers and the uninsured, about half the offenders were dissatisfied.

Generally speaking there seemed to be less dissatisfaction with the finding than with the sentence, and it was the penalty that was the main target of criticism. Inconsistency was the most common criticism: a typical comment was from an offender who had been sentenced for driving under the influence: 'Why fine me £50 and disqualify me for two years for a slight collision with one car, and fine – [another offender just reported in the local paper] a few pounds more and disqualify for three years when he hit three cars and did not stop or report? Surely my offence does not compare as closely with his as the two sentences would suggest?' Another uninsured offender observed: 'Why fine me £3 and disqualify me for three months when the lorry driver who was convicted of an identical offence before me was fined £4 and disqualified for fourteen days only? It doesn't make sense.'

It is not possible to evaluate comments of this kind without full knowledge of the facts of each case. But there is no doubt that the courts do come in for strong criticism on the grounds of inconsistency in sentencing, especially with regard to motoring cases.

Of the twenty-nine offenders who had not, in their view, been treated fairly, all but two thought the sentence quite disproportionate to the offence, particularly the penalty of disqualification. But when all 43 cases are compared with the 653 cases in the documentary study, only one offender could be said to have been dealt with more severely than other similar offenders. The case where there did seem to have been harsh treatment concerned an elderly driver, aged 70, who had been involved in two slight collisions; he stopped after one of them only, and reported neither. He was fined a total of £70 and disqualified until he had taken a further test. This was a rather pathetic case of old age; the respondent denied any crime, and broke down three times during the interview while he was describing the events. He said that, as a pensioner, he could ill afford the 'huge' fine, and although this was perhaps doubtful (he had his own business), his means were clearly not such that he could meet it without hardship. Given these facts, disqualification seemed to be the obvious penalty for the offender, and perhaps it was not necessary to penalize him so heavily by fine as well; in any case he had undertaken not to drive again.

Although comparisons are notoriously difficult, this case brings to mind another (mentioned on p. 247 above), in which a baronet of approximately the same age as the offender just described was concerned in an incident in which two were killed and several injured; yet he was fined only £10, and disqualified pending a further driving test.

Another point of interest that emerged from the interview with this elderly respondent was that he had been advised by his doctor and his solicitor not to attend court, and the case was dealt with in his absence. Had the bench seen the defendant they would probably have been less severe. Indeed, this is an example of the undesirability of trying cases in the absence of the accused.

However, this offender at least had the benefit of legal assistance, but it was quite surprising how many respondents did not even seek it. Excluding the uninsured, for whom it may not have been of much avail, no fewer than twelve were without legal advice or representation: of these, ten were convicted for dangerous driving, and the remaining two for drunken driving. One of the latter was the offender who could not stand bright lights (see p. 281 above), and he might well have fared very differently with a skilled defence; undoubtedly he would have been advised against a guilty plea, since he believed himself to be quite fit to drive. The other respondent who had no legal aid and who was convicted of drunken driving was also dealt with outside the District. He said that he was arrested shortly after midnight, in London, driving without lights; he was taken to the police

284

station, charged with drunken driving, and put in the cells. He was not allowed, he said, to telephone his home or his solicitor, or his doctor. He was taken next day to a stipendiary magistrates' court, and put in a cell with a housebreaker who assured him that he would get 'three months' prison'. In the event he was fined £50 and disqualified for a year, having been advised by the police to plead guilty 'as it would go better for me if I did'. Now it may well be that this case was really what the accused himself described as 'a fair cop', but there are aspects of the way in which it was handled that seem to call for criticism if the offender's account is true. And, since he did not think himself hard done by, there is no reason to doubt his veracity; moreover, he was one of the more responsible and better educated respondents. He had no previous convictions.

Most of the dangerous drivers who were not defended were youngsters who said that they could not afford it; several of them were in fact members of motoring organizations, but it had not occurred to them to use the facilities for legal aid to which they were entitled. Clearly some offenders, after hearing the prosecution's case, wished that they had not pleaded guilty so that they could have contested it; and it seemed that they had not really appreciated the disadvantages entailed in the course that they took. One offender – a motor cyclist who had quite a good defence – tried to defend himself in court, but the result was a rather pathetic display by the young man, who was clearly out of his intellectual depth.

From what they said, many of these offenders, especially the younger ones, apparently went to court without really appreciating the probable consequences of conviction. The resultant blow was often a shock, especially when the penalty of disqualification for six months or more became a reality. Offenders rarely complained about having been fined, except where the amount was over £50; three of the young working-class offenders said that their fines did not matter because their parents would pay most of the money. But disqualification hit very hard in every case, and it was clearly the punishment that no one relished. It was not merely that it was inconvenient to be unable to drive; disqualification also meant in most cases a much longer journey to and from work, and in two instances the loss of jobs because they were no longer accessible; the more enthusiastic motor cyclist was deprived of leisure-time enjoyment as well. But perhaps most uncomfortable of all was the ever-present and powerful temptation to drive while disqualified, an urge that became stronger as time wore slowly on and memory of court and offence faded. Three offenders admitted frankly that they could not stand it, and they drove in the hope that 'if anything happened' (other than an injury to someone) they could say that they had not been driving. From all accounts the temptation to drive must be very great, especially for people who use a vehicle regularly and rely upon it, as many do, when they live a long way from work. Perhaps this explains why only two of the forty-three respondents thought that driving while disqualified could be regarded as a crime; for most of those who had been disqualified it was an understandable lapse which they did not feel able to condemn – although it amounted also to driving uninsured, which the offenders were much more ready to criticize as potentially antisocial. It was noticeable that few respondents realized that in committing one offence, such as driving when disqualified, they were automatically committing another.

A common line of criticism among the respondents was that magistrates were too old and were 'out of touch' with motoring problems. Two complainants were moved to make this criticism only – as far as could be determined – because there was an elderly lady on the bench: it was assumed that, being a woman and being elderly, she *must* be out of touch – perhaps an example of the manner in which the minds of accused persons leap to rather prejudiced conclusions.

Thirty of the offenders – a substantial majority – thought that benches were much too severe with motoring offenders, and were so prejudiced against motorists and motor cyclists that they were doing more harm than good by giving rise to increasing bitterness and resentment against the law; ten thought that the courts' handling of cases was 'about right'; and three felt that the courts were much too lenient and should be more severe with offenders of all kinds.

Some offenders were critical also of the manner in which summary proceedings were conducted, especially when magistrates came to a decision without retiring: 'It was all buttoned up long before I ever came into court,' one offender said, 'they never bothered to retire, but just looked at each other and the chairman said "guilty"; it was a farce.' Another was sharply critical of the practice whereby applications for the removal of disqualification were heard by the justices who made the order of disqualification; he inferred that they must be prejudiced towards upholding their original order.

Whereas there seems to be something in the first criticism – since justice must not only be done, but be seen to be done – the second point does not really stand up to examination since only the justices who heard the case originally would know why they acted as they did; they would therefore be in the best position to evaluate the police recommendation that always accompanies applications of this kind.

Interviews with Forty-three Offenders

The police are given the opportunity to recommend or oppose all applications for the removal of a disqualification order; they will therefore make preliminary inquiries about the offender's conduct, and then submit a report to the justices accordingly. This is a necessary procedure when licences are suspended in the interests of public safety; however, there is a sense of injustice among offenders when one application is successful and another is not. The following example from the offenders who were interviewed shows that there can be grounds for this sense of injustice.

The offender in question had been convicted, outside the Police District, for driving under the influence of drink, for which he was fined £25 and disqualified for eighteen months. As a foreman roundsman, driving was part of his job, and he had to be taken 'inside' because of his suspension; but his employer was sympathetic and he did not seem to suffer any financial loss or reduction in status. After six months he applied for the removal of his disqualification, and it was said on his behalf that he was a teetotaller and of unimpeachable conduct; the justices removed the ban accordingly. Yet this respondent admitted at interview that he had driven several times while disqualified, and that it was the practice of his group of friends to enjoy themselves outwitting the police on minor breaches of the motoring law. He told with glee how the police, when arresting him for drunken driving, had failed to see that his road fund licence was for a goods vehicle: 'That's how efficient they are,' he said. He then went on to say that he and his friends had run a sweep on how long they could drive with an out-of-date licence in the holder without being stopped by the police. He also boasted of his prowess as a drinker, and admitted to driving at speeds around 80 mph in his 'hotted up' car just before he was stopped by the police; but he denied that he was drunk, and held that his driving was perfectly safe. In all, this respondent's attitude did not indicate that he was likely to be a suitable applicant for the removal of a disqualification order at any time, and his success in this respect must have caused some amusement – or cynicism – in his circle of friends. There were four previous non-motoring offences recorded against him.

Another criticism of the courts was made by the respondents convicted of dangerous driving: they were quite unable to see any difference between what they had done and what others convicted of 'without due care' had done. Endless examples were quoted of marked differences in the disposal of the two kinds of offence; probably the fact that they coexist and overlap does much to augment the impression of inconsistency, and hence unfairness, that exists.

Typical of the confusion about these two offences was the case of a young

The Interview Study

army officer who, in daylight, was taking a short cut across a disused airfield in order to reach a main road. He was talking to his wife, and turned onto what he thought was the main runway of the airfield; but it was the main road, and his car was hit almost instantaneously by an approaching lorry, whose driver could not stop in time on the wet and skiddy surface. Both the officer and his wife were hurt, and their car was completely wrecked. He was charged with dangerous driving, and was fined £10 without disqualification. This respondent fully accepted his guilt, but he was very puzzled as to why he had been charged with the more serious 'danger' if the offence was 'worth' only £10: a normal penalty for 'due care'. Oddly enough, this man might have been less astonished had he been fined more heavily. His case was dealt with in another District, and there were no previous convictions.

SOCIAL CONSEQUENCES OF CONVICTION

Earlier in this chapter there was some discussion about whether these offenders regarded themselves in any way as criminals, but it is of equal, and perhaps greater, interest to inquire about the attitudes of other people towards the convictions, as imagined by the offenders themselves. Hence it was put to them that, had they been convicted for stealing or burglary, some sort of stigma might have been attached to them, and some kind of social repercussions might have followed; they were then asked whether anything like that had happened as a result of their publicized conviction for the motoring offence. And in order to enable respondents to answer with some degree of truth, interviews were never carried out until at least two days – and more usually seven – after the publication of their cases; so they had a little time in which to experience 'public opinion'.

The offenders were later classified rather crudely according to whether there had been much, some, or no adverse effect on their personal relations with others, which they thought to be attributable to their conviction. *Table 64* presents the results. It will be seen that the majority of the offenders said that the conviction had made no difference at all to their relations with others, and most of these added that they had received much sympathy from fellow-sufferers who had experienced the attentions of the police and the courts. One dangerous driver of the upper-middle class put it in typical terms: 'I found that it was like joining a sort of club. One only had to mention the affair in any group and others immediately spoke of their own experiences, rather as people talk about their illnesses.' And another said: 'I suppose people think about not stopping after hitting someone else's

288

car as a bit like walking away and saying nothing after being given too much change in a shop. It's a great temptation and nobody really blames you for falling for it.' And another: 'Nothing matters much these days, people live and let live and mind their own business more than they did; I don't think anyone would have pointed at me if I'd been sent to prison' (this man had been convicted for drunken driving). One of the dangerous drivers – a professional driver – put his view in terms of social class: 'As usual, from the working class you get nothing but sympathy and they know how things are; it's the other bastards who point and hint.'

Table 64

SOCIAL CONSEQUENCES OF CONVICTION

Offence	*Offenders who had experienced adverse effect on personal relations*			
	Much	*Some*	*None*	*Total*
Driving under the influence	1	5	5	11
Dangerous driving	1	5	7	13
Failing to stop	0	1	6	7
Failing to insure	2	2	8	12
Total	4	13	26	43

Apparently those who experienced the least adverse reaction were the offenders convicted for failing to stop after damaging other cars, of whom only one said that he had been 'stared at' and 'whispered about' since he had been 'in the papers'. Indeed the apparent tolerance shown by all the respondents towards this kind of offence was surprising, and it is epitomized by the 'wrong change' analogy mentioned above. Most respondents believed that the victim's insurance company would make good the damage – which was, anyhow, unintentional – and that stopping would only make matters more unpleasant and complicated for everyone concerned; but it is interesting that two respondents who had had their parked cars damaged by hit-and-run drivers took a very different line, and rated this offence as both cowardly and 'crooked'. Moreover, none of the failing to stop group had been involved in bad instances of the offence, and the press reports were very bald and unsuggestive in each case.

The press report is, of course, of major importance in influencing an offender's public relations, and every respondent emphasized this. All who said that there had been adverse reactions blamed the press report, and two offenders were threatening to sue the local papers for defaming them, thought it was hard to see on what grounds they could have done so (both were under 21, and it is suspected that they were of dubious local reputation). But in other cases where there was a feeling that the press had been unfair the reaction was understandable, especially when the inebriated conversations of the drunken drivers with the police were reported, after a guilty plea had removed any opportunity for the accused persons to deny or modify the account of what they had said. There was also the inevitable criticism that, whereas in some cases all the facts were reported, in others, in which the penalties hinted at something more heinous, the press account was no more than a few lines. This happened in one instance in which the maximum fine for driving under the influence had been imposed: the offender's occupation was not mentioned, and the account of the proceedings was confined to name and sentence only. In another case the incident was reported in full, but the offender's occupation was not mentioned. Presumably the aim was to avoid scandal and to minimize the social consequences of conviction for the offender, but it was not known whether it was the court or the newspaper that was exercising discretion in the matter. Whichever it was, as one respondent put it, 'It makes you think!'

Only four respondents had experienced much social reaction from conviction. One was a professional man, with no previous convictions, who had been convicted for drunken driving; his case was reported widely in the national press, and although all his business associates and friends had, he said, been 'kindness itself', he had received two very abusive and unpleasant anonymous telephone calls during the early hours of the morning following publication of the case, and there had been a lot of local gossip which had caused him and his wife great distress – their reaction was understandable, for this was one respondent who was deeply contrite about his offence. On the other hand, he also said that he had received a few sympathetic letters, including one from someone he had not met, who ended his letter with a request for employment – not as a chauffeur.

Another offender with a 'clean record' who said that he had suffered was one of the young dangerous drivers – he had hoped to join the police force but his conviction had 'finished all that'. He also claimed that some friends had 'taken the mickey out of him', but on the whole there was much sympathy for him in his plight (this could not be called a bad case).

The two uninsured offenders had previous non-motoring convictions and were both somewhat notorious locally; it was clear that they had been the object of gossip for unruliness before the occurrence of these particular offences, which thus reinforced impressions already existing. They complained of being 'pointed at and looked down on', and of difficulty in getting jobs which enabled them to work with cars or motor cycles which, they claimed, were their main interests. This last is not too easy to understand, unless other factors were involved, since several of the respondents were employed in garages and did not lose their jobs because of their offences; on the contrary, it seemed that employers in the motor trade were sympathetic and tolerant.

Among others who experienced some social repercussions from their offences were two of the three serving soldiers who were interviewed. One had ridden a friend's motor cycle without insurance and had, he said, been reported by a particularly zealous NCO who was always 'out to get who he could'; this was the same NCO who was the offender in one of the 653 cases reviewed above (p. 227). It is not thought that this respondent was aware of the NCO's record; if he was, he did not say so. The respondent made the point that his case was, in his view, prejudiced by his having to appear in court with a military escort (he was under close arrest for being absent without leave), which would imply that he was a 'bad lot'. He also felt that the offender in the services invariably had more than a fair share of punishment since he was brought up on a military charge and given another punishment on the same set of facts for which the civil court had dealt with him. In fact, as far as he was concerned this was not a valid complaint, since the military authority was penalizing him for absence only; it is possible, however, that cognizance was taken of the motoring offence, because he had been removed from trade training as a driver – not unreasonably, it may be thought. The complaint of the other serviceman had more substance, for he was an acting NCO himself and lost his rank because of the court case; it is in this sense that the serviceman is apt to suffer two penalties – again, not unreasonable if the NCO rank is a purely disciplinary one and is held on condition that its holder is of exemplary conduct. This 20-year-old soldier had been the object of a chase by the police at speeds up to 80 mph in the early hours, after he had taken a friend's car for an outing to London when in a fit of drink-stimulated boredom. He was fined £40 and disqualified for a year which, with the loss of rank, was a severe penalty for a young married man with two children.

The overall impression was that it was the offender convicted of driving under the influence whose reputation was most likely to suffer in consequence, and it was clear that all those who had been convicted on this charge expected some social repercussions, even if they had not in fact experienced any. That this offence carried more stigma than most other motoring offences has been mentioned already, since so many respondents singled it out for special mention when considering motoring offences as 'crimes'. This general attitude was certainly reinforced in the course of an interview with an offender who had a previous conviction for being drunk while in charge of a car. He considered that his first conviction had made him a target for the police and that they had arrested him on the second occasion purely 'on spec'; his accent had, he said, led an over-zealous officer to think him to be drunk, and the bantering way he had treated the officer had caused annoyance which was 'worked off' in charging him. He claimed that, since his conviction, his friends had 'pulled his leg' endlessly, and that he had been ridiculed in the town because some people thought he must be a drunkard. Nevertheless, he made much of his prowess as a drinker and of that of his father before him, and he did not do much to dispel the impression that he liked to drink. Like most of the other men convicted of this offence he was very much the extravert, and a likeable, sociable character. As a commercial traveller his disqualification had hit him very hard indeed, and when seen he was much concerned about his job – yet another example of the very serious consequences of more than a few weeks' disqualification for many motoring offenders.

Indeed the published consequences – the fine and the disqualification – do not often indicate the real effects of conviction. Costs, as mentioned already, are apt to be between £10 and £50 in a serious motoring case; then there is the legal fee, which may be at least ten guineas (though those who are members of motoring organizations, and make use of the facilities, get these services free); furthermore, if damage has been caused the 'no-claim bonus' is automatically lost; and finally, the first £5 or £10 of repairs to the vehicle have to be paid. One offender, fined £50 for driving under the influence, calculated the total cost of his conviction to be £225: owing to a long disqualification he had to sell his car, and 'dropped' £100 on it, and he paid his legal costs himself. Another offender – a dangerous driver – was fined only £10, but replacement of car and clothing, in addition to the costs of the case, amounted to £120, which, when he itemized the outlay, seemed if anything to be an underestimate. Several disqualified drivers had to pay increased fares to work, two had to employ drivers and one had to rent a room because he could not commute. It is no wonder that nearly every offender said that disqualification was the penalty that really hurt.

ADDITIONAL CONVICTIONS

Obtaining details of additional convictions posed some ethical difficulties. The respondents had been promised that nothing would be done that would enable the police to identify them as informants; hence it would have been improper to approach the local police for details of their records, since this would have meant disclosing the names and addresses of the respondents. It would then have been easy for the police to 'put two and two together', had they wished to do so. It was therefore decided to check on their records through the Home Office Research Unit, which has access to Criminal Record Office files; this means that many offences may not be included – especially motoring offences – but it is better than nothing, and it preserves the respondents' anonymity as far as the local police are concerned. The results of the check are presented in *Table 65*.

Table 65

INTERVIEWS WHO HAD CRO RECORDS

Offence for which respondent was interviewed	Number of additional non-motoring convictions recorded at the CRO				Total offenders with non-motoring convictions
	I	2	3	4	
Driving under the influence	—	—	—	I	I
Driving dangerously	I	2	—	I	4
Failing to stop	I	—	—	—	I
Failing to insure	I	I	I	I	4
Total	3	3	I	3	10

At least ten of the forty-three respondents (23·2 per cent) had additional non-motoring convictions recorded in CRO files; a strikingly similar proportion to that found among the 653 offenders in the documentary study, of whom it will be remembered that 18·2 per cent had CRO files and just over 23 per cent had convictions recorded at *either* the CRO *or* the local police station.

Three of the respondents had additional motoring convictions: two had been convicted for insurance offences and one for being 'drunk in charge'. Also it is of interest that the additional offences of all but one of the ten offenders included offences against property; other offences recorded were those of assault and of the possession of offensive weapons.

CONCLUSIONS

From a sociological standpoint this small sample of serious offenders seems to be strikingly similar in composition to the larger group of 653. And

293

perhaps the most remarkable similarity is that the proportion of offenders who had additional non-motoring convictions – 23 per cent – tallies almost exactly in the two populations. The fact that the groups are alike means that further doubt is cast on the two key hypotheses – that the serious motoring offender is otherwise an 'upright law-abiding citizen', and that most motoring offenders come from the white-collar classes.

Assessment of personality was extremely difficult, having regard to the fleeting acquaintanceship with the respondents and the interviewer's lack of psychiatric training. It was possible to infer from their answers to questions on driving ability that most respondents tended to be sensitive and also over-confident about their capacity to handle a vehicle; but there was not enough evidence to justify any conclusions about the presence of pathological traits. The most that could be done was to record, after the interview, any reservations about the respondent's stability; these were based upon such evidence as signs of excessive tension, the repeated mention of personal vendettas which could be indicative of an unusually suspicious attitude, boasting about physical or sexual prowess to an extent that would be unusual to a comparative stranger, and frequent self-contradiction about which the respondent showed no apparent concern. On this basis there were reservations about seventeen of the forty-three respondents. When the CRO check was completed, five of these seventeen offenders were found to have additional non-motoring convictions; that is, they constituted half the number of offenders in the group who had CRO files. Perhaps this may be regarded as a slender corroboration of the assessment made.

The offenders who were interviewed were by no means an inept or unintelligent group: only four were suspected of being of limited intelligence, and only one of the forty-three was unable to cope with conversation about the handling and maintenance of cars or motor cycles. Their knowledge was not surprising because they were, generally speaking, quite experienced drivers: all but six had been driving for over two years, and nineteen could be rated as enthusiasts.

Their attitudes towards the law and to what they had done were, in the majority of cases, distinguished by a seemingly sincere belief that motoring misbehaviour is not in a criminal sphere. Although it is true that fifteen respondents were contrite, only three were prepared to apply the label 'criminal' to their behaviour, and when they did so they gave the impression that they were making a conscious exaggeration.

It was obvious that most of the respondents considered the law to be highly discretionary, and thought that discretion had been exercised by the police against the offender when it need not have been; also there was the strongly held belief that it paid the police officer to secure a conviction, in that it improved his standing with his superiors and his prospects of promotion. It was noticeable, too, that offenders thought that the police and the justices were 'in league' against the motoring offender, and that their cases were decided before they appeared in court. This was apparent especially among the young respondents, who seemed to have no difficulty in ignoring the numbers of offenders who are *not* convicted; they had apparently decided that the police and the courts were against them, and they seemed to be adamant. Moreover, there was considerable misunderstanding among most respondents about the relationship between the police and the justices – giving the impression that such topics had not been included in their education.

The younger offenders were at some disadvantage also in that they seemed to know little about their rights, and rarely considered it worth while to take legal advice. This was true of some older men, too, and none of those who said that they had been pressed by the police to plead guilty thought that this was an infringement of their rights; rather, they were annoyed that a 'bargain' had not been honoured, in the sense that they had not been let off with a very light sentence and that the police evidence had not been limited in scope.

It may be asked why some of these people did not think it worth while to take legal advice: it seemed that in all twelve cases the main factor was financial, and the respondent thought that he would be faced with a heavy expense. This was especially true of the young working-class respondents; yet some were members of the Automobile Association and did not know that legal services could thereby be obtained gratis. This particular point may partially explain the preponderance of working-class offenders in the research population: perhaps the white-collar offender turns more readily to legal assistance and so is more likely to secure an acquittal. However, there is no means of following up this possibility unless people who have been acquitted can be included in a research study; and even then it could not be said with any certainty that an individual's social status had been the main factor in deciding the outcome of a case. Hence objective research must be confined to the convicted.

Finally it is clear that the social consequences of conviction for a serious motoring offence are not by any means severe; what hardship there was among those who were interviewed was generally the result of disqualification. The penalty of disqualification from driving undoubtedly has an impact on the life of the offender, especially when he uses his vehicle to get to and from his place of employment. Its effects were most evident in the case of offenders in the lower occupational groups, whose work involves travelling in the early morning, or at rush hours, or at inconvenient times for shift periods. As one of the managers put it: 'Disqualification is a nuisance to me, but it doesn't really matter as I can always get a taxi or one of the firm's fleet if I need a car.' Perhaps manual workers therefore have the strongest temptation to drive while disqualified, and this may be one reason why they are so numerous among offenders convicted for this offence.

In the event this small interview survey yielded more information than was expected; and the respondents cooperated to a remarkable extent considering the informal and spontaneous approach. It is regretted that time and money did not permit an inquiry of this kind on a much larger scale.

PART FOUR

Conclusions

A Final Assessment of the Evidence

The aim of this final chapter is to make some assessment of the achievements of this study. But first it is important to recall the limitations of the evidence adduced. A great deal of it is statistical, but the statistics of motoring offences have been shown to be peculiarly confusing, and they do not present a completely objective and reliable picture. Nor, by the strictest standards of social investigation, are the police records as objective as a research worker would like; they rarely included the full case for the defence, they relied greatly on the *impressions* of witnesses, and they were concerned more with the circumstances of the offence than with the personal characteristics of the offender. It was therefore necessary to make inferences about the offenders from a distance, and although the credibility of these inferences was checked by interview, the subjects seen were not the same persons as those in the documentary study; moreover, the sample of forty-three was too small to be a satisfactory check.

The resultant material is therefore a mixture of fact and impression, with rather more of the latter than is desirable; but it provides enough information to show whether the hypotheses under examination can be supported. Beyond that point, what is offered is, at best, a comprehensive and unprejudiced interpretation of the available evidence, and at least something better then mere speculation.

THE HYPOTHESES RE-EXAMINED

Let us now reconsider the basic hypotheses in the light of the evidence from the research.

(a) *The serious motoring offender, unlike the majority of other offenders found guilty of criminal offences, e.g. offenders against property, is a respectable citizen whose behaviour apart from his offence is reasonably in accord with the requirements of law and order.*

Against this hypothesis it was found that 151 of the 653 offenders in the documentary study and 10 of the 43 offenders in the interview group had additional convictions for non-motoring offences; i.e. about 23 per cent of

Conclusions

both groups. This proportion is substantially in excess of even the most pessimistic estimate of the proportion of persons that could be expected to have criminal records in a random sample of the population of England and Wales (see p. 210 above). The findings against the hypothesis are strengthened still further if all the offenders who were 'known to the police' as suspected persons are included in this regard, since this would make the total of persons in whom the police had cause to be interested for reasons other than motoring behaviour 211, or 32.3 per cent of the 653 offenders. (Unfortunately it was not possible to secure information about minor offences, or about status as suspected persons, in respect of the 43 interviewees.)

So the truth of this hypothesis is questionable; and the case against it seems to be substantial enough to change any stereotype that might be founded upon it.

(b) *The majority of serious motoring offences are derived from accidents, and there is nothing in the offender's personality or background that predisposes him to break the law.*

If an accident is a chance event that happens so quickly and suddenly that it is beyond anyone's control to prevent it, then it is clear that this hypothesis is disproved. For only about 14 per cent of the 653 offences could possibly be called inadvertent accidents in this sense, and even this estimate is stretching credulity to its limits. In the great majority of cases the offences were largely of the offenders' own making, and the most obvious explanation seemed to be expediency in the absence of any constraints upon behaviour. In 11 per cent of the 653 cases and 21 per cent of the 43 offenders who were interviewed there was evidence of selfish, and even ruthless, self-interest, but it was not possible to infer personality disturbance in more than 25 per cent of the 653 and 39 per cent of the 43 offenders. Though the inferences with regard to personality traits may be an overestimate in the interpretation of qualitative data, they could equally be an underestimate, since so very little was ever recorded about the offenders themselves. The lack of data is a consequence of the almost total lack of interest in motoring offenders as persons: as far as could be judged from the police records, it was not thought necessary to make any inquiries about an individual's way of life in these cases unless there was to be a trial by jury. Nor did it arouse any comment if age and occupation were not disclosed, as happened in several cases. Information of this kind has importance for purposes other than research, since it seems that benches often fix fines and disqualification orders with due regard for what they know of the offender; and usually, it appears, what they know is just as much as the defendant himself or his solicitor is prepared to tell them.

It must be assumed, therefore, in the absence of evidence to the contrary, that the majority of these serious motoring offenders were normal people who succumbed to temptation when circumstances were favourable and it was expedient to take a chance. So perhaps there is something in the normal personality that predisposes a driver to break the law. Whatever it is, its presence is much more evident in males than in females, since the analysis of the national statistics shows a predominance of males over females of between 18:1 and 22:1, and in the Police District the ratio was nearly 12:1. The real significance of these figures is hard to assess, because the relative proportions of each sex at risk are unknown. Munden (1962, p. 2) produced a ratio of six males to one female from his sample of insurance policy holders, but this is almost certainly an underestimate since many females – probably more than males – are likely to be driving on someone else's policy. Hence the ratio of three to one (found in a recent analysis (1962) by the County Treasurer whose area coincided with the Police District) is probably nearer to the real state of affairs. Females reached noticeable proportions only among the hit-and-run drivers, and there seems to be some justification for calling this the 'feminine' offence among those that were studied.

The difference between the sexes in their relative propensity to break the law on the roads is important, because it shows that motoring offenders have a characteristic in common with offenders in other fields of criminal activity, where males predominate to a marked degree. Further support for the view that there are considerable differences between the sexes in driving behaviour was given by a report in the *Daily Telegraph* (2 July 1962) of a motor insurance underwriter's intention to offer discounts on premiums where the policy holder or the 'named driver' was a woman.

This hypothesis is further disproved by the very high incidence, among the offences studied, of failing to insure against third-party risks. For this offence only a 10 per cent sample of the offenders resident in the District was included, and if they had been expanded to their full population they would have constituted an overwhelming majority in the research. Yet only 2·7 per cent of these offences were derived from accidents and it could not possibly be said that this, the most common of the serious offences, was brought about by providence. On the contrary, it can be regarded as a typical form of economic crime, which, although sometimes committed through inadvertence, is more usually quite deliberate and calculated.

Conclusions

(c) *The offender convicted of a serious motoring offence does not regard himself as a criminal, nor does he think himself to be regarded as such by the rest of society.*

This hypothesis could be tested directly only from the interview survey, in which it was found that three of the forty-three respondents used the term 'criminal' about themselves, and even then it was hard to believe that they really meant it. None of the others thought the term in the least appropriate to his behaviour, though they all found great difficulty in defining it; it seemed that only offences involving severe injury or dishonesty were considered criminal, though, when pushed to it, nineteen respondents applied the term to the drunken driver. The social repercussions of conviction were negligible in all but four cases, and none of these offenders was affected at all severely; in the thirteen cases where some repercussions were reported the reason was evidently the reputation of the offender, and the motoring offence was just another increment to a body of existing opinion.

It seemed that there was little or no inclination among the police or the public to apply the term criminal or any social stigma to these motoring offenders. The police had a clear-cut but indefinable concept of a distinction between what they called crime – meaning usually offences handled by the CID – and motoring offences, a concept which was, generally speaking, shared by members of the public. It is also interesting that the offenders interviewed who had criminal records were careful to distinguish between motoring offences and what they called 'real crime', which they defined as 'breaking, burglary, and assault'.

These conclusions are confirmed to some extent by Martin (1962, p. 129), in his study *Offenders as Employees*. A sample of ninety-seven firms answered a question regarding the effect of certain offences (including serious driving offences) on an offender's chances of employment, if it were known that he had committed one of them. The results showed that 'serious driving offences were regarded in a completely different light from all other "criminal" offences. It seems likely that they would only be regarded as a bar to employment if the job itself involved driving. So marked is this attitude that one may even wonder whether, in its way, it may not be just as irrational as the aversion towards sex offences. Among some who have studied traffic offences there is a school of thought that a man drives as he lives; if there is anything in this, then the bad driver may be more of an employment risk (even in a non-driving job) than is popularly supposed.'

Hence this hypothesis seems to be adequately supported by the evidence.

302

A Final Assessment of the Evidence

(d) *If the Registrar-General's classification of occupational groups is taken as a criterion of social class, serious motoring offenders will be distributed widely over the range of occupations, in contrast to the majority of other offenders convicted of indictable offences (or those akin thereto), who tend to come mostly from the manual groups.*

As Chapter 2 showed, it was extremely difficult to deal with this hypothesis as it stood, because there was no reliable picture of the occupational distribution of the population with which to compare the distribution of the offenders. Hence it was decided to simplify the hypothesis to state that

. . . *the majority of serious motoring offenders will be found to come from non-manual occupations, in contrast to the majority of other offenders convicted of indictable offences (or those akin thereto), who tend to come mostly from manual occupations.*

With 62 per cent of the 653 offenders and 60 per cent of the interviewees coming from manual occupations there seems to be no doubt that the modified hypothesis is nullified. And if the sample of insurance offenders were expanded to its actual size, the proportion of manual workers would be even higher.

The data also cast more than reasonable doubt on the original hypothesis, since, if the Registrar-General's classification is used for comparison, it is found that the semi-skilled and the unskilled occupations are considerably over-represented among the offenders. Forty-four per cent of the 653 and 49 per cent of the interviewees were in these groups, in contrast to an expected 29 per cent, which is the comparable proportion in the population of England and Wales. Moreover, these figures emerged from a District where manual workers are fewer than in the country overall, and white-collar workers more numerous. There is, in fact, a slight over-representation of the highest occupational group among the offenders, as might be expected from the high proportion of this group in the District; but, on the other hand, the remaining white-collar workers, who might practicably be called the 'middle class', produced a much lower proportion of offenders than would be expected.

In sum, though it may be true to say that more people from the white-collar and skilled manual occupations are found among motoring offenders than among offenders of other kinds, it remains that the majority – indeed the great majority – of serious motoring offenders are from the so-called 'working class'. When the six classes of offence are considered discretely, manual workers predominate in all save one – drunken driving; and even in that group, 46 per cent of the offenders were in manual occupations.

Conclusions

(e) *The typical serious motoring offender is 'the motorist' – the driver of a private car. These drivers form the majority, in contrast to drivers of public-service vehicles, drivers of goods vehicles, and motor cyclists.*

This hypothesis was nullified very early in the research by the national statistics which, when weighted according to the proportions of the respective vehicles on the roads, showed that the motor cyclist is the typical serious motoring offender of today, and that his typical offence is failing to insure. Indeed, this offence has done more than any of the other five to send the incidence of offences up during the period 1954 to 1959. Next came drivers of private cars, with drivers of goods vehicles a long way behind, and drivers of public-service vehicles almost non-existent as offenders. The motor cyclists' lead was maintained even when failing to insure and driving while disqualified – two offences to which motor cyclists seem especially prone – were omitted from the calculations. It may be that it was the self-discipline of the professional driver that kept him out of trouble, relatively speaking, since his representation among the offenders studied was about equal to the estimated proportion of professionals in the country as a whole.

(f) *Serious motoring offenders are not concentrated in any particular age group.*

Strictly speaking, this hypothesis does not hold: the most usual age among the 653 offenders was 26, and there was a marked concentration of offenders in the age group 21 and under 30. The bias towards youth was due to the high proportion of youngsters among the insurance and driving while disqualified groups; if the sample of insurance offenders were expanded to its real total, the mode for the 653 offenders could be as low as 21 years (range 17 to 81 years). The drunken drivers were much older (most usual age, 46), and so were those convicted for failing to stop (mode 52), of whom 17 per cent were over 60. The ages of the dangerous drivers were distributed widely from 17 to 80 years, but the mode was quite young at just under 25; 54 per cent were under 30, including all the motor cyclists in this offence group. Of the latter, 47 per cent were under 21, in comparison with 10·8 per cent of the private car drivers and 13 per cent of the lorry drivers.

(g) *Having been found guilty and punished for one offence of a serious nature, the motoring offender does not repeat the offence.*

This hypothesis must be rejected, since 134 of the 653 offenders had repeated the same kind of offence or committed another equally heinous.

304

A Final Assessment of the Evidence

About one-third of the driving while disqualified group had additional convictions for the same offence, and one-tenth of the drunken drivers had been convicted for either driving under the influence or being drunk in charge of a vehicle. Twelve per cent of the 653 had four or more additional motoring convictions on their records and they would seem legitimately to qualify for the label 'recidivist'. Habitual offenders were especially common in the driving while disqualified group, often after they had been disqualified from driving for periods of more than one year. There is apparently a compulsive element in this offence which is not checked by long periods of disqualification – these may, in fact, do more harm than good.

(h) *Given the opportunity to do so, the serious motoring offender will usually elect to be tried before a jury.*

In fact, only 8 per cent of those who were eligible to elect trial by jury did so. The majority agreed to summary trial, and the interviews, in corroborating this finding, suggested a number of reasons for it: e.g. less publicity, lower costs, less delay, and a reduced risk of being sent to prison if convicted. There was no evidence to suggest that those who elected trial were treated more or less severely than was usual in the magistrates' courts, nor did the cases seem out of the ordinary. The most noticeable thing about the offenders who chose to go before a jury was the low proportion of manual workers among them. Perhaps this is because manual workers are less able to afford a legal contest, but the interviews suggested also that they might be unaware that they are entitled to legal aid through their motoring organizations; most of them were members of the organizations, but it rarely occurred to them to use the facilities provided.

Lest it be thought that this is an attempt to absolve the jury system from the accusations of perversity made against it from time to time, it should be stressed that this research is concerned mostly with the convicted offender. There were, however, some perverse acquittals seen in the police records, and press reports of cases leave no doubt that they are not rare.

(i) *The treatment of serious motoring offenders by the courts is much more lenient than the treatment of offenders charged with offences against the person or against property, or with sex offences.*

There is evidence of lenient sentencing among the motoring cases that have been studied, but most of the facts that are relevant to this hypothesis are to be found in the *Criminal Statistics* for England and Wales. It seems to be beyond question that this hypothesis stands. Analysis of the official statistics (see Chapter 5 above) showed that the proportion of motoring

Conclusions

offenders who were sent to prison was consistently lower than the comparable proportions of offenders against property or the person. The difference was especially striking with regard to cases of motoring manslaughter, and causing death by dangerous driving (as it became after 1956). Up to 1956 100 per cent of these offenders were sent to prison; since then the proportion has gradually fallen, from 44 per cent in 1957 to 31 per cent in 1960. However, for 'other manslaughter' offences (i.e. excluding cases of diminished responsibility and the survivors of suicide pacts) over the same period, the courts sent over 80 per cent of those found guilty to prison (the percentage in 1957 was only 62, but that was an abnormal year in this respect). It is curious that the grave view of taking life implied in a prison sentence is not extended to motoring offenders who cause death, though it does seem to hold in the case of airline pilots and master mariners, and perhaps above all in the case of train drivers. In comparison with non-motoring offenders, fines were imposed much more extensively on motoring offenders, and probation orders were rare. Also it should be noted that disqualification is a penalty that is almost exclusive to the motoring offender, although certain statutory bodies have power to revoke the licences of airline pilots and master mariners.

Assessment of the equity of sentencing can be only tentative when it is based mainly on the records of cases. As to whether there were differences in the treatment of offenders according to their occupational group or social class, it may be noted that 93 per cent of those who were sent to prison were from the manual groups; this was mainly owing to the fact that a large number of manual workers were convicted for driving while disqualified. It did appear, however, that one offender (an army officer) escaped prison for this offence for no other reason than to protect his status. There was also a noticeable tendency to be severe when an offender was revealed as a man with several non-motoring convictions. In some cases there was no scruple about producing evidence of the earlier convictions, although in most it was usual to regard them as irrelevant. The only other observable tendency was to impose heavier fines on those in the top half of the occupational scale than on those in the bottom half.

(j) *The courts rarely use their power to order a serious motoring offender to take another driving test.*

To test this hypothesis there are only the data from this research, since details of re-tests are not given in the official statistics. Of the 653 offenders in the documentary study and the 43 who were interviewed, further driving tests were ordered in only seven cases, all of them elderly persons: four of them convicted of dangerous driving and three of failing to stop (these three were convicted also of careless driving, and the re-tests were ordered for that offence). The evidence therefore supports the hypothesis.

When orders for re-tests are made, they are linked to the penalty of disqualification, to which they add a constructive and reformative element. Unless provision is also made for the retraining and re-testing of the driver, disqualification is limited to deterrence and retribution. It cannot prevent offences, because it does not necessarily stop offenders from driving if they choose to take the risk – which they often do, it seems, if the period of suspension exceeds one year. The evidence suggests, therefore, that longer periods of disqualification should be applied with much more discrimination, to cases where the first consideration must be to protect the public from drivers who are a 'menace' on the roads. For other offenders, a shorter period of suspension, coupled with a re-test, might prove a more effective solution.

So much for the ten basic hypotheses which it was possible to examine. It should now be possible to formulate a very generalized stereotype of the motoring offender or, more properly, the serious motoring offender. On the evidence adduced he (the offender is typically a male) would be a young man in his early twenties, following a manual occupation, either semi-skilled or unskilled. He would most probably be a motor cyclist, and there would be a chance of nearly one in three that he would be known to the police either as a suspected person or as a previously convicted non-motoring offender. It is, however, unlikely that there would be anything specially pathological about his mental state, and he would recognize that he had broken the law; but it is doubtful if he would be in the least ashamed of having done so – on the contrary, he would probably regard himself as unlucky for having been caught, while others usually 'get away with' the same kind of conduct.

But this is speculation of a kind that is hardly appropriate in a serious study, which was designed to defeat such practices. Let us therefore complete this chapter with a discussion of some general points which arise from the research as a whole rather than from any particular hypothesis.

TOWARDS A SENTENCING POLICY

Analysis of the cases reviewed has shown that the sentence received for a serious motoring offence was largely a matter of chance, and it is impossible to see how the amount of a fine or the length of a period of disqualification

Conclusions

was determined. Fines aim to punish and deter; but disqualification, as already discussed, may be supposed to seek to effect some reform. The criteria that are employed in deciding on the length of the period of suspension are therefore worthy of serious study. The matter is of even greater importance, from the driver's point of view, now that the Road Traffic Act, 1962, has increased the number of offences for which the courts must disqualify unless there are 'special reasons' for not doing so. In addition to six offences for which disqualification is mandatory for a period of not less than twelve months, disqualification for not less than six months is also compulsory on a third or subsequent conviction for a further twenty offences. This suggests that substantial periods of suspension are envisaged.

Disqualification has thus become the main weapon of the courts against the motoring offender, and it should be employed as justly and efficiently as possible. The need for a fair and effective sentencing policy is not, of course, confined to motoring cases, and a considerable amount of research has been carried out with this aim in view. The prediction tables of Mannheim and Wilkins (1955) have already been mentioned (p. 16 above). These particular tables were constructed after a systematic study of a sample of Borstal boys had indicated that certain objective criteria (e.g. previous convictions, employment record) were associated with success or failure after Borstal training; given the necessary information about the offender, his suitability for Borstal training could then be assessed.

If a similar study were undertaken of a large sample of motoring offenders, it might be possible to establish that certain criteria were critical, in the sense that they indicated those who were likely to become persistent offenders – then an appropriate sentence could be determined. Moreover, it would be helpful to know the answer to the question: 'Given certain information about the offender, what is the optimum period of disqualification that might bring about a change for the better in his attitude?' In passing sentence it would still be necessary to take into consideration such factors as the need to deter others, but by seeking the answers to questions like this we may hope to achieve more rational and constructive sentencing.

Another means by which the treatment of motoring offenders can be systematized is the 'points system' used in Canada and the United States: offending drivers are given 'demerit points', scaled to specific offences; if the number of points acquired during a given period exceeds the permitted total, automatic disqualification follows. For example, in Ontario a warning letter is sent to all drivers who receive six demerit points, informing them that if they get nine points they will have to attend at the Driver Control Branch of the police 'to discuss driving problems, and to give reasons why

A Final Assessment of the Evidence

their licences should not be suspended'. If they survive this interview, a further three points separate them from an automatic disqualification for three months. Commenting on the first six months of the operation of the scheme, the Minister of Transport for Ontario claimed that fatal accidents had declined from 45·2 per million drivers to 38·9. Such a scheme has its attractions because it makes for consistent penalties; and it is worth noticing (with regard to the wisdom of imposing long periods of disqualification) that the period of suspension is usually three months (*Toronto Globe and Mail*, 28 October 1959).

Nevertheless, whatever attractive method of treatment may be devised, justices dealing with serious motoring cases will be operating in a vacuum unless they can obtain reports on the offenders' mental and physical fitness to drive; and this information is especially important if it is true that driving is a function of personality. Hence the value of the psychiatric clinics available to the Chicago courts, which, incidentally, provide services also for licensing authorities and for the employers of large numbers of drivers. Moreover, these are practical research centres which can supply the courts with valuable data on the psychology of driving, especially deviant driving.

No facilities comparable to those offered by these clinics are available in Britain, and the information at the disposal of justices is appallingly limited. For example, there is the curious practice of excluding non-motoring convictions from the list of previous convictions given to the bench. Regarded objectively, this practice has nothing to commend it since it obscures the offender's real character, and it underscores more clearly than almost anything else the dichotomy that exists between motoring offences and what those who enforce and administer the law call crime. No doubt the insistence that the two kinds of offence are distinct has arisen mainly because of the numerous trivial motoring offences that come before the courts, which make it difficult to separate the sheep from the goats. But justices need to have full details of an offender's criminal record in order to determine a fair sentence. It may be noted that they can be given such information in writing, instead of having it read out in open court, so that they can use it with discretion: the public revelation of a single offence that occurred in the offender's distant past would not then be necessary in trivial cases.

THE ATTITUDE OF THE POLICE

As things stand now, it is the police who decide how much justices shall know about an offender. And indeed it is the police who have the most

309

Conclusions

decisive influence on the whole chain of events in motoring cases, from the precipitating incident onwards. They decide whether to warn, prosecute, or do nothing, and the way that they present a case will affect the degree of seriousness with which it is treated. So it is of fundamental importance in considering this problem to get into perspective the attitude of the police towards motoring offenders.

The results of this inquiry leave little doubt about their general attitude: the police do not, on the whole, see even *serious* motoring offenders as criminals. Hence their evident reluctance to prosecute unless the case is nearly flawless, especially where drunken driving is concerned. In fact there seems to be little or no substance in the belief that the police prosecute to get easy convictions, or to impress superiors in order to achieve promotion; indeed, the paper work alone is enough to deter them from such practices. The *Royal Commission on the Police* (1962, *Final Report*, p. 107) also found that suspicions of this kind were 'groundless'.

There were few reasons for suspecting police motives in the District in which this research was carried out, but the same cannot be said of some of the other forces that were encountered in the course of the study. One force in particular was concerned in cases in which offenders had been induced to plead guilty, and in which there was a clear failure to allow defendants to speak to their doctors or lawyers; nor were the defendant's rights explained as they should have been. It often occurred to the writer how very easy it could be for a defendant who was confused with drink, fright, or both to become so pliable that he might convict himself needlessly. It is, however, hard to see how this possibility can be avoided, although the police are already well aware of the defendant's rights, and of the risks they would run in trying to influence an offender's plea. The defendant's protection also depends on the willingness of his solicitor or doctor to advise him, and such help is generally forthcoming if the accused asks for it. There is, however, one exception: when the arrest is for drunken driving or being drunk in charge late at night. In these circumstances an accused driver is very much on his own and dependent on police propriety – which did not, as far as the District police were concerned, appear to be lacking.

There is, indeed, a strong aura of 'fair play' about the whole relationship between the police and the driver. It is epitomized by the almost endless controversy as to the propriety of employing police patrols in plain clothes, and with cars or motor cycles that would be indistinguishable as police vehicles. For some curious reason (which may not be unconnected with the powerful influence of the motoring organizations) the use of such patrols is

A Final Assessment of the Evidence

objected to because it would imply that motoring offenders are like criminals in that subterfuge is needed to deal with them. Yet the facts suggest that if the police approached the problem of the serious motoring offender with the same vigour that they now show in dealing with what they call crime, the roads of Britain might be made much safer and more pleasant.

REVISION OF THE LAW

However, the motoring organizations, in their *Memorandum to the Royal Commission on the Police* (1960), implied that a thorough and determined attempt to enforce the present law would worsen relations between the police and the motoring public. And, indeed, the existing law is vague and ambiguous to the point of appearing to be fair to no one. To this author (who has no legal qualifications) it seems to be a bad law, and the first essential is its complete renovation – a task that might be helped towards accomplishment if recourse were had to the findings of the *Royal Commission on Transport* (1928–29), many of which are applicable today. Even so, it may well be time for another inquiry into the problems of revising a law which now affects such a large proportion of the population.

From a criminologist's standpoint, the growth of the motoring law is of much interest. The attempt to legislate for every possible contingency in this area of conduct has resulted inevitably in an increasing tendency to rule that motoring offences are absolute prohibitions, since motives are almost impossible to unravel in most cases of motoring misbehaviour; but the effect is mainly to frustrate and irritate the many defendants who are convinced that their behaviour was not only justified but unavoidable. Another unfortunate consequence has been the bringing into court of a vast number of trivial and minor offenders with whom the public can easily identify and sympathize; these offenders help to maintain in the public eye an image of the motoring offender as a 'technical offender' – and this stereotype shelters an antisocial type of individual who benefits from the tolerance accorded to the 'smaller fry'.

There are in fact so many trivial offences that a driver can commit, that an appearance in court becomes a fairly ordinary event to which no significance is attached – it is no more than an inconvenience and an irritant. And it is unlikely that people will regard motoring offences with a proper sense of proportion until this kind of court appearance is reduced. Perhaps set fines, such as were authorized under the Road Traffic Act, 1960, would offer some solution to the problem if they were extended to a wider range of minor motoring offences. But if this solution were adopted there would

Conclusions

have to be a system, such as that of the demerit points found in parts of America and Canada, under which the lawless driver who committed a succession of minor offences could be brought before the courts.

SOME THEORETICAL CONSIDERATIONS

Finally, can criminology offer any explanation of the pattern of behaviour that has emerged from this research? Of the motoring offenders studied, 32 per cent were known to the police for reasons unconnected with motoring behaviour; the remainder seem to have been 'ordinary' people who had no previous crimes recorded against them or whose only previously recorded crimes were also motoring offences.

First, however, let us deal with the view that the main factor responsible for bad motoring behaviour is the inadequacy of the roads, with their numberless hazards made infinitely more dangerous by the great increase in traffic density. A persuasive exponent of this idea is the County Surveyor for Dorset, J. J. Leeming, who considers that the chaotic and unfair road traffic laws combine with archaic and bad highway systems to encourage, and even compel, drivers to commit offences (Leeming, 1960). In other words, drivers are the victims of a system that militates against them. This argument is not without substance, and Leeming quotes some convincing examples of cases in which drivers have been found guilty of careless, or even dangerous, driving, when it was not the driving or the vehicle, but the road itself, that was dangerous. Furthermore, he suggests that the contribution of road conditions to motoring offences is so vast and complex that it is beyond the capacity of the police to estimate it, and that traffic duties should be transferred from the police to a traffic corps under the highway authority.

To exclude roads and driving behaviour from the jurisdiction of the police would imply that motoring offences are essentially 'technical', and would confirm them in their 'apartness' from the criminal law, thus encouraging a climate of toleration within which they might continue to increase. On the other hand, it would be useful for an effective and continuous liaison to be established between the police and the highway engineers, so that the state of the road could be carefully assessed as a factor in incidents. However, a review of all the cases in this study does not suggest that any of them should have been dropped or dismissed for the reasons put forward by Leeming. This is not, of course, to say that the offence might not have happened had the road been of a different design, especially where the danger was caused by overtaking in such a way as to imperil

312

oncoming traffic, since incidents of this kind could not occur on a proper dual carriageway. But in every case there was evidence that the offender failed to take precautions that should have been obvious to any motorist, and that he more or less ignored the danger at the time.

It is apposite here that only eight of the forty-three interviewees thought road conditions to be a major reason for the increase in traffic offences in recent years – or even for their own offence. Nevertheless, a study of careless driving cases might reveal many instances in which it was the highway authority – or even the Minister of Transport – who should have been before the court.

To turn now to two theories concerning the behaviour of motoring offenders, which may, in fact, overlap: according to the first, serious motoring offenders constitute an abnormal minority among drivers, who are predisposed to commit offences because of abnormal traits in their personalities; the second view suggests that they are normal people who, when they committed their offence, made what seemed to them to be the most advantageous response to an expected and familiar group situation.

The dilemma posed by these alternatives is familiar to criminologists, since it is found in studies of all but the very extreme groups of criminals. That is to say, are criminals an abnormal minority in society, whose personalities make normal adjustment impossible under most conditions; or are they normal personalities, who are conditioned to fit into an abnormal (criminal) subculture? In general terms, these two viewpoints might be called, respectively, the 'psychiatric' and the 'sociological' approaches.

The first explanation might be tenable if it appeared that the subjects of this research *were* an abnormal minority. With regard to their minority status, it is not known what proportion of licence holders have been convicted of a serious motoring offence at any time; but it is known that, at the present high offence rates, about 3 per cent of all drivers are thus convicted annually. That some offenders are abnormal should now be self-evident, but it cannot be estimated with confidence how many can be so described; nor will this be possible until much more interest is taken in these offenders as individuals.

The second theory is tenable if we accept the roads of Britain as part of the social environment, and those who use them as a cross-section of interacting individuals that is typical of society itself. This conception does not seem to be unreasonable now that the motor vehicle is no longer a luxury but has become a necessity in an increasing proportion of families. Thus, just as delinquent or criminal subcultures exist in society-at-large, so might a delinquent or criminal subculture be found among road users.

Conclusions

It might or might not consist of the same people, since different criminal groups have their own characteristic patterns of behaviour which they may not manifest in all spheres of social activity, but only when conditions are favourable for the commission of the kind of offence to which they are prone. For example, the selfish and utterly ruthless burglar may be a model driver because he does not want to attract the attention of the police – especially when using his car for business. It is likely, however, that some of the individuals in the criminal subculture among road users would be found also in other subcultures of deviant behaviour, because basically antisocial traits might be brought out by driving. In other words, it is suggested that serious motoring offenders may form a criminal subculture within the community of road users or, perhaps more realistically, one of the many types of criminal subculture that exist in British society today.

If this is so we might look for illumination at one of the main sociological theories in criminology: that of E. H. Sutherland (Sutherland and Cressey, 1955, pp. 74–97). Briefly, this theory suggests that most criminal activity is behaviour which is learned from a delinquent environment, in which it is the normal and expected response from normal individuals. Learning in this environment is not necessarily an imitative process; one does not have to associate with, or identify with, criminals to be tempted to behave like them: one might do so after having been a victim of criminal behaviour. However, in most developed contemporary societies such as our own, an individual can be influenced by persons who 'define the legal codes as rules to be observed', or by persons who define them as rules to be violated; consequently there is what Sutherland calls 'culture conflict' in relation to the legal codes. The individual has, therefore, a realistic idea of the law and its constraints, and his behaviour will depend on whether there is 'an excess of definitions favourable to the violation of the law over definitions unfavourable to violating the law'. In other words, whenever there is an excess of conditions that are favourable to a delinquent response it will very likely be made, and when conditions are unfavourable it may well not be made. This is Sutherland's principle of 'differential association'.

It is evident that drivers learn their behaviour from other drivers; moreover, the attitudes that an individual adopts from other people are largely determined by his own disposition. Hence a driver who is greatly influenced by persons unfavourable to the law and the highway code is unlikely to be influenced by, for example, road safety propaganda. When many drivers are disregarding the law there will be strong pressure on individuals to do the same: take, for instance, the experience of the Minister of Transport (see p. 107 above) when driving along a three-lane one-way

314

road on which there was a speed limit of 40 mph. It is also apposite that many of the young offenders who had come before the courts for driving without insurance or while they were disqualified had responded to an irresistible pressure from 'mates' to go out as usual none the less. As one young respondent in the interview study said: 'Round here nobody bothers about driving uninsured so it's hard to keep out of it and so be called a goody-goody.' And another: 'Everyone in the gang rides very fast; they call you "chicken" if you don't.' Yet another: 'The girls are often the worst. I was doing 100 mph with one on my pillion and she kept on saying go faster.' And one of the drunken drivers, a professional man, said: 'I knew it was risky to drive as I'd had more than I could take, but my friends were urging me to get the car out and drive into the town for supper, so I took the chance.'

These seem to be the normal responses of people who were put under great pressure to break the law, and pressures of this kind are in the range of experience of most adults. So much so that many serious motoring offenders – and, indeed, many non-offending drivers also – might think it erroneous to regard such pressures in the same light as those that impel people to behave in other 'more criminal' ways. But it is questionable whether this view is tenable when it is realized how strong group pressure can be on the individual to conform to the group's approved ways of behaving. As Sutherland (1955, p. 78) put it, 'if there is isolation from anti-criminal patterns' the response to such pressure may well be a criminal act.

According to this theory, then, the present study would suggest that a group of people, the majority of whom were apparently normal citizens, submitted to delinquent pressures when they were applied; and the question is why all but 32 per cent of them should have responded only in the realm of motoring behaviour and not, so far as is known, in other ways. One answer would be that 'the excess of definitions' (especially social sanctions) was unfavourable to a violation of the law in other spheres of activity, but it was favourable in the motoring situation. Hence a latently delinquent pattern of behaviour found its outlet in driving when the conditions for its expression were favourable.

Thus these serious motoring offenders, belonging to a criminal subculture among road users, will have the same attitude towards the laws that affect their code as is found among individuals in other criminal subcultures. Moreover, this conception of the serious motoring offender is not to be discounted on the ground that over two-thirds of the offenders studied could be considered more or less normal people in a psychiatric sense, for

Conclusions

an equally large proportion of normal people might be found in most other criminal subcultures. Indeed, Miller (1960) has suggested that delinquent traits are present in many outwardly normal and 'respectable' persons whose reputations are without blemish. One can be a criminal without being manifestly abnormal as a personality.

As Sutherland's theory of differential association appears to have such a distinct relevance to the problem under discussion, it is of interest to consider his views on the treatment of offenders also. He stressed the futility of passing sentence on individuals, and then returning them unchanged to the same subcultural environment or situation that nurtured the crime (1955, p. 602). Yet this happens in nearly all motoring cases, whether serious or not, and there is hardly ever any positive effort to bring about the offender's reform. The only principles of punishment that appear to be applied are those of retribution and deterrence; prevention is achieved in a partial sense by disqualification or, very rarely, by imprisonment, but reformation is almost completely ignored. If genuine prevention and positive reformation are to be achieved, it will be necessary to facilitate the offender's assimilation into a law-abiding group which he could respect and with which he could readily identify. A period of probation, during which there could be intensive and stimulating training at a level appropriate to the offender's experience, might achieve this end. For example, it should not be too expensive or complicated to set up in police districts a kind of 'attendance centre' for errant drivers, where they could be given lectures on driving and road safety; and where they could receive dual instruction, and be positioned in 'black spots' to note and criticize the driving of others. They could repay this in kind by cleaning police vehicles.

But, as Sutherland pointed out (ibid. p. 604): 'The source of pressure on the criminal whose change is sought must lie within the group. The group must not rely upon the criminal to change himself.' When related to our present discussion this means that the culture of which the delinquent subculture is a part (i.e. the motoring community of which the serious offenders are a part) must try to change the attitudes of the criminal element so that its needs are no longer satisfied by the possession of a delinquent set of norms. To achieve this it will be essential, *inter alia*, to establish a concept of good driving that in itself constitutes a challenge – a challenge within the context of a law which is easily understood and whose *raison d'être* is self-evident.

A Final Assessment of the Evidence

Should this be thought to be too ambitious, it might be apposite again to consider the problem (referred to in Chapter 1 above) faced by the Royal Air Force early in the second world war, when it became urgently necessary to reconcile the dash and enthusiasm of young pilots in machines of increasing speed and power with the need to avoid unnecessary wastage, in accidents, of lives and aircraft which were vital to the war effort. The solution was found in an intensive campaign to persuade pilots that disciplined and accurate flying was essential to effectiveness in operations, and that this could be achieved only by mastery of the machine. In other words, *the good pilot was master of himself and of his aircraft whatever its speed and power*, and this idea was pressed home in attractive pamphlets and current literature showing how the 'aces' of the time and of the previous war achieved their successes by aiming at superlative polish and perfection in flying. At the other end of the scale there was created the amusing but very effective stereotype of 'Pilot Officer Prune', of vacuous expression and bed-raggled, yet exhibitionistic, appearance, whose every illustrated action (in cartoon and poster) was a menace to himself and to others, from forgetting to lower the wheels before landing to low flying in and out of the balloon barrages during enemy raids. This stereotype was readily applied to the careless and the stupid with suitably pungent embellishment by the laconic and derisory term 'clot': an appellation that was about the worst insult that could be hurled at any pilot.

How effective the campaign was is a matter of opinion, for many other factors contributed to the increase in 'professional pride' among aircrew that has culminated in the high sense of discipline and the perfectionism that are manifest among airline and service pilots today. But it seemed to the author, who was in charge of a flying training unit at the time, that the whole campaign was a powerful stimulus that rapidly caught the imagination. So it is a pity that Prune expired with the war, for it would be interesting to see how effective his stereotype could be when dressed and mounted appropriately to achieve 'the ton' in a built-up area, or when shown in typical situations in a variety of vehicles.

There is, unfortunately, not much literature on the methods employed in dealing with aircrew during the war. But an excellent account by Paterson (1955) shows how attitudes towards careless flying were changed by the infiltration of new ideas into squadrons through a number of 'exemplars' who were already of high prestige among the pilots. Perhaps distinguished racing drivers could influence the ordinary motorist and motor cyclist similarly.

That the climate is not unripe for such approaches is suggested by the

317

Conclusions

following extract from a leading article in *The Autocar* (8 June 1962), 'Unwritten Law for Safety':

'Public opinion is the most powerful and even the only effective weapon there is against irresponsibility and its consequences on the roads. That public opinion can act in this way is illustrated by a parallel from the past. Many years ago drunkenness was a serious social problem, yet very little was achieved to reduce it while the attitude taken, even in mixed company, was one of 'some men are like that and one has got to put up with it'. However, as soon as general opinion swung another way and it became a disgrace to be seen drunk in public, the great majority of offenders very quickly mended their ways.

Similar examples are to be found in schools and barracks. Practically all the rules in the book, laid down by authority, may be broken by individuals without a word of protest from their fellows. Let one of them break the unwritten rule, or fail to observe the recognized code of behaviour, and at once the offender becomes an outsider, shunned and unhelped by the rest.

Now the question remains of how to awaken public opinion to the wrongs and rights of behaviour on the roads, and how, as a result, to imbue the individual with the necessary reluctance to overstep the mark. This seems to call for some clever psychological approach that appears to have been singularly lacking in all the safety propaganda with which we have been bombarded so far.'

As may be inferred from this article, a substantial body of highly responsible motorists and motor cyclists view the anarchical and dangerous conduct of the delinquents with concern and distaste. For nothing is more galling to the keen and competent driver than to be grouped with such people. Perhaps it would behove the motoring organizations to campaign themselves for a tightening up of standards for the granting and retention of driving licences; to encourage motorists and motor cyclists to join clubs (which do much to increase care and competence); and generally to foster a concept of professionalism and pride in driving which would make safe and skilful driving in a clean and well-maintained vehicle the ambition of all concerned.

So much for *one* way of dealing with the subcultural problem. But it seems unlikely that it would be effective with regard to the abnormal personalities who are certainly to be found among serious motoring offenders, even if at the moment their number is incalculable. They present a problem which will be solvable only when its real nature is understood –

318

and this calls for a wholly different approach to the apprehension and treatment of the serious motoring offender than that which now obtains; that is to say, he must be regarded as an individual whose conduct reflects his personality and his way of life.

A final thought demands expression. It is that this study of serious motoring offenders and their offences has presented nothing more in reality than a normal social environment in which criminal behaviour is found to be perpetrated by a criminal element, compounded of normal and abnormal individuals. As such it is a microcosm of the society in which we live, and it offers a field of investigation which the sociologist and the criminologist cannot afford to continue to ignore.

Appendices

Appendix A

COPE-CHAT CARD RECORD AND KEY FOR MOTORING OFFENDERS

ITEM	KEY	
Age		
14 and under 17	Top	A
17 and under 21	T	B
21 and under 30	T	C
30 and under 50	T	D
50 and over	T	E
Sex		
If female	T	F
Occupational group		
Professional and higher administrative	T	G
Managerial and executive	T	H
Lower non-manual grades	T	I
Skilled manual	T	J
Semi-skilled manual	T	K
Unskilled manual	T	L
Previous convictions		
Motoring: 0	T	M
1	T	Mc
2	T	N
3	T	O
4	T	P
5	T	Q
6/10	T	R
over 10	T	S
Other: 0	T	T
1	T	U
2	T	V
3	T	W
4	T	X
5/10	T	Y
over 10	T	Z
Offence (principal charge on which found guilty)		
Causing death by dangerous driving	Right	1
Dangerous and reckless driving	R	2
Driving under the influence	R	3

323

Appendix A

ITEM	KEY	
Driving while disqualified	R	4
Failing to stop	R	5
Failing to insure	R	6
If offence charged:		
with alternatives	R	7
with other motoring offences	R	8
with other offences	R	9
On indictment	R	10
Accused elected trial	R	11
Charge reduced at trial	R	12
Trial in higher court	R	13

Year of trial

1957	R	14
1958	R	15
1959	R	16

Sentence of court

Absolute or conditional discharge	Bottom	1
Fined	B	2
Probation	B	3
Prison	B	4
Disqualified	B	5
Other disposal	B	6
Driving re-test	B	7
Accused appealed against finding or sentence	B	8

Type of vehicle driven by accused

Public-service vehicle	B	9
Goods vehicle	B	10
Private car	B	11
Motor cycle	B	12

Date of offence

January	B	13
February	B	14
March	B	15
April	B	16
May	B	17
June	B	18
July	B	19
August	B	20
September	B	21
October	B	22
November	B	23
December	B	24

Appendix A

Appendix B

1. *Name:*   *Age:*   *Occupation:*
2. Offence of which convicted, court and date.

Offence and attitude to it

3. What were the circumstances of the offence?
   Type of vehicle driven.
   Was it offender's own property?
   Offender's apportionment of blame.

4. How does offender think he was treated by the police and the court?
   Does he think the punishment fair?
   Does he think it brands him as a criminal?
   How does he think the case will affect his reputation among neighbours, workmates, and friends?

5. Generally speaking, does he think that motoring offenders are treated fairly by the police and the courts? Are courts too lenient or too severe?

6. Does he think that *any* motoring offender should be labelled as a criminal? Obtain reasons for answering in affirmative or negative.

Driving experience and attitudes to driving

7. How many years a licence holder? Number of miles driven annually.

8. When was test taken, how many times, and by whom was it administered?

9. Membership of motoring organizations or clubs.

10. Does he read motoring literature? Check for detailed knowledge.

11. Interest in motor sports? Attendance at meetings?

12. How does he rate his driving? (As good as most, better than most, or below the average.) Is he satisfied with his driving? Does he intend to make any changes in his driving behaviour since the offence?

13. Does he think that the number of motoring convictions in England and Wales is greater than it should be. If so, why does he think so, and where does the fault lie? (E.g. police over-zealous, road system unable to take traffic.)

Appendix C

ITEM	KEY	
Age		
14 and under 17	Top	A
17 and under 21	T	B
21 and under 30	T	C
30 and under 50	T	D
50 and over	T	E
Sex		
If female	T	F
Occupational group		
Professional and higher		
administrative	T	G
Managerial and executive	T	H
Lower non-manual grades	T	I
Skilled manual	T	J
Semi-skilled manual	T	K
Unskilled manual	T	L
Previous convictions		
Motoring: 0	T	M
1	T	Mc
2	T	N
3	T	O
4	T	P
5	T	Q
6/10	T	R
over 10	T	S
Other: 0	T	T
1	T	U
2	T	V
3	T	W
4	T	X
5/10	T	Y
over 10	T	Z
Offence (principal charge on which found guilty)		
Causing death by dangerous driving	Right	1
Dangerous and reckless driving	R	2

327

Appendix C

Driving under the
influence   R   3
Driving while disqualified   R   4
Failing to stop   R   5
Failing to insure   R   6

Attitude to offence

Contrite   R   7
Indifferent   R   8
Shameless   R   9

Attitude to police

Favourable   R   10
Indifferent   R   11
Hostile   R   12

Attitude to sentence

Just   R   13
Unjust   R   14
Pressure to plead guilty?
(clip for yes)   R   15
Elected trial?
(clip for yes)   R   16

Effect on personal relations

Much   Bottom   1
Some   B   2
None   B   3
Press report unfair or
inaccurate   B   4

Are motoring offenders criminal?

All   B   5
Some   B   6
None   B   7

Rating as driver

Better than most   B   8
Good as most   B   9
Below average   B   10

Driving experience

Over 5 years   B   11
2 years and under 5   B   12
Under 2 years   B   13
Provisional licence   B   14

Vehicle owner   B   15

Vehicle

Goods   B   16
Private car   B   17
Motor cycle   B   18

Appendix C

ITEM	KEY	
Member of motoring organization (yes)	B	19
Enthusiast (yes)	B	20

Mechanical aptitude

Good	B	21
Average	B	22
Poor	B	23

Impression of intelligence

Average or above	B	24
Low	B	25

Assessment of personality

Appears normal	B	26
Reservations about normality	B	27

Evidence of drink

(not drunk in charge cases)	B	28

Sentence of court

Fined	B	29
Disqualified	B	30

Was there an accident?

Another vehicle	L	1
Pedestrian	L	2
Other	L	3

Police division

A	L	7
B	L	8
C	L	9
D	L	10
E	L	11
F	L	12
G	L	13
H	L	14
CRO check completed	L	15

Appendix D

Sir,

I am appearing before you on. . . . . for driving a motor bike on . . . . . I am, Sir, a married man with three children and I was with my wife on that day. The reson Im sending you this letter if Im found guilty of this charge. I hope Im not but at the present it is only my word against that of the police and my wife is trying to see people I saw on that day. If given a chance by been put on probation or a find or conditional discharge Im shore that I will be able to clear my name and find the person who done this in my name. If any of them could be given me I would be very gratefull. If not could you please adjorn for 28 days so I can clear my name. I have just come out of the Army but just befor I was sent to prison my wife and three children was being turned out.

For the past $3\frac{1}{2}$ years I have only lived with my wife and children for 5 or 6 months because we could not get a place together. She lives with her mother but owing to a misunderstanding Im not allowed over there house and its been like that for about 3 years. But now that Im 21 on my release from prison the Council are getting me a job with a house in a new town and we can be together. I can find out who done it and clear my name. It is only over my wife being turned out that Im in prison now. They had nowhere to go and I had just over 10 weeks to find a place but rents was too much. The only thing I could do was to buy this little van, repair it and sell it at a profit to put down a deposit on a caravan but it did not work as I had to test the brakes and steering and so drove it up my road and was reported to the police and sent to prison. When all this happened the person changed his mind and did not buy the van and I still have it. But cant you see Sir that this was not done for fun there was no other thing I could do and as you see Im paying hard for the good I tried to do. I pray that you can give me a chance as my wifes mother cant have her any longer. . . .

As you see Sir all our future lays in your hands as might never get the chance of a house of our own again.

References

ARCHBOLD. (1962). *Criminal Pleading, Evidence & Practice.* 35th edition by T. R. Fitzwalter Butler and Marston Garsia. London: Sweet & Maxwell.

AUTOMOBILE ASSOCIATION AND ROYAL AUTOMOBILE CLUB STANDING JOINT COMMITTEE (1960). *Memorandum to the Royal Commission on the Police.*

BLOM-COOPER, L. (1960). 'The Case of Gypsy Smith.' *Brit. J. Crim.,* vol. I, pp. 171-3.

BRODY, L. (1941). *Personal Factors in the Safe Operation of Motor Vehicles.* New York: Center for Safety Education.

BURGESS, E. W. (1950). Discussion of Hartung, 'White Collar Offences in the Wholesale Meat Industry in Detroit,' and Hartung's reply. *Amer. J. Sociol.,* vol. 56, pp. 32-4.

CANTY, ALAN (1940). 'The Case Study Method of Rehabilitating Drivers.' *J. Soc. Psychol.,* vol. 12, p. 272.

CANTY, ALAN (1942). 'The Youthful Problem Driver.' *Defenses against Crime Yearbook.* New York: National Probation Association.

CANTY, ALAN (1953). 'The Structure and Function of the Psychopathic Clinic, Recorder's Court, Detroit, Mich.' *Ohio State Law J.,* vol. 14, pp. 142-53.

CANTY, ALAN (1956). 'Problem Drivers and Criminal Offenders.' *Canadian Services Medical J.,* vol. VII, pp. 136-43.

CARR-SAUNDERS, A. M., and JONES, C. (1958). *Social Conditions in England and Wales.* London: Oxford Univ. Press.

CHANDLER, K. N., and TANNER, J. C. (1958). 'Estimates of Total Miles run by Motor Vehicles in G.B. in 1952 and 1956.' *J. R. Stat. Soc.,* vol. 121, pp. 420-37.

CHRISTIAN ECONOMIC AND SOCIAL RESEARCH FOUNDATION (1959). *Drunken Driving and Drunk-in-Charge Offences.* London.

CHRISTIAN ECONOMIC AND SOCIAL RESEARCH FOUNDATION (1960). *Publicans and Drunkenness.* London.

CLARKE, B. (1949). *Drivers who have Accidents.* Unpublished research paper. London.

COLE, G. D. H. (1955). *Studies in Class Structure.* London: Routledge & Kegan Paul.

CRIMINAL STATISTICS, ENGLAND AND WALES (Annual). Home Office. London: HMSO.

CULPIN, M. (1937). 'The Psychology of Motoring.' *The Practitioner,* vol. CXXXIX, pp. 213-17.

DAVIS, D. R. (1948). *Pilot Error.* London: HMSO.

DREW, G. C., et al. (1959). *The Effect of Small Doses of Alcohol on a Skill Resembling Driving.* Medical Research Council Memorandum 38. London: HMSO.

DUNBAR, H. F. (1944). Cited by McFarland (1955).

EDGERTON, H. A. (1951). Cited by McFarland (1955).

EMMETT, B. P. (1952). Appendix to Trenaman, J.P., *Out of Step.* London: Methuen.

ENO FOUNDATION (1948). Cited by McFarland (1955).

331

References

GIBBENS, T. C. N. (1958). 'Car Thieves.' *Brit. J. Delinq.*, vol. VIII, pp. 257–65.

GOODHART, A. L. (1953). *English Law and the Moral Law*. London: Stevens.

GREIG, D. R. (1955). *The AA's Approach to Road Safety*. London: Automobile Association.

GRYGIER, T. G. (1956). *The Dynamic Personality Inventory*. London: National Foundation for Educational Research.

HALL, J. R., and MOSER, C. A. (1954). In D. V. Glass (Ed.), *Social Mobility in Britain*. London: Routledge & Kegan Paul.

HARTUNG, F. E. (1950). 'White Collar Offences in the Wholesale Meat Industry in Detroit.' *Amer. J. Sociol.*, vol. 56, pp. 25–32.

HEATH, E. D. Jr. (1955). *Relationship between Driving Records, Selected Personality Characteristics and Biographical Data of Traffic Offenders and Non-offenders*. New York: Center for Safety Education.

HOOD, ROGER (1962). *Sentencing in Magistrates' Courts*. London: Stevens.

HOSKINS, P. (1961). 'Crime Reporting and its Role.' *The Times Lit. Supp.*, 23 June.

JOHNSON, N. L., and GARWOOD, F. (1957). 'An Analysis of the Claim Records of a Motor Insurance Company.' *J. Inst. Actuaries*, vol. 83, p. 365.

KENNY, C. S. (1962). In Turner (Ed.), *Outlines of Criminal Law*. London: Cambridge Univ. Press.

LAUR, A. R. (1939). Cited by McFarland (1955).

LEEMING, J. J. (1960). 'A New Approach to Road Accidents.' *Traffic Engineering and Control*, vol. 2, p. 100.

LODGE, T. S. (1953). 'Criminal Statistics.' *J. Roy. Stat. Soc.*, vol. 116, pp. 283–97.

MCFARLAND, R. A. (1955). *Human Variables in Motor Vehicle Accidents*. Boston: Harvard School of Public Health.

MCFARLAND, R. A., and MOORE, R. C. (1957). 'Human Factors in Highway Safety.' *New Eng. J. Med.*, vol. 256, pp. 792–9, 837–45, 890–7.

MCFARLAND, R. A., and MOSELEY, A. L. (1954). *Human Factors in Highway Transport Safety*. Boston: Harvard School of Public Health.

MANNHEIM, H. (1946). *Criminal Justice and Social Reconstruction*. London: Routledge & Kegan Paul.

MANNHEIM, H. (1960). Review of Wootton, *Social Science and Social Pathology*. *Jewish J. Sociol.*, vol. II, p. 57.

MANNHEIM, H., and WILKINS, L. T. (1955) *Prediction Methods in Relation to Borstal Training*. London: HMSO.

MARTIN, J. P. (1962). *Offenders as Employees*. London: Macmillan.

MIDDENDORFF, WOLF (1959). *Soziologie des Verbrechens*. Düsseldorf/Köln: Diederichs.

MILLER, E. (1960). 'Delinquent Traits in Normal Persons.' *Brit. J. Delinq.*, vol. X, pp. 170–7.

MOORE, R. L. (1956). 'Accident Proneness and Road Accidents.' *J. Inst. Auto. Assessors*, vol. 8, pp. 32–7.

MOSER, C. A. (1958). *Survey Methods in Social Investigation*. London: Heinemann.

MOYNIHAN, D.P. (1960). 'Public Health and Traffic Study.' *J. Crim. Law, Criminol. and Police Sci.*, vol. 51, p. 93.

References

MUNDEN, J. M. (1962). 'Some Analysis of Car Insurance Rates.' *Asdin Bulletin*, Vol. II, 2, September.

OFFENCES RELATING TO MOTOR VEHICLES (Annual). Home Office. London: HMSO.

PARKER, J. W. (1953). Cited by McFarland (1955).

PATERSON, T. T. (1955). *Morale in War and Work*. London: Max Parrish.

REPORT OF THE COMMISSIONERS OF PRISONS (Annual). Home Office. London: HMSO.

ROYAL COMMISSION ON MOTOR CARS (1906). Cd. 3080. London: HMSO.

ROYAL COMMISSION ON TRANSPORT (1929). *First Report*. Cmd. 3365. *Minutes of Evidence*, 1928. London: HMSO.

ROYAL COMMISSION ON THE POLICE (1962). *Final Report*. Cmnd. 1728. London: HMSO.

SELLING, L. S. (1941). 'The Psychopathology of the Hit and Run Driver.' *Amer. J. Psychiatry*, vol. 98, pp. 93–8.

SELZER, M. (1961). 'Personality versus Intoxication as a Critical Factor in Accidents caused by Alcoholic Drivers.' *J. Nerv. Ment. Disease*, vol. 132, pp. 298–303.

SILVEY, J. (1961). 'The Criminal Law and Public Opinion.' *Crim. Law Review*, pp. 349–58.

STACK, M. V., and WALKER, D. B. (1959). *Motorized Drunkenness*. London: London Diocesan CETS.

SUMNER, W. G. (1906). *Folkways*. Boston: Ginn.

SUTHERLAND, E. H., and CRESSEY, D. R. (1955). *Principles of Criminology*. New York: Lippincott.

TAYLOR, G. (1961). 'Prison? It's a Picnic.' *Today*, 14 Jan.

TILLMANN, W. A., and HOBBS, G. E. (1949). 'The Accident Prone Automobile Driver.' *Amer. J. Psychiatry*, vol. 106, pp. 321–31.

UNIVISION (1960). Survey by Staff of Univision Ltd., London. Published in *The Observer*, 31 July 1960.

WATERSON, J. H. L. (1961). 'Religion and Road Safety.' *Theology*, June, p. 228; July, p. 271.

WILKINSON, G. S. (1960). *Road Traffic Offences* London: Solicitors' Law Stationery Society.

WILLIAMS, C. (1961). 'The Criminal Law and Public Opinion.' *Crim. Law Review*, pp. 359–67.

WILLIAMS, G. (1961). *Criminal Law*. 2nd edn. London: Stevens.

WOOTTON, B. (1957). 'Who are the Criminals?' *Twentieth Century*, August, pp. 138–48.

WOOTTON, B. (1959). *Social Science and Social Pathology*. London: Allen & Unwin.

Index

Index